Imaging of Gynecologic Malignancy: The Current State of the Art

Editor

ARADHANA M. VENKATESAN

RADIOLOGIC CLINICS
OF NORTH AMERICA

www.radiologic.theclinics.com

Consulting Editor
FRANK H. MILLER

July 2023 • Volume 61 • Number 4

ELSEVIER

1600 John F. Kennedy Boulevard • Suite 1800 • Philadelphia, Pennsylvania, 19103-2899

http://www.theclinics.com

RADIOLOGIC CLINICS OF NORTH AMERICA Volume 61, Number 4
July 2023 ISSN 0033-8389, ISBN 13: 978-0-323-94035-1

Editor: John Vassallo (j.vassallo@elsevier.com)
Developmental Editor: Karen Justine S. Dino

Radiologic Clinics of North America (ISSN 0033-8389) is published bimonthly by Elsevier Inc., 360 Park Avenue South, New York, NY 10010-1710. Months of issue are January, March, May, July, September, and November. Periodicals postage paid at New York, NY and additional mailing offices. Subscription prices are USD 544 per year for US individuals, USD 1107 per year for US institutions, USD 100 per year for US students and residents, USD 643 per year for Canadian individuals, USD 1415 per year for Canadian institutions, USD 739 per year for international individuals, USD 1415 per year for international institutions, USD 100 per year for Canadian students/residents, and USD 315 per year for international students/residents. To receive student and resident rate, orders must be accompanied by name of affiliated institution, date of term and the signature of program/residency coordinatior on institution letterhead. Orders will be billed at individual rate until proof of status is received. Foreign air speed delivery is included in all *Clinics* subscription prices. All prices are subject to change without notice. **POSTMASTER:** Send address changes to *Radiologic Clinics of North America*, Elsevier Health Sciences Division, Subscription Customer Service, 3251 Riverport Lane, Maryland Heights, MO63043. **Customer Service: Telephone: 1-800-654-2452** (U.S. and Canada); **1-314-447-8871** (outside U.S. and Canada). **Fax: 1-314-447-8029. E-mail: journalscustomerservice-usa@elsevier.com (for print support); journalsonlinesupport-usa@elsevier.com (for on-line support).**

Reprints. For copies of 100 or more of articles in this publication, please contact the Commercial Reprints Department, Elsevier Inc., 360 Park Avenue South, New York, New York 10010-1710. Tel.: +1-212-633-3874; Fax: +1-212-633-3820; E-mail: reprints@elsevier.com.

Radiologic Clinics of North America also published in Greek Paschalidis Medical Publications, Athens, Greece.

Radiologic Clinics of North America is covered in *MEDLINE/PubMed (Index Medicus), EMBASE/Excerpta Medica, Current Contents/Life Sciences, Current Contents/Clinical Medicine, RSNA Index to Imaging Literature, BIOSIS, Science Citation Index,* and *ISI/BIOMED*.

Contributors

CONSULTING EDITOR

FRANK H. MILLER, MD, FACR, FSAR, FSABI
Lee F. Rogers, MD Professor of Medical
Education, Chief, Body Imaging Section,
Medical Director, MRI, Professor, Department
of Radiology, Northwestern Memorial Hospital,
Northwestern University Feinberg School of
Medicine, Chicago, Illinois, USA

EDITOR

ARADHANA M. VENKATESAN, MD
Professor of Radiology, Term Tenure, Director
of Translational Research, Department of
Abdominal Imaging, Division of Diagnostic
Imaging, The University of Texas MD Anderson
Cancer Center, Houston, Texas

AUTHORS

GIACOMO AVESANI, MD, MSc
Dipartimento di Diagnostica per Immagini,
Radioterapia Oncologica ed Ematologia,
Fondazione Policlinico Universitario "A.
Gemelli" IRCCS, Italy

OLGA R. BROOK, MD
Department of Radiology, Beth Israel
Deaconess Medical Center, Boston,
Massachusetts, USA

KYLE M. DEVINS, MD
Instructor of Radiology, Harvard Medical
School, Department of Pathology,
Massachusetts General Hospital, Boston,
Massachusetts, USA

NICOLE HINDMAN, MD
Professor of Radiology and Surgery,
Department of Radiology, NYU Grossman
School of Medicine, New York, New York, USA

MEGAN C. JACOBSEN, PhD
Assistant Professor, Division of Diagnostic
Imaging, Department of Imaging Physics, The
University of Texas MD Anderson Cancer
Center, Houston, Texas, USA

AOIFE KILCOYNE, MBBCh, BAO
Instructor, Department of Radiology,
Massachusetts General Hospital, Harvard
Medical School, Boston, Massachusetts, USA

ANN H. KLOPP, MD, PhD
Professor, Department of Radiation Oncology,
The University of Texas MD Anderson Cancer
Center, Houston, Texas, USA

MATTHEW LARSON, MD, PhD
Department of Radiology, University of
Wisconsin-Madison School of Medicine and
Public Health, Madison, Wisconsin, USA

SUSANNA I. LEE, MD, PhD
Associate Professor, Department of Radiology,
Massachusetts General Hospital, Harvard
Medical School, Boston, Massachusetts, USA

PETRA LOVREC, MD
Department of Radiology, Loyola University
Medical Center, Maywood, Illinois, USA

MICHELA LUPINELLI, MD
Department of Radiology, Morgagni-Pierantoni Hospital, Forlì, Italy; Department of Radiology, Università Cattolica Del Sacro Cuore, Rome, Italy

EKTA MAHESHWARI, MD
Assistant Professor, Division of Abdominal Imaging, Department of Radiology, University of Pittsburgh Medical Center, Pittsburgh, Pennsylvania, USA

KATHERINE E. MATUREN, MD, MS
Clinical Professor of Radiology and Obstetrics/Gynecology, Michigan Medicine, University of Michigan, University Hospital, Ann Arbor, Michigan, USA

MELISSA MCGETTIGAN, MD
Moffitt Cancer Center, University of South Florida College of Medicine, Tampa, Florida, USA

CHRISTINE MENIAS, MD
Mayo Clinic Radiology, Scottsdale, Arizona, USA

CAMILLA NERO, MD, PhD
Dipartimento di Scienze Della Salute Della Donna, del bambino e di sanità pubblica, Fondazione Policlinico Universitario A. Gemelli IRCCS, Università Cattolica Del Sacro Cuore, Rome, Italy

STEPHANIE NOUGARET, MD, PhD
Montpellier Cancer Research Institute, University of Montpellier, INSERM, U1194, Department of Radiology, Montpellier Cancer Institute, Montpellier, France

ESTHER OLIVA, MD
Professor of Pathology, Harvard Medical School, Department of Pathology, Massachusetts General Hospital, Boston, Massachusetts, USA

TAEMEE PAK, MD
Assistant Professor, Department of Radiology, The University of Texas Southwestern Medical Center, Dallas, Texas, USA

CAMILLA PANICO, MD
Dipartimento di Diagnostica per Immagini, Radioterapia Oncologica ed Ematologia, Fondazione Policlinico Universitario "A. Gemelli" IRCCS, Italy

KRUPA PATEL-LIPPMANN, MD
Assistant Professor, Department of Radiology and Radiological Sciences, Vanderbilt University, Medical Center North, Nashville, Tennessee, USA

ROBERT PETROCELLI, MD
Clinical Assistant Professor, Department of Radiology, NYU Grossman School of Medicine, New York, New York, USA

ALI PIRASTEH, MD
Departments of Radiology and Medical Physics, University of Wisconsin-Madison School of Medicine and Public Health, Madison, Wisconsin, USA

CAROLINE REINHOLD, MD, MSc
Professor, Department of Radiology, McGill University Health Center, Montreal, Quebec, Canada

DOUGLAS ROGERS, MD
Department of Radiology and Imaging Sciences, University of Utah, Salt Lake City, Utah, USA

MOLLY E. ROSELAND, MD
Clinical Assistant Professor of Radiology, Michigan Medicine, University of Michigan, University Hospital, Ann Arbor, Michigan, USA

LEONARDO RUNDO, PhD
Department of Information and Electrical Engineering and Applied Mathematics (DIEM), University of Salerno, Salerno, Italy

ELIZABETH A. SADOWSKI, MD
Professor, Departments of Radiology and Obstetrics and Gynecology, University of Wisconsin-Madison School of Medicine and Public Health, University of Wisconsin Hospital and Clinics, Madison, Wisconsin, USA

MICHELLE D. SAKALA, MD
Department of Radiology, University of Michigan, Ann Arbor, Michigan, USA

EVIS SALA, MD, PhD, FRCR, FRCP
Dipartimento di Diagnostica per Immagini, Radioterapia Oncologica ed Ematologia, Fondazione Policlinico Universitario "A. Gemelli" IRCCS, Università Cattolica Del Sacro Cuore, Rome, Italy

MARTINA SBARRA, MD
Unit of Diagnostic Imaging, Fondazione Policlinico Universitario Campus Bio-medico, Roma, Italy

MADELEINE SERTIC, MBBCh, BAO
Instructor, Department of Radiology,
Massachusetts General Hospital, Harvard
Medical School, Boston, Massachusetts, USA

AKRAM SHAABAN, MBBCh
Department of Radiology and Imaging
Sciences, University of Utah, Salt Lake City,
Utah, USA

KIMBERLY L. SHAMPAIN, MD
Clinical Assistant Professor of Radiology,
Michigan Medicine, University of Michigan,
University Hospital, Ann Arbor, Michigan, USA

ANUP S. SHETTY, MD
Mallinckrodt Institute of Radiology,
Washington University School of Medicine, St
Louis, Missouri, USA

ERICA B. STEIN, MD
Clinical Associate Professor of Radiology,
Michigan Medicine, University of Michigan,
University Hospital, Ann Arbor, Michigan, USA

ARADHANA M. VENKATESAN, MD
Professor of Radiology, Term Tenure,
Department of Abdominal Imaging, Division of
Diagnostic Imaging, The University of Texas
MD Anderson Cancer Center, Houston, Texas,
USA

ASHISH P. WASNIK, MD
Clinical Professor of Radiology, Michigan
Medicine, University of Michigan, University
Hospital, Ann Arbor, Michigan, USA

MAGGIE ZHANG, MD, PhD
Department of Radiology, University of
Michigan, Ann Arbor, Michigan, USA

**KONSTANTINOS ZORMPAS-PETRIDIS,
BSc, MSc, PhD**
Division of Radiotherapy and Imaging, The
Institute of Cancer Research, London, United
Kingdom

MARIA ZULFIQAR, MD
Mayo Clinic, Scottsdale, Arizona, USA

Contents

> Epithelial ovarian neoplasms (EON) constitute the majority of ovarian cancers. Among EON, high-grade serous carcinoma (HGSC) is the most common and most likely to present at an advanced stage. Radiologists should recognize the imaging features associated with HGSC, particularly at ultrasound and MR imaging. Computed tomography is used for staging and to direct care pathways. Peritoneal carcinomatosis is common and does not preclude surgical resection. Other less common malignant EON have varied appearances, but share a common correlation between the amount of vascularized solid tissue and the likelihood of malignancy.

> Ovarian malignant germ cell tumors are a diverse set of masses originating from the primitive gonadal germ cells, often in young females. They have useful imaging and clinical features, including serum tumor marker elevation, that may aid the radiologist at the time of diagnosis, and also during follow-up. Accurate and timely diagnosis is essential, as standard-of-care therapies lead to a high rate of cancer remission.

> Ovarian sex cord-stromal tumors (OSCSTs) are a rare group of ovarian neoplasms that can be benign or malignant. They are classified into pure sex cord tumors, pure stromal tumors, and mixed SCST. The most common malignant OSCSTs are adult granulosa cell tumors. In contrast to the more common ovarian epithelial malignancies, OSCSTs present in younger patients, often at early stages, with better prognoses. Imaging features are variable, and pathology is required for diagnosis. However, certain tumors demonstrate characteristic imaging appearances that can be useful in narrowing the differential diagnosis.

> Endometrial cancer is the most common gynecologic cancer in the United States and Europe, with an increasing incidence rate in high-income countries. MR imaging is recommended for treatment planning because it provides critical information on the extent of myometrial and cervical invasion, extrauterine spread, and lymph node status, all of which are important in the selection of the most appropriate therapy. This article highlights the added value of imaging, focused on MR imaging, in the assessment of endometrial cancer and summarizes the role of MR imaging for endometrial cancer risk stratification and management.

Uterine sarcomas are a group of rare uterine tumors comprised of multiple subtypes with different histologic characteristics, prognoses, and imaging appearances. Identification of uterine sarcomas and their differentiation from benign uterine disease on imaging is of critical importance for treatment planning to guide appropriate management and optimize patient outcomes. Herein, we review the spectrum of uterine sarcomas with a focus on the classification of primary sarcoma subtypes and presenting the typical MR imaging appearances.

Cervical cancer remains a significant contributor to morbidity and mortality for women globally despite medical advances in preventative medicine and treatment. The 2018 Internal Federation of Gynecology and Obstetrics committee modified their original 2009 staging scheme to incorporate advanced imaging modalities, where available, to increase the accuracy of staging and to guide evolving treatments. Having a robust understanding of the newest staging iteration, its consequences on treatment pathways, and common imaging pitfalls will aid the radiologist in generating valuable and practical reports to optimize treatment strategies.

Vaginal and vulvar malignancies are rare gynecologic malignancies but can be associated with high morbidity and mortality if undiagnosed and untreated. Advanced imaging modalities such as MRI enable assessment of the local extent of disease and evaluation for regional or distant spread. Accurate identification and description of the primary lesion and sites of involvement as well as detection and localization of suspicious lymph nodes are critical in guiding appropriate management. Additionally, radiologists should be aware of potential mimickers on imaging and the differential diagnoses for vaginal and vulvar lesions.

Several recent guidelines have been published to improve accuracy and consistency of adnexal mass imaging interpretation and to guide management. Guidance from the American College of Radiology (ACR) Appropriateness Criteria establishes preferred adnexal imaging modalities and follow-up. Moreover, the ACR Ovarian-Adnexal Reporting Data System establishes a comprehensive, unified set of evidence-based guidelines for classification of adnexal masses by both ultrasound and MR imaging, communicating risk of malignancy to further guide management.

MR imaging is the modality of choice for the pre-treatment evaluation of patients with gynecologic malignancies, given its excellent soft tissue contrast and multiplanar capability. However, it is not without pitfalls. Challenges can be encountered in the assessment of the infiltration of myometrium, vagina, cervical stroma, and parametria, which are crucial prognostic factors for endometrial and cervical cancers.

Other challenges can be encountered in the distinction between solid and non-solid tissue and in the identification of peritoneal carcinomatosis for the sonographically indeterminate adnexal mass.

Matthew Larson, Petra Lovrec, Elizabeth A. Sadowski, and Ali Pirasteh

Patients with gynecologic malignancies often require a multimodality imaging approach for initial staging, treatment response assessment, and surveillance. MRI imaging and PET are two well-established and widely accepted modalities in this setting. Although PET and MRI imaging are often acquired separately on two platforms (a PET/computed tomography [CT] and an MRI imaging scanner), hybrid PET/MRI scanners offer the potential for comprehensive disease assessment in one visit. Gynecologic malignancies have been one of the most successful areas for implementation of PET/MRI. This article provides an overview of the role of this platform in the care of patients with gynecologic malignancies.

Megan C. Jacobsen, Ekta Maheshwari, Ann H. Klopp, and Aradhana M. Venkatesan

Pelvic imaging is integral to contemporary radiotherapy (RT) management of gynecologic malignancies. For cervical, endometrial, vulvar, and vaginal cancers, three-dimensional imaging modalities aid in tumor staging and RT candidate selection and inform treatment strategy, including RT planning, execution, and posttherapy surveillance. State-of-the-art care routinely incorporates magnetic resonance (MR) imaging, 18F-fluorodeoxyglucose-PET/computed tomography (CT), and CT to guide external beam RT and brachytherapy, allowing the customization of RT plans to maximize patient outcomes and reduce treatment-related toxicities. Follow-up imaging identifies radiation-resistant and recurrent disease as well as short-term and long-term toxicities from RT.

Camilla Panico, Giacomo Avesani, Konstantinos Zormpas-Petridis, Leonardo Rundo, Camilla Nero, and Evis Sala

Ovarian cancer, one of the deadliest gynecologic malignancies, is characterized by high intra- and inter-site genomic and phenotypic heterogeneity. The traditional information provided by the conventional interpretation of diagnostic imaging studies cannot adequately represent this heterogeneity. Radiomics analyses can capture the complex patterns related to the microstructure of the tissues and provide quantitative information about them. This review outlines how radiomics and its integration with other quantitative biological information, like genomics and proteomics, can impact the clinical management of ovarian cancer.

PROGRAM OBJECTIVE

The objective of the *Radiologic Clinics of North America* is to keep practicing radiologists and radiology residents up to date with current clinical practice in radiology by providing timely articles reviewing the state of the art in patient care.

TARGET AUDIENCE

Practicing radiologists, radiology residents, and other healthcare professionals who provide patient care utilizing radiologic findings.

LEARNING OBJECTIVES

Upon completion of this activity, participants will be able to:
1. Describe how imaging is useful in the surveillance of gynecologic malignancies.
2. Discuss the integral role image guided radiotherapy plays within gynecologic care.
3. Recognize the impact imaging has in clinical management of ovarian cancer and the assessment of disease extent.

ACCREDITATION

The Elsevier Office of Continuing Medical Education (EOCME) is accredited by the Accreditation Council for Continuing Medical Education (ACCME) to provide continuing medical education for physicians.

The EOCME designates this journal-based CME activity for a maximum of 12 *AMA PRA Category 1 Credit*(s)™.Physicians should claim only the credit commensurate with the extent of their participation in the activity.

All other healthcare professionals requesting continuing education credit for this enduring material will be issued a certificate of participation.

DISCLOSURE OF CONFLICTS OF INTEREST

The EOCME assesses conflict of interest with its instructors, faculty, planners, and other individuals who are in a position to control the content of CME activities. All relevant conflicts of interest that are identified are thoroughly vetted by EOCME for fair balance, scientific objectivity, and patient care recommendations. EOCME is committed to providing its learners with CME activities that promote improvements or quality in healthcare and not a specific proprietary business or a commercial interest.

The planning committee, staff, authors, and editors listed below have identified no financial relationships or relationships to products or devices they or their spouse/life partner have with commercial interest related to the content of this CME activity:

Giacomo Avesani, MD; Olga R. Brook, MD; Kyle M. Devins, MD; Nicole Hindman, MD; Lynette Jones, MSN, RN-BC; Aoife Kilcoyne, MB BCh BAO; Ann H. Klopp, MD, PhD; Kothainayaki Kulanthaivelu; Matthew Larson, MD, PhD; Susanna I. Lee, MD, PhD; Petra Lovrec, MD; Michela Lupinelli, MD; Katherine E. Maturen, MD, MS; Melissa McGettigan, MD; Christine Menias, MD; Camilla Nero, MD; Stephanie Nougaret, MD, PhD; Esther Oliva, MD; Taemee Pak, MD; Camilla Panico, MD; Krupa Patel-Lippmann, MD; Robert Petrocelli, MD; Caroline Reinhold, MD, MSc; Douglas Rogers, MD; Molly E. Roseland, MD; Leonardo Rundo, PhD; Elizabeth Sadowski, MD; Michelle D. Sakala, MD; Martina Sbarra, MD; Madeleine Sertic, MB BCh, BAO; Akram Shaaban, MBBCh; Kimberly L. Shampain, MD; Anup S. Shetty, MD; Erica B. Stein, MD; Aradhana M. Venkatesan, MD; Ashish P. Wasnik, MD; Maggie Zhang, MD, PhD; Konstantinos Zormpas-Petridis, PhD; Maria Zulfiqar, MD

The planning committee, staff, authors, and editors listed below have identified financial relationships or relationships to products or devices they or their spouse/life partner have with commercial interest related to the content of this CME activity:

Ali Pirasteh, MD: Researcher: GE HealthCare

Evis Sala, MD, PhD, FRCR, FRCP: Ownership Interest: Lucida Medical; Researcher & Speaker's Bureau: GE HealthCare, Canon USA, Inc.

UNAPPROVED/OFF-LABEL USE DISCLOSURE

The EOCME requires CME faculty to disclose to the participants:
1. When products or procedures being discussed are off-label, unlabelled, experimental, and/or investigational (not US Food and Drug Administration [FDA] approved); and
2. Any limitations on the information presented, such as data that are preliminary or that represent ongoing research, interim analyses, and/or unsupported opinions. Faculty may discuss information about pharmaceutical agents that is outside of FDA-approved labelling. This information is intended solely for CME and is not intended to promote off-label use of these medications. If you have any questions, contact the medical affairs department of the manufacturer for the most recent prescribing information.

TO ENROLL

To enroll in the *Radiologic Clinics of North America* Continuing Medical Education program, call customer service at 1-800-654-2452 or sign up online at http://www.theclinics.com/home/cme. The CME program is available to subscribers for an additional annual fee of USD 340.00.

METHOD OF PARTICIPATION

In order to claim credit, participants must complete the following:

1. Complete enrolment as indicated above.
2. Read the activity.
3. Complete the CME Test and Evaluation. Participants must achieve a score of 70% on the test. All CME Tests and Evaluations must be completed online.

CME INQUIRIES/SPECIAL NEEDS

For all CME inquiries or special needs, please contact elsevierCME@elsevier.com.

RADIOLOGIC CLINICS OF NORTH AMERICA

Preface

Imaging of Gynecologic Malignancy: The Current State-of-the-Art

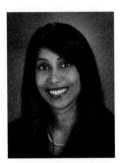

Aradhana M. Venkatesan, MD
Editor

Gynecologic malignancies are among the most common cancers worldwide. They encompass a broad spectrum of malignancies affecting the female genital and reproductive tract. As such, they are frequently encountered in clinical radiology practice. A fundamental understanding of the role of imaging and the characteristic imaging findings associated with these malignancies is of critical importance to the practicing radiologist in order to maintain diagnostic accuracy.

In this issue of *Radiologic Clinics of North America*, we present the spectrum of gynecologic malignancies that are encountered in radiologic practice, with an emphasis on cervical, uterine, ovarian, vaginal, and vulvar neoplasms. Current imaging guidelines for adnexal mass imaging are also summarized as well as practical pearls and pitfalls in gynecologic MR imaging that are directly applicable to daily practice. Each of these comprehensive articles is paired with valuable case-based imaging examples. Also described in this issue are recent innovations in the realm of PET/MR imaging, image-guided radiotherapy for gynecologic malignancies, and advanced radiomics analyses and their implications for treatment monitoring and clinical management. As such, these comprehensive, contemporary articles provide practical information for daily practice as well as important, data-driven perspectives on where we stand currently and what the future may bring to contribute to the field.

I am very grateful for the expertise and dedication of the talented authors who have contributed to this issue. Many of these authors are internationally known experts in their field, and I am deeply appreciative of the time they have dedicated to this work. I would also like to thank *Radiologic Clinics of North America* for selecting this important topic to promote. This issue provides vital information that is of value to any radiologist or radiology trainee working to augment or refresh their knowledge and understanding of the current state-of-the-art in gynecologic malignancy imaging.

Aradhana M. Venkatesan, MD
Department of Abdominal Imaging
Division of Diagnostic Imaging
The University of Texas MD Anderson Cancer Center
1400 Pressler Street, MSC 1182
FCT 15.6074
Houston, TX 77030, USA

E-mail address:
avenkatesan@mdanderson.org

Imaging of Gynecologic Malignancy: The Current State of the Art

Malignant Epithelial Tumors of the Ovary
Pathogenesis and Imaging

Katherine E. Maturen, MD, MS[a,b,]*, Kimberly L. Shampain, MD[b],
Molly E. Roseland, MD[b], Michelle D. Sakala, MD[b], Maggie Zhang, MD, PhD[b],
Erica B. Stein, MD[b]

KEYWORDS

- Ovarian neoplasm • Serous carcinoma • Mucinous ovarian carcinoma
- Clear cell ovarian carcinoma • Endometrioid ovarian carcinoma • Epithelial ovarian neoplasm
- Ovarian cancer • Tubal carcinoma

KEY POINTS

- The most common and most deadly epithelial ovarian neoplasm is high-grade serous carcinoma, which usually presents with advanced-stage disease.
- High-grade serous carcinoma arises from small solid precursors within the fallopian tubes and is not a simple cyst at any stage of its development.
- Peritoneal carcinomatosis is a common presentation in high-grade serous carcinoma and does not preclude surgical resection.

INTRODUCTION

Ovarian cancer is an important public health problem. Overall, it is the most lethal gynecologic cancer and the fifth leading cause of cancer death in women, with approximately 20,000 new cases expected in the United States in 2022.[1] Despite these impacts, and resulting clinical attention and research, there is no evidence-based strategy for early detection.[2] However, ovarian cancer mortality has decreased by approximately 2% to 3% per year this century, attributed to a combination of decreased incidence and improved therapies.[1]

The term "ovarian cancer" encompasses several very different histologies. Among all ovarian and tubal malignancies, 90% are epithelial tumors and provide the focus for this review. Masses arising from germ cell and stromal elements are more commonly benign (such as teratoma and fibroma, respectively), but they do have malignant counterparts, which are each explored in a separate chapter in this edition.

Radiologists who understand the natural history and characteristic growth patterns of this group of diseases will be equipped to perform appropriate risk stratification of adnexal lesions, stage cancer when a diagnosis is established, assess treatment response, and recognize tumor recurrence. Advanced imaging techniques play an increasingly important role in therapeutic decision-making for women with gynecologic cancers.

EPITHELIAL HISTOLOGIES AND GRADING

Table 1 enumerates the major subtypes of malignant epithelial ovarian neoplasm (EON).[3] Serous tumors are the most common.[4,5] The incidence of primary ovarian mucinous tumors was historically overestimated, because adnexal metastases from gastrointestinal primary tumors were

[a] Department of Obstetrics & Gynecology, University of Michigan; [b] Department of Radiology, University of Michigan, 1500 East Medical Center Drive, Ann Arbor, MI 48109, USA
* Corresponding author.
E-mail address: kmaturen@umich.edu
Twitter: @katematuren (K.E.M.); @kimshampainMD (K.L.S.); @homeostatic (M.E.R.); @msakalaMD (M.D.S.); @manzhang01 (M.Z.); @ericasteinMD (E.B.S.)

Radiol Clin N Am 61 (2023) 563–577
https://doi.org/10.1016/j.rcl.2023.02.003
0033-8389/23/© 2023 Elsevier Inc. All rights reserved.

Table 1
Important subtypes of ovarian epithelial malignancy

Subtype		Proportion of Malignant OEN	Clinical Presentation	Serum Tumor Markers	Approximate Five-Year Survival	Unique Imaging Features
Serous	High grade	63%	Stage III to IV most common, postmenopausal abdominal bloating, and pelvic mass	CA-125 HE4	40%	Papillary solid components, hypervascular soft-tissue masses obscuring pelvic tissue planes, intratubal masses, and omental cake Psammomatous calcifications
	Low grade	2%	Approximately 50% of patients have locoregional disease and 50% advanced at presentation	CA-125 HE4	70%	
Mucinous		10%	>80% stage I, carcinomatosis is uncommon but advanced disease may feature pseudomyxoma peritonei	CA-125 CA-19–9 CEA	80% to 90%	Large multilocular masses with thickened irregular septations, mucinous contents, and eggshell calcifications
Clear cell		10%	Most stage I to II	CA-125 CA-19–9	95% for locoregional disease	Approximately 70% arise in endometriosis
Endometrioid		10%	Most stage I to II	CA-125 HE4	85% for locoregional disease	40% arise in endometriosis
Carcinosarcoma		5%	Stage III most common, slightly older than HGSC cohort	CA-125	30%	Not distinctive, variable cystic and solid components depending on histology
Brenner tumor		<1%	Only 1% of Brenner tumors are malignant but these are aggressive; benign forms may secrete excess estrogen	CA-125	30%	Low signal on T2WI, mimics fibroma/thecoma, synchronous with other benign (or rarely malignant) ovarian neoplasm such as mucinous cystadenoma in 30% of cases

erroneously classified as ovarian in origin.[5] Clear cell and endometrioid carcinomas often, but not always, arise in endometriosis.[6] Brenner tumors are overwhelmingly benign and were previously called transitional cell tumors because of their histologic resemblance to urothelium.[7,8] Any of these subtypes may coexist in a mixed-type epithelial tumor such as seromucinous tumor, or mingle with mesenchymal elements in a carcinosarcoma. Previously known as malignant mixed Mullerian tumor (MMMT), carcinosarcoma may contain a variety of cell types and has aggressive clinical behavior.[9] Carcinosarcoma may be more difficult to target with chemotherapy due to its combination of cell types.[10] Distinctive imaging features and clinical considerations will be detailed in separate sections.

EONs are pathologically classified as benign, borderline, low grade, or high grade. However, this is not a stepwise progression, and carcinogenesis is thought to proceed along two distinct pathways (Fig. 1). Benign epithelial tumors, including cystadenomas and cystadenofibromas, are formed along Type I pathway. Much more common than malignant EON, these lesions are predominantly or entirely cystic, often unilocular, and have minimal or no enhancing soft-tissue components[11] (Figs. 2–4). Histologically, most cystadenomas and cystadenofibromas are essentially inclusion cysts and entirely lack monoclonal epithelial proliferation, suggesting that they are not actually neoplasms.[12,13] Cystadenomas grow slowly and may become very large yet remain benign; mucinous cystadenomas grow slightly faster than serous.[14,15] Importantly, cystadenomas and cystadenofibromas are not precursor lesions for high-grade epithelial ovarian cancers.[16]

Borderline tumors are a distinct neoplastic subtype that is histologically malignant, yet limited to the surface of the ovary, without deep invasion of the ovarian stroma.[17,18] Although most malignant EON affect postmenopausal women, borderline tumors are often seen in women in their 20s and 30s. Many borderline serous tumors have a highly characteristic morphology of frondlike, papillary tissue, either within a cyst or arising exophytically from the ovarian surface (Figs. 5 and 6). Preoperative recognition of a likely borderline histology enables appropriate presurgical patient counseling and consideration of a fertility-sparing approach (leaving the uterus and at least one ovary in situ).[19] Borderline tumors may form peritoneal implants, but these implants are superficial and do not affect the long-term excellent prognosis.[5] Borderline epithelial tumors are not considered true malignancies.

Many mucinous cancers have low-grade histology, but most serous cancers are high grade. High-grade cancers show larger and more highly vascularized soft-tissue components by imaging and gross pathology, with greater cellular atypia and mitotic rate under the microscope. Unlike other common abdominal malignancies such as colorectal cancer, EONs do not follow a progression of sequential mutations from metaplasia to adenoma and carcinoma. As illustrated in Fig. 1, high-grade serous cancers have a distinct cellular lineage along Type II pathway and do not grow from low-grade cancers in most cases. We will consider this process and its imaging implications in more detail in the following section.

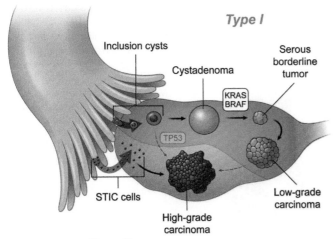

Type I

Inclusion cysts

Cystadenoma

KRAS
BRAF

Serous borderline tumor

TP53

STIC cells

Low-grade carcinoma

High-grade carcinoma

Type II

Fig. 1. Schematic of the two primary pathways of tubo-ovarian carcinogenesis. In Type I pathway, inclusion cysts are the precursor lesion. Many cystadenomas are actually large inclusion cysts. Genetic mutations rarely lead to intracystic development of borderline and low-grade tumors, but almost never result in high-grade carcinoma. In Type II pathway, the precursor lesion is STIC that arises in the distal fallopian tube, is shed onto the ovarian surface, and develops directly into predominantly solid high-grade cancers. (*Adapted from* Kurman, R.J. and M. Shih, The origin and pathogenesis of epithelial ovarian cancer: a proposed unifying theory. Am J Surg Pathol, 2010. 34(3): p. 433-43.)

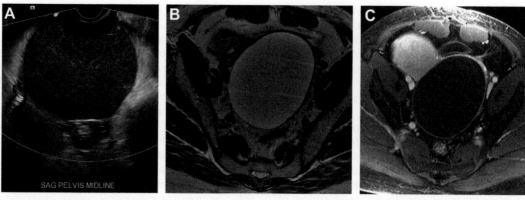

Fig. 2. Mucinous cystadenoma in a 32-year-old with palpable mass. (*A*) Color Doppler TVUS shows a unilocular cyst with speckled pattern of internal echoes resembling an endometrioma, and no soft-tissue components, ACR O-RADS US score 2. The internal echoes on US are due to mucin. (*B*) Axial T2WI reveals a unilocular thin-walled cyst. (*C*) Axial post-contrast T1WI shows a smooth, thin enhancing wall. ACR O-RADS MR score 3. On MR imaging, the internal fluid is simple, with no shading on T2WI or hyperintense signal on T1WI as would be expected in an endometrioma.

EPIDEMIOLOGY AND PATHOGENESIS OF EPITHELIAL OVARIAN NEOPLASMS

The single most important risk factor for epithelial ovarian cancer is age, with 50% of cases affecting women over 65.[5] Worldwide, ovarian cancer is most common in Europe and North America. This may in part be nutritional, with a small increased risk of ovarian cancer in obese women, though much less significant than the increased risk of endometrial cancer posed by excess body fat. Women in economically developed countries also tend to have fewer children, which may be the more important factor. There is substantial evidence that a woman's total number of lifetime ovulations is directly proportional to her ovarian cancer risk. This "incessant ovulation" theory was first posed more than 50 years ago[20] yet remains imperfectly explained, though potentially related to repeated cycles of tissue damage and repair. What is clear is that prevention of ovulation by pregnancy, breastfeeding, or oral contraceptives reduces lifetime risk of ovarian cancer.

Genetic syndromes including breast cancer gene (BRCA) and Lynch syndrome are also associated with increased risk. Usually serous type, BRCA-associated cancers occur in younger women than sporadic ovarian cancer and tend to be more chemoresponsive. Cancers associated with Lynch syndrome have a higher predominance of endometrioid and clear cell types. Women with these high-risk genetic mutations are often treated with risk-reducing bilateral salpingo-oophorectomy (RRSO) at age 40 or after childbearing is completed, with an 80% to 100% reduction in their lifetime ovarian cancer risk.[21,22] Endometriosis and repeated or chronic pelvic inflammatory disease are additional risk factors for malignant EON.

High-grade ovarian cancer may be more properly termed "tubo-ovarian" cancer, given the increasing recognition of precursors called serous tubal intraepithelial carcinomas (STIC). Because STICs are usually only a few millimeters in size, they are rarely detected by current imaging techniques. Although there is no known cancer

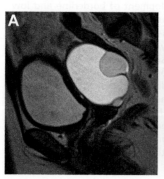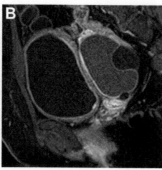

Fig. 3. Mucinous cystadenoma in a 42-year-old with incidental mass. Sagittal MR imaging images show multiple locules of varying signal intensity on (*A*) T2WI and (*B*) T1WI post-contrast. Enhancing septations are thin and smooth. ACR O-RADS MR score 3.

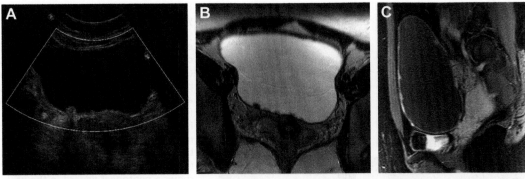

Fig. 4. Serous cystadenofibroma in a 30-year-old with pelvic fullness. (*A*) Transabdominal color Doppler image shows a large unilocular cyst with numerous papillations lacking demonstrable vascularity along the posterior wall, ACR O-RADS US score 5 due to >4 papillary projections. (*B*) Axial T2WI shows very low signal within these papillations, matched by low signal on DWI (not shown). (*C*) Sagittal post-contrast T1WI shows nodular enhancement of numerous papillations. ACR O-RADS MR score 2 due to "dark/dark" pattern in fibrous tissue nodules.

precursor lesion from ovarian epithelium, STICs are found in up to 70% of women with malignant EONs and are often incidentally detected in RRSO specimens from women with high-risk genetic mutations.[16] STICS develop into high-grade epithelial carcinomas, and are not cystic at any point in their life cycle. This is the key pathway for the development of aggressive epithelial carcinomas, as depicted in **Fig. 1**. This Type II pathway gives rise to high-grade serous ovarian, tubal, and primary peritoneal carcinoma, which are histologically identical and treated with the same approach.[5,23] To save lives by early detection,

we need to develop the capacity to detect STICs and prevent their evolution into carcinoma.

MALIGNANT EPITHELIAL OVARIAN NEOPLASMS: CLINICAL AND IMAGING FEATURES

Radiologists are not pathologists, and our gynecologic oncology colleagues do not expect or rely on us to make histologic diagnoses by imaging. In addition to imaging, clinical presentation, demographics, and tumor markers also contribute to the differential diagnosis.[24] However, some malignant EON tissue types have highly characteristic morphologies and can be suggested

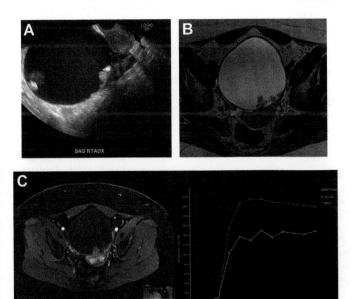

Fig. 5. Serous borderline tumor in a 36-year-old with incidental mass. (*A*) Sagittal TVUS shows a large unilocular cyst with numerous papillary projections; no demonstrable internal vascularity on color Doppler (not shown). ACR O-RADS US Score 5 (*B*) Axial T2WI shows frond-like intracystic projections. (*C*) Brisk enhancement within papillary soft tissue, with intermediate-risk time–intensity curve (white curve) compared with myometrium (green curve). ACR O-RADS MR score 4.

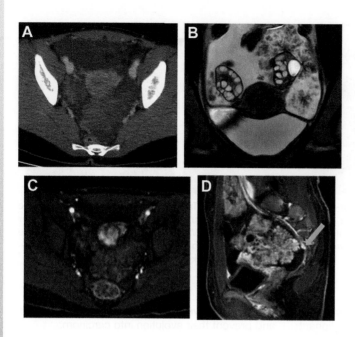

Fig. 6. Serous borderline tumor in a 26-year-old with incidental mass. (A) Axial contrast-enhanced CT (CECT) shows bilateral adnexal masses with frond-like architecture, in a background of ascites. (B) Oblique axial T2WI shows delicate papillary and branching soft tissue arising exophytically from both ovaries. (C) Axial T1WI 30 s after contrast administration illustrates enhancement of both masses, visually less than myometrium but full DCE series was not performed. (D) Sagittal delayed post-contrast T1WI shows a peritoneal deposit in the posterior pelvis (arrow). ACR O-RADS MR Score 5 due to peritoneal disease. She was treated with a fertility-sparing surgical approach and remains disease free at 5 years.

preoperatively, aiding surgical planning and patient counseling. These are also the most common subtypes of malignant EON.

Serous Carcinoma

Clinical context

High-grade serous carcinoma (HGSC) is often insidious, with early symptoms of pelvic pain or fatigue sometimes dismissed by patients or physicians. Most patients are post-menopausal. Serous carcinoma rapidly spreads within the peritoneal space and is bilateral in >50% of cases. Intraperitoneal soft-tissue masses and ascites cause abdominal bloating and gastrointestinal symptoms, whereas physical examination reveals pelvic masses and fixed organs. Serum cancer antigen 125 (CA-125) is elevated in nearly all women with HGSC, and has a positive predictive value of >80% for ovarian malignancy in postmenopausal women.[24] However, mild elevation is nonspecific and can be associated with some benign conditions and virtually all epithelial neoplasms.

HGSC is treated with a combination of surgery and chemotherapy. At the time of initial staging, clinical and imaging findings, performance status, and serum CA-125 all factor into an important initial decision. Debulking includes bilateral salpingo-oophorectomy, hysterectomy, pelvic and para-aortic lymph node dissection, omentectomy, and peritoneal stripping/washing as indicated. Optimal debulking removes all tissue deposits > 1 cm. Some patients undergo immediate surgical debulking, whereas others with more extensive disease are treated with three to six cycles of platinum-based neoadjuvant chemotherapy before interval debulking. Adjuvant chemotherapy follows surgery.

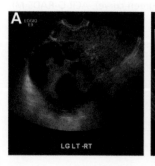
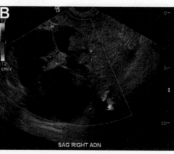

Fig. 7. High-grade serous carcinoma in a 55-year-old with incidental mass. (A) TVUS shows nodular soft tissue studding cyst walls and septations, with large adjacent solid component with irregular margin. (B) Color Doppler confirms internal vascularity. ACR O-RADS US score 5.

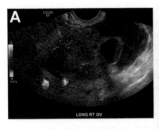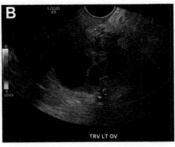

Fig. 8. High-grade serous carcinoma in a 72-year-old with pelvic pain. Color Doppler TVUS images (*A*, *B*) illustrate confluent soft tissue obscuring both ovaries with abundant vascularity (Color Score 4) on color Doppler, and pelvic ascites. ACR O-RADS US score 5.

Low-grade serous carcinoma is a rare subset of serous carcinoma, which may present in younger women and may be more properly termed a Type I cancer given its association with cystadenoma and borderline tumor.[25] Low-grade serous cancer rarely causes systemic symptoms but may be detected as a palpable mass. It is less aggressive but also less chemoresponsive than HGSC, probably due to its relatively slow mitotic rate and cell growth. Thus, neoadjuvant therapy is less common and upfront surgery is usually favored.[26] Patients may undergo long-term hormonal therapy for maintenance and disease suppression.

Imaging pearls

Simple adnexal cysts are not cancer and do not develop into high-grade cancers. Cystic masses with solid components are more likely to be neoplastic, with the risk of malignancy increasing with the quantity of soft tissue and vascularity of solid elements. The American College of Radiology (ACR) Ovarian-Adnexal Reporting and Data System Ultrasound (O-RADS US) and MR imaging frameworks, discussed in detail elsewhere in this issue, provide an evidence-based approach to risk stratification of adnexal observations.[27,28] The term "complex cyst" is discouraged in favor of more precise descriptors. Ultrasound (US) is the most appropriate initial imaging study for clinically suspected adnexal mass.[29] Serous carcinomas are usually mixed cystic and solid, with highly vascular soft-tissue elements and one or a few locules. These elements may include frondlike or papillary branching masses as in borderline tumors, but also irregular or nodular thickened septations (**Fig. 7**), or large solid elements (**Fig. 8**). Because early intracoelomic spread is common, US may show bilateral adnexal masses and/or uterine involvement; thus, delineating the organ of origin can be challenging.

When US findings are indeterminate, or a mass is incompletely imaged by US, contrast-enhanced pelvic MR imaging increases specificity for malignancy.[30,31] Solid components in serous carcinoma may be papillary, irregular, or confluent as described above by US, with intermediate signal on T2-weighted image (T2WI) and clear

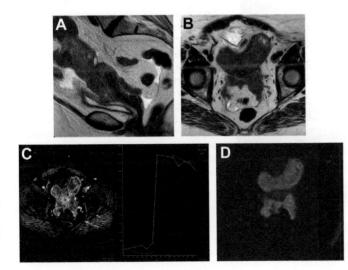

Fig. 9. High-grade serous carcinoma in a 69-year-old with early satiety. Sagittal (*A*) and axial (*B*) T2WI illustrate confluent intermediate signal soft tissue involving both adnexal regions, the uterine fundus, and the posterior cul de sac, obscuring delineation between organs. (*C*) High-risk time–intensity curve within the mass, mirroring that of the myometrium. (*D*) Obvious restricted diffusion on DWI within the confluent soft tissue. ACR O-RADS MR score 5.

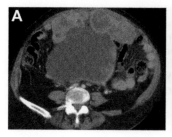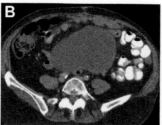

Fig. 10. High-grade serous carcinoma in a 57-year-old before and after neoadjuvant platinum-based chemotherapy. (A) Axial CECT before therapy shows bulky omental disease and a cystic and solid pelvic mass. (B) Following chemotherapy, the omental disease is substantially decreased and the solid elements of the pelvic mass have regressed. Decreased tumor volume increases the likelihood of optimal surgical debulking.

restricted diffusion. HGSCs enhance briskly after contrast administration, with greater enhancement than outer myometrium at 30 to 40 s following injection or a high-risk time–intensity curve on dynamic contrast-enhanced sequences[28] (Fig. 9).

Computed tomography (CT) is not an appropriate modality for adnexal lesion characterization, although many masses are incidentally detected when CT is ordered for other suspected diagnoses. Nonsimple appearing fluid contents, solid tissue, irregular margins, or ascites are indications for additional lesion characterization with US or MR imaging.[32] CT provides important staging information to direct the initial clinical pathway, whether toward upfront debulking or neoadjuvant chemotherapy (Fig. 10).[33] Stage I tumor is confined to ovaries, Stage II tumor involves one or both ovaries with pelvic extension (below the pelvic brim), Stage III involves the extrapelvic peritoneal space or retroperitoneal nodes, and Stage IV reflects distant metastatic disease.

Often, CT is helpful to identify sites of disease, such as omental metastases or an enlarged lymph node, for potential confirmatory biopsy before surgery. A recent international consensus guideline provides an imaging lexicon for ovarian cancer staging, intended to improve interreader concordance and report clarity.[34] Radiologists should be aware of specific disease sites associated with suboptimal debulking, including right subdiaphragmatic deposits, lesser sac disease, and retroperitoneal nodes superior to the renal veins[35] (Fig. 11). Radiologists often combine serosal, mesenteric, and omental tumor deposits together as "peritoneal carcinomatosis," but in the setting of ovarian carcinoma, these sites should be specifically distinguished. Omental disease is readily removed at omentectomy, but serosal and mesenteric disease may limit optimal debulking or increase surgical complexity and should be specifically identified.

After completion of surgery and chemotherapy, patients are monitored clinically and by serial measurement of serum CA-125.[26] Imaging is not a standard part of surveillance after successful treatment and is generally ordered only when

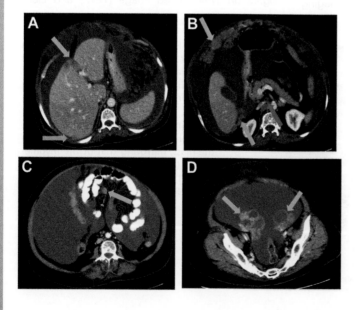

Fig. 11. High-grade serous carcinoma in a 75-year-old with bloating. Axial CECT images show (A) ascites and tumor deposition along the falciform ligament (yellow arrow) and along the posterior right hemidiaphragm (blue arrow), (B) omental cake (yellow arrow), and extensive tumor in Morison's pouch (blue arrow) as well as high retroperitoneal nodes (orange arrow), (C) mesenteric nodule (arrow) and (D) bilateral hypervascular cystic and solid adnexal masses. Several of these findings were thought likely to limit optimal debulking and neoadjuvant therapy was given.

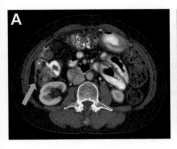 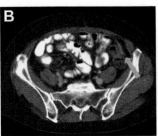

Fig. 12. Recurrent high-grade serous carcinoma in a 68-year-old with rising serum CA-125. Axial CECT images show new nodular soft-tissue plaques (*arrows*) along peritoneal surfaces adjacent to (*A*) right and (*B*) left colon.

recurrence is suspected. CT and 18F-fluoro-2-deoxy-D-glucose (^{18}FDG) PET/CT are most appropriate in this clinical setting, although pelvic or abdominal MR imaging may be appropriate for tissue characterization of lesions that are incompletely assessed by other modalities, or to provide greater anatomic detail when surgery or targeted radiotherapy are considered.[33] In HGSC, intraperitoneal and pelvic soft-tissue recurrences are common. Tumor deposits may be subtle, and radiologists should carefully evaluate serosal surfaces, particular in dependent locations (**Fig. 12**). Intraparenchymal recurrences within liver and spleen are less common than surface deposits. Ascites and nodal recurrences are also possible.

Low-grade serous carcinoma may be an indolent process for decades in some women. Sometimes called "psammocarcinoma," low-grade serous carcinoma has a unique pattern of calcified intraperitoneal metastases due to the presence of psammoma bodies (**Fig. 13**).

Mucinous Carcinoma

Clinical context

In contrast to serous carcinomas, mucinous carcinomas form along Type I pathway and are more common in premenopausal women. They are rarely associated with BRCA mutations. Mucinous carcinomas tend to be large and unilateral, with an average size of 18 cm, but more than 80% are limited to Stage I at the time of diagnosis.[36] Thus, symptoms of pain and abdominal distension relate to the size of the pelvic mass rather than

associated carcinomatosis. Serum CA-19 to 9 and CA-125 may be elevated. If CEA is significantly elevated, this may favor a gastrointestinal primary tumor with ovarian metastasis.

Intact removal of the ovarian mass is the goal of surgery, which may in some cases be performed with a fertility-sparing approach. Most mucinous tumors are benign, so intraoperative frozen section is used to guide the extent of resection based on diagnosis of malignancy. If there is no spillage of mucinous contents or visible peritoneal tumor, lymph node dissection is not necessary due to the low frequency of nodal involvement. The appendix is visually assessed and removed if abnormal.

Mucinous tumors confined to the ovary may not require adjuvant chemotherapy. Women with more advanced diseases may be treated with several different chemotherapy regimens, some of which are derived from gastrointestinal cancer therapies.[26] As in serous carcinomas, routine surveillance imaging is not performed after successful treatment, and patients are monitored for recurrence clinically and with tumor markers.

Imaging pearls

Imaging appropriateness guidelines are identical for all subtypes of EON, detailed in the above section on serous cancers. US is usually the preferred initial modality. In contrast to HGSCs with their abundant solid tissue, the most common appearance of a mucinous carcinoma is a large multilocular cyst with thickened, nodular walls and septations (**Fig. 14**). Internal mucin contents may

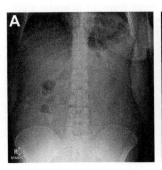 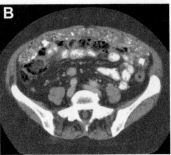

Fig. 13. Low-grade serous carcinoma with psammomatous calcifications in a 63-year-old with BRCA-1 mutation and prior right mastectomy. (*A*) Coarse and eggshell intraperitoneal calcifications are evident on abdominal radiograph, localized to the omentum on (*B*) axial CECT.

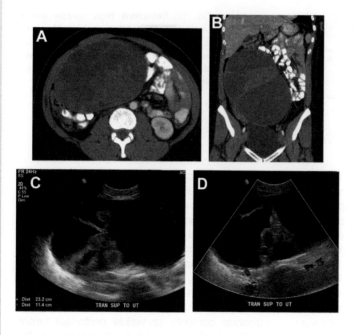

Fig. 14. Mucinous cystadenocarcinoma in a 45-year-old with abdominal discomfort. (*A*) Axial and (*B*) coronal CECT images show a large, smooth-walled multilocular mass with thick, irregular septations. (*C*) Grayscale and (*D*) color Doppler images show analogous findings, with large hypovascular solid components. ACR O-RADS US score 4.

be evident as nonsimple fluid with tiny internal echoes at US (see **Fig. 2**).

MR imaging is helpful for full coverage of larger multilocular lesions, identification of solid elements, and risk stratification using enhancement kinetics. Primary anatomic origin of tumor may be difficult to evaluate by US and CT, and MR imaging may provide additional localization information. Internal mucin may appear simple in some patients, but in other cases may show a streaming appearance on T2WI or a "stained glass" heterogeneity of signal in fluid contents on T1-weighted image (T1WI) and T2WI. Solid components show restricted diffusion and an intermediate or high-risk time–intensity curve[37] (**Fig. 15**).

CT is not used for lesion characterization but is indicated for staging. Radiologists should carefully evaluate the contralateral ovary, peritoneal space, and potential gastrointestinal primary sites such as stomach, appendix, and pancreas. As above, nodal disease is uncommon. In the small subset of patients with advanced disease, peritoneal involvement may have the unique appearance of pseudomyxoma peritonei, where gelatinous mucin

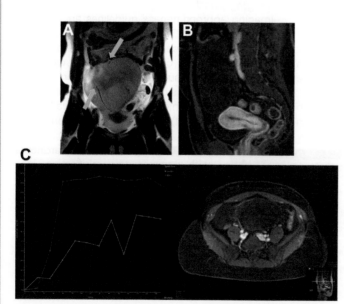

Fig. 15. Low-grade mucinous cystadenocarcinoma in a 52-year-old with abdominal pain. (*A*) Coronal T2WI shows a multilocular cyst with a ruptured wall along the right lateral margin (*arrows*), with mucin spilling into the abdomen. (*B*) Post-contrast sagittal T1WI shows enhancement of numerous fine septations. (*C*) Intermediate-risk time–intensity curve from an irregular thickened septation anteriorly (white curve) compared with myometrium (green curve). ACR O-RADS MR score 4.

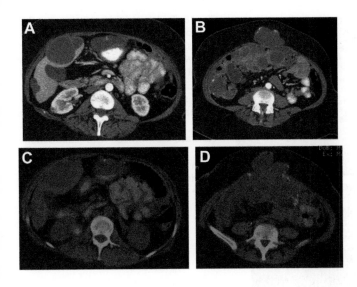

Fig. 16. Pseudomyxoma peritonei due to advanced mucinous ovarian carcinoma in a 55-year-old with abdominal distension. Axial CECT images (*A, B*) show low-density mucin locules with eggshell calcifications exhibiting mass effect on liver and bowel, and protruding from an umbilical hernia. [18]FDG PET/CT fusion images (*C, D*) at the same levels show no significant avidity in the hypocellular mucin deposits.

deposits exert mass effect on solid organs with scalloped margins, rather than layering dependently like simple fluid (**Fig. 16**).

Following surgical resection with or without adjuvant therapy, recurrent disease is relatively uncommon but may present as small locules of intraperitoneal mucin at CT or MR imaging. Notably, these mucin accumulations are hypocellular and may be associated with false-negative results on [18]FDG PET/CT (see **Fig. 16**).

Clear Cell and Endometrioid Carcinomas

Clinical context
Clear cell and endometrioid cancers form along Type I pathway and are typically present in perimenopausal and post-menopausal patients. Both have a strong association with endometriosis, particularly when it is long-standing. In fact, even in patients without clinically recognized endometriosis, endometrial cells shed onto the ovary are the suspected cell of origin, perhaps via retrograde menstruation. This hypothesis is supported by the observation that tubal ligation is protective against clear cell and endometrioid EON of these specific cell types.[16] Both subtypes are associated with Lynch syndrome and synchronous endometrial cancers.

Most patients have the locoregional disease at presentation, with a higher propensity for advanced-stage disease in clear cell carcinoma.

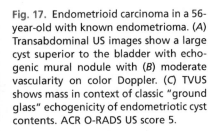

Fig. 17. Endometrioid carcinoma in a 56-year-old with known endometrioma. (*A*) Transabdominal US images show a large cyst superior to the bladder with echogenic mural nodule with (*B*) moderate vascularity on color Doppler. (*C*) TVUS shows mass in context of classic "ground glass" echogenicity of endometriotic cyst contents. ACR O-RADS US score 5.

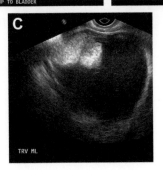

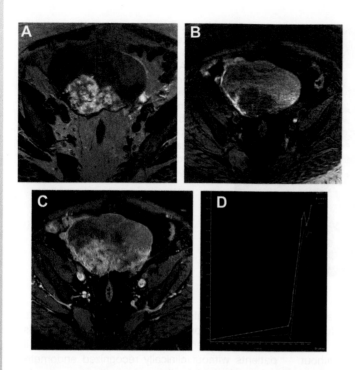

Fig. 18. Endometrioid carcinoma in a 77-year-old with remote history of endometriosis. (A) Axial T2WI shows unilocular cyst with "T2 shading" and large high signal solid component posteriorly. (B) Axial pre-contrast T1WI confirms very high signal within this large endometrioma with solid mass. (C) Posterior mass enhances avidly on T1WI post-contrast, confirmed with subtractions (not shown). (D) High-risk time–intensity curve (white curve) mimics myometrium (green curve). ACR O-RADS MR score 5.

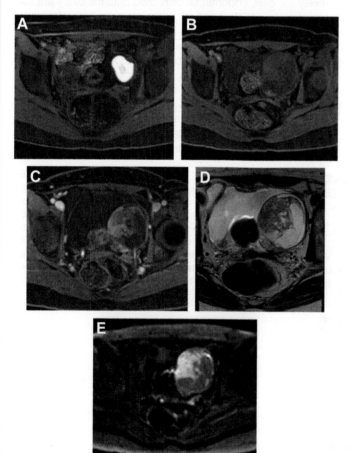

Fig. 19. Clear cell carcinoma arising from endometriosis in a 42-year-old. (A) Axial pre-contrast T1WI with fat saturation 5 years before diagnosis of malignancy showed a left adnexal endometrioma with classic high signal. (B) Axial pre-contrast T1WI with fat saturation reveals a new cystic mass with (C) enhancing solid components. (D) Axial T2WI shows solid tissue with intermediate signal (higher than skeletal muscle) and (E) distinct restricted diffusion on DWI at $b = 1000$. ACR O-RADS MR score 5.

CA-125 may be elevated with both cell types, whereas elevated HE4 is uniquely associated with endometrioid histology and elevated CA 19 to 9 with clear cell histology. Clear cell tumors are also associated with thromboembolic events.[5]

Neoadjuvant chemotherapy is rarely a factor in patients with these histologies, most of whom have Stage I disease. The surgical approach is similar to other EON, with the extent of debulking dependent upon intraoperative observations. Early-stage endometrioid cancer may be clinically observed, but clear cell carcinoma is usually treated with adjuvant platinum-based chemotherapy.[26]

Imaging pearls

Both clear cell and endometrioid tumors are well-vascularized solid masses at US and MR imaging and are difficult to distinguish from one another by imaging. The association with endometriosis is a unique feature observed in both histologies. These tumors may arise as a vascularized nodule within an endometrioma (Figs. 17 and 18), as a solid mass adherent or adjacent to a pelvic endometrioma or glandular deposit (Fig. 19), or even as a solid mass associated with endometriotic deposits in the body wall or elsewhere. Not all clear cell and endometrioid tumors are associated with endometriotic fluid, but when present it is highly characteristic. When endometriotic fluid is present, it is important to use subtraction imaging to distinguish enhancing soft tissue from fluid with inherent hyperintense signal on T1WI.

As with other cell types, US and MR imaging are primary modalities for initial risk assessment, whereas CT is used for staging and assessment of clinically suspected recurrence. [18]FDG PET/CT may be appropriate in the setting of recurrent disease.

DISCUSSION

In summary, the most common and most deadly epithelial ovarian carcinoma is high-grade serous cancer (HGSC), and radiologists who are well-versed in the diagnosis and management of this disease are poised to contribute to patient care. HGSC arises from tubal precursors called STICs along Type II pathway, not from benign or multilocular cysts. Most HGSC presents with advanced-stage disease, but unlike other abdominal malignancies, peritoneal spread does not preclude surgical resection of HGSC. Other epithelial ovarian malignancies arising from Type I pathway (mucinous, clear cell, endometrioid) are much less common, and more likely to present with early-stage disease.

US and MR imaging have primary roles in characterization and risk stratification of adnexal masses. CT is indicated for staging and assessment of clinically suspected recurrence. [18]FDG PET/CT may be helpful in the setting of suspected recurrence but is notably limited for mucinous histology. Radiologists who approach ovarian cancer from a disease-focused perspective can better integrate information from multiple modalities and map it onto standardized management pathways, contributing to clinical decision-making at diagnosis, staging, treatment, and beyond.

CLINICS CARE POINTS

- Simple adnexal cysts are rarely neoplastic, and when neoplastic they are benign or low-grade tumors.

- Risk of malignancy increases with the size and number of any vascularized soft-tissue elements in an adnexal mass. ACR O-RADS US and MR imaging systems can be used for evidence-based risk stratification by imaging.

- Serous carcinomas are the most common subtype of epithelial ovarian neoplasm and the most common ovarian cancer overall, with aggressive clinical behavior and <40% disease specific 5-year survival.

- High-grade serous carcinoma commonly presents with peritoneal carcinomatosis. In this setting, the task of the radiologist is to identify difficult-to-resect areas within the peritoneal space or retroperitoneum, to guide management toward neoadjuvant therapy versus immediate debulking surgery.

- All epithelial ovarian tumors may be associated with elevated serum cancer antigen 125 (CA-125). Markedly elevated serum CA-125 suggests high-grade serous cancer. Image-guided biopsy of the omental tumor or retroperitoneal nodes is often a confirmatory test before initiation of therapy.

- After completion of surgery and chemotherapy, current guidelines do not include routine imaging surveillance. If a previously treated patient with ovarian cancer is being imaged, the context is probably an elevated tumor marker or a new sign or symptom. Therefore, the pretest probability of recurrence is high.

DISCLOSURE

The authors have nothing to disclose.

ACKNOWLEDGMENTS

The authors would like to thank medical illustrator Danielle Dobbs of the University of Michigan Radiology Media Group.

REFERENCES

1. Cancer Facts and Figures. Atlanta: American Cancer Society; 2022.
2. Expert Panel on Women's, Imaging:, Kang SK, Reinhold C, Atri M, et al. ACR appropriateness criteria((R)) ovarian cancer screening, J Am Coll Radiol, 2017;14 (11S): S490–S499.
3. Peres LC. Cushing-Haugen KL. Köbel M. et al. Invasive epithelial ovarian cancer survival by histotype and disease stage, J Natl Cancer Inst, 2019; 111(1):60–68.
4. Taylor EC, Irshaid L, Mathur M. Multimodality imaging approach to ovarian neoplasms with pathologic correlation. Radiographics 2021;41(1):289–315.
5. Barakat RRB, Markman M, Randall ME. Principles and practice of gynecologic oncology. Philadelphia: Lippincott Williams & Wilkins, Wolters Kluwer; 2013.
6. Matias-Guiu X, Stewart CJR. Endometriosis-associated ovarian neoplasia. Pathology 2018;50(2): 190–204.
7. Costeira FS, Felix A, Cunha TM. Brenner tumors. Br J Radiol 2022;95(1130):20210687.
8. Montoriol P.F., Hordonneau C., Boudinaud C., et al., Benign Brenner tumour of the ovary: CT and MRI features, Clin Radiol, 76 (8), 2021, 593–598.
9. Rauh-Hain JA, Diver EJ, Clemmer JT, et al. Carcinosarcoma of the ovary compared to papillary serous ovarian carcinoma: a SEER analysis. Gynecol Oncol 2013;131(1):46–51.
10. Hollis RL, Croy I. Churchman M. et al. Ovarian carcinosarcoma is a distinct form of ovarian cancer with poorer survival compared to tubo-ovarian high-grade serous carcinoma, Br J Cancer, 2022;127 (6):1034–1042.
11. Okamoto Y, Tanaka YO, Tsunoda H. et al. Malignant or borderline mucinous cystic neoplasms have a larger number of loculi than mucinous cystadenoma: a retrospective study with MR, J Magn Reson Imaging, 2007;26(1):94–99.
12. Seidman JD, Mehrotra A. Benign ovarian serous tumors: a re-evaluation and proposed reclassification of serous "cystadenomas" and "cystadenofibromas". Gynecol Oncol 2005;96(2):395–401.
13. Rashid S, Arafah MA, Akhtar M. The Many Faces of Serous Neoplasms and Related Lesions of the Female Pelvis: A Review. Adv Anat Pathol 2022;29(3): 154–67.
14. Frederick RP, Patel AG, Young SW, et al. Growth Rate of Ovarian Serous Cystadenomas and Cystadenofibromas, J Ultrasound Med, 2021; 40(10):2123–2130.
15. Suh-Burgmann E, Nakhaei M, Gupta S, et al. Ovarian Cystadenomas: Growth Rate and Reliability of Imaging Measurements, J Ultrasound Med, 2022; 41(9):2157–2167.
16. Kurman RJ, Shih Ie M. The origin and pathogenesis of epithelial ovarian cancer: a proposed unifying theory. Am J Surg Pathol 2010;34(3):433–43.
17. Tsuboyama T, Sato K, Ota T, et al. MRI of Borderline Epithelial Ovarian Tumors: Pathologic Correlation and Diagnostic Challenges, Radiographics, 2022; 42(7):2095–2111.
18. Li K, Yu L, Shi H, et al. Role of MRI in characterizing serous borderline ovarian tumor and its subtypes: Correlation of MRI features with clinicopathological characteristics. Eur J Radiol 2022;147:110112.
19. Stein EB, Hansen JM, Maturen KE. Fertility-Sparing Approaches in Gynecologic Oncology: Role of Imaging in Treatment Planning. Radiol Clin North Am 2020;58(2):401–12.
20. Fathalla MF. Incessant ovulation–a factor in ovarian neoplasia? Lancet 1971;2(7716):163.
21. Finch A, Beiner M, Lubinski J, et al. Salpingo-oophorectomy and the risk of ovarian, fallopian tube, and peritoneal cancers in women with a BRCA1 or BRCA2 Mutation. JAMA 2006;296(2):185–92.
22. Schmeler KM, Lynch HT, Chen L, et al. Prophylactic surgery to reduce the risk of gynecologic cancers in the Lynch syndrome. N Engl J Med 2006;354(3): 261–9.
23. Kroeger PT Jr, Drapkin R. Pathogenesis and heterogeneity of ovarian cancer. Curr Opin Obstet Gynecol 2017;29(1):26–34.
24. Rao S, Smith DA, Guler E, et al. Past, Present, and Future of Serum Tumor Markers in Management of Ovarian Cancer: A Guide for the Radiologist, Radiographics, 2021; 41(6):1839–1856.
25. Moujaber T, Balleine RL, Gao B, et al. New therapeutic opportunities for women with low-grade serous ovarian cancer, Endocr Relat Cancer, 2021;29(1): R1–R16.
26. NCCN, Ovarian Cancer/Fallopian Tube Cancer/Primary Peritoneal Cancer, in National Comprehensive Cancer Network Guidelines, Clinical Practice Guideline, Version 5.2022, NCCN.org, LCOC-3.
27. Andreotti RF, Timmerman D, Strachowski LM, et al. O-RADS US Risk Stratification and Management System: A Consensus Guideline from the ACR Ovarian-Adnexal Reporting and Data System Committee, Radiology, 2020;294(1):168–185.
28. Sadowski EA, Thomassin-Naggara I, Rockall A, et al. O-RADS MRI Risk Stratification System: Guide for Assessing Adnexal Lesions from the ACR O-RADS Committee, Radiology, 2022;303(1):35–47.
29. Expert Panel on Women's Imaging:, Atri M., Alabousi A, Reinhold C. ACR Appropriateness Criteria((R))

Clinically Suspected Adnexal Mass, No Acute Symptoms, J Am Coll Radiol, 2019;16(5S):S77-S93.

30. Sadowski EA, Stein EB, Thomassin-Naggara I, et al. O-RADS MRI After Initial Ultrasound for Adnexal Lesions: AJR Expert Panel Narrative Review, AJR Am J Roentgenol, 2022;220(1):6–15.

31. Guo Y, Phillips CH, Suarez-Weiss K, et al. Inter-reader Agreement and Intermodality Concordance of O-RADS US and MRI for Assessing Large, Complex Ovarian-Adnexal Cysts, Radiol Imaging Cancer, 2022;4(5): e220064.

32. Patel MD, Ascher SM, Horrow MM, et al. Management of Incidental Adnexal Findings on CT and MRI: A White Paper of the ACR Incidental Findings Committee, J Am Coll Radiol, 2020;17(2):248–254.

33. Expert Panel on Women's Imaging:, Kang SK, Reinhold C, Atri M, et al. ACR Appropriateness Criteria((R)) Staging and Follow-Up of Ovarian Cancer, J Am Coll Radiol, 2018;15(5S):S198–S207.

34. Shinagare AB, Sadowski EA, Park H, et al. Ovarian cancer reporting lexicon for computed tomography (CT) and magnetic resonance (MR) imaging developed by the SAR Uterine and Ovarian Cancer Disease-Focused Panel and the ESUR Female Pelvic Imaging Working Group, Eur Radiol, 2022;30(5): 3220–3235.

35. Suidan R.S., Ramirez P.T. Sarasohn D.M., et al., A multicenter prospective trial evaluating the ability of preoperative computed tomography scan and serum CA-125 to predict suboptimal cytoreduction at primary debulking surgery for advanced ovarian, fallopian tube, and peritoneal cancer, Gynecol Oncol, 2014;134(3):455–461.

36. Marko J, Marko KI, Pachigolla SL, et al. Mucinous Neoplasms of the Ovary: Radiologic-Pathologic Correlation, Radiographics, 2019;39(4):982–997.

37. Wengert GJ, Dabi Y, Kermarrec E, et al. O-RADS MRI Classification of Indeterminate Adnexal Lesions: Time-Intensity Curve Analysis Is Better Than Visual Assessment, Radiology, 2022;303(3):566–575.

Malignant Germ Cell Tumors of the Ovary
Clinical and Imaging Features

Douglas Rogers, MD[a],*, Christine Menias, MD[b], Akram Shaaban, MBBCh[a]

KEYWORDS

- Ovarian malignant germ cell tumor • Ultrasound • CT • MR • Dysgerminoma • Immature teratoma
- Yolk sac tumor

KEY POINTS

- An adnexal mass in younger females should raise suspicion for ovarian malignant germ cell tumors (OMGCTs).
- Evaluation of serum tumor markers (particularly alpha-fetoprotein, beta-human chorionic gonadotropin, and lactate dehydrogenase) can confirm the diagnosis in many cases.
- OMGCTs may be associated with carcinoid syndrome, hyperthyroidism, choriocarcinoma syndrome, virilization, precocious pseudo-puberty, and pseudo-Meig's syndrome.
- Macroscopic fat in an ovarian mass is not pathognomonic for mature teratoma; recognize the distinguishing features between mature and immature teratoma.
- OMGCTs are extremely sensitive to chemotherapy, allowing for fertility-sparing surgeries and conservative debulking with high remission rates.
- Growing teratoma syndrome may occur when metastases are growing despite adequate chemotherapy and normalization of tumor markers—mature teratoma is not responsive to chemotherapy.

INTRODUCTION

Germ cell tumors (GCTs) are a heterogeneous group of lesions that derive from primordial ovarian germ cells. These are the most common primary ovarian neoplasms, and the second most common that involve the ovary behind epithelial tumors.[1] GCTs constitute 20% to 25% of ovarian neoplasms due to the high prevalence of benign mature teratomas. Approximately 5% of ovarian GCTs are malignant, accounting for 2.6% of malignancies that involve the ovary.[2] Cellular subtypes of ovarian malignant germ cell tumors (OMGCTs) are listed in **Box 1**.

Unlike epithelial neoplasms, OMGCTs are more common in young females, and occur more often in Black and Asian females.[3] Clinically, OMGCTs are much larger at diagnosis due to their more rapid growth, commonly presenting with abdominal pain

and palpable mass, and ∼10% present acutely with adnexal torsion or tumor rupture/hemorrhage. Endocrine manifestations may occur depending on tumor type, due to secretion of beta-human chorionic gonadotropin (bHCG; precocious pseudo-puberty), serotonin (carcinoid syndrome), or thyroid hormone (struma ovarii). Paraneoplastic effects have been described, including sarcoid-like reaction (which may confound staging with PET avid lymph nodes and pulmonary nodules), and rare antibody-mediated syndromes (such as anti-NMDA receptor encephalitis).[4] Imaging and serum tumor markers are the mainstays of diagnosis for these tumors.[2]

Serum Tumor Markers

A young female presenting with a pelvic mass, elevated alpha-fetoprotein (AFP), or bHCG is virtually

[a] Department of Radiology and Imaging Sciences, University of Utah, 30 N Medical Dr, Salt Lake City, UT 84132, USA; [b] Mayo Clinic Radiology, 13400 E Shea Boulevard, Scottsdale, AZ 85259, USA
* Corresponding author.
E-mail address: Douglas.rogers@hsc.utah.edu

Radiol Clin N Am 61 (2023) 579–594
https://doi.org/10.1016/j.rcl.2023.02.004
0033-8389/23/© 2023 Elsevier Inc. All rights reserved.

Box 1
Cellular classification of ovarian germ cell tumors

Dysgerminoma

Yolk sac tumor

Mixed germ cell tumor

    Embryonal carcinoma

    Polyembryoma

Choriocarcinoma

Teratoma:

    Immature

    Mature with malignant transformation

    Monodermal/highly specialized:

        Struma ovarii

        Carcinoid

        Other (neuroectodermal/ependymoma)

---

diagnostic of OMGCT. Lactate dehydrogenase (LDH) is an additional nonspecific marker that is elevated in most tumor subtypes (~88%).[2] These markers are useful for monitoring during therapy and post-treatment surveillance (**Table 1**).

Table 1
Serum tumor markers in ovarian malignant germ cell tumors

	AFP	bHCG	LDH
Dysgerminoma	−	±	+
Yolk sac tumor	↑↑	−	+
Choriocarcinoma	−	↑↑	±
Mixed germ cell tumor	±	±	±
Immature teratoma	±	−	±

Abbreviations: AFP, alpha fetoprotein; bHCG, human chorionic gonadotropin; LDH, lactate dehydrogenase.

Although serum AFP may be mildly elevated in the setting of embryonal carcinoma and polyembryoma components within mixed germ cell tumors (MGCTs), significant AFP elevation is indicative of at least a component of yolk sac tumor (YST). Substantial bHCG elevation indicates at least a component of choriocarcinoma, although mild elevations of bHCG may be seen with dysgerminomas due to scattered multinucleated syncytiotrophoblastic giant cells. Less commonly, embryonal carcinoma or polyembryoma components of an MGCT produce low levels of bHCG.[2] Serum squamous cell carcinoma antigen is useful if malignant degeneration of a mature teratoma is suspected, and a thyroid panel is useful if struma ovarii is suspected.

DYSGERMINOMA

The ovarian equivalent to testicular seminoma, dysgerminomas are the most common OMGCT, accounting for 37.5% of cases (**Box 2**).[2] They have a wide range of incidence (7 months to 70 years), but usually occur in adolescence or early adulthood (~10% in the first decade).[5] There is an increased incidence of disorders of sexual development such as gonadal dysgenesis due to malignant degeneration of gonadoblastoma.

Box 2
Dysgerminoma pearls

- Typically lobulated solid mass with intervening fibrovascular septa
- Prominent vascular pedicle
- Typically young females
- Histologic equivalent to testicular seminoma
- May have elevated LDH, ALP, and mildly elevated bHCG
- Can arise from gonadoblastoma in disorders of sexual development
- Most common OMGCT to primarily involve bilateral ovaries (~10%)
- Often associated with a mature teratoma

Since dysgerminomas typically are large at diagnosis (>15 cm), patients present with a palpable abdominal mass, pain, and sometimes with abnormal vaginal bleeding. Pure dysgerminomas usually do not secrete hormones; however, ~5% may produce bHCG.[2] There may also be nonspecific elevation of LDH and alkaline phosphatase (ALP).

Imaging

The classic appearance of dysgerminoma is that of a large, well-defined solid adnexal mass composed of multiple lobules with intervening fibrovascular septations, and a prominent vascular pedicle with tortuous vessels (**Fig. 1**). Enhancement is heterogeneous and typically less than myometrium; however, the fibrovascular septations may avidly enhance and show color Doppler vascularity (**Fig. 2**). Variable degrees of stromal edema predominantly affect the septations,

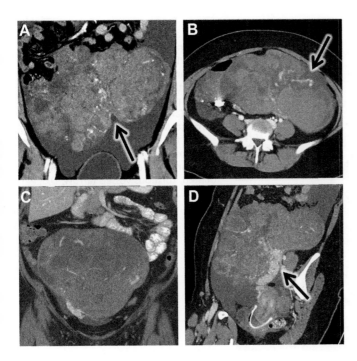

Fig. 1. Dysgerminoma. Four different cases of ovarian dysgerminoma are featured on coronal (A), axial (B), coronal (C), and sagittal oblique (D) CECT. These are predominantly solid and heterogeneously enhancing, with multiple lobules that are separated by fibrovascular septations (arrow, A,B). Large vascular pedicles with tortuous vessels are a typical feature of dysgerminomas (arrow, D). Axial and coronal CECT shows a large, multilobulated heterogeneously enhancing left adnexal mass with adjacent ascites. The mass has a prominent vascular pedicle (arrow, A), and low attenuation septations between the lobulations (arrow, B).

leading to thickening, decreased computed tomography (CT) attenuation, and T2 hyperintensity on MR imaging (Fig. 3).[5] Areas of hemorrhage and/or necrosis may be present. Speckled calcifications have been associated pathologically with coexisting precursor gonadoblastoma.[2,5]

Uncommonly, dysgerminomas may appear as a multiloculated cystic mass with septations and papillary projections, mimicking an epithelial neoplasm. Dysgerminomas are the most likely OMGCT to be bilateral in up to 10% of cases, and are often seen in association with a mature teratoma (Fig. 4).[2]

YOLK SAC TUMOR

Previously known as "endodermal sinus tumors," YSTs are the third most common OMGCT, accounting for 16% of cases (Box 3). They are most common between 18 and 25 years old, and

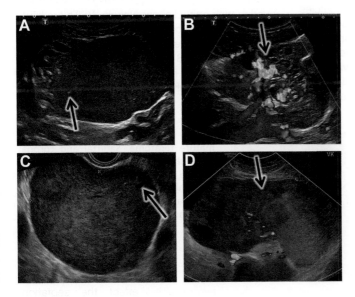

Fig. 2. Dysgerminoma. Four different cases of dysgerminoma are shown on pelvic ultrasound (A, B,D are transabdominal technique, C is transvaginal). These show predominantly solid masses that may contain echogenic foci (arrow, A), an enlarged vascular pedicle on color Doppler (arrow, B), cystic spaces (arrow, C), and additional, increased vascularity on color Doppler along the fibrovascular septations between tumor lobules (arrow, D).

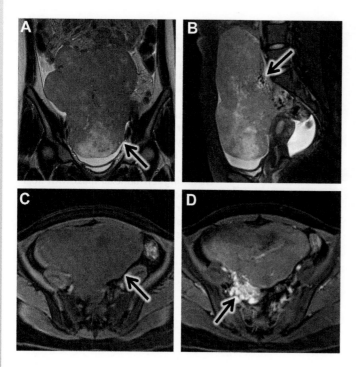

Fig. 3. Dysgerminoma. Coronal T2 MR shows a large, circumscribed heterogeneous pelvic mass (*arrow, A*). Sagittal T2 MR with fat saturation shows the lobulated and heterogeneous mass with T2 hypointense flow voids, corresponding to the prominent vascularity within the lesion (*arrow, B*). Axial T1 pre and post-contrast MR with fat saturation (*C,D*) shows the heterogeneously enhancing right ovarian mass with a prominent vascular pedicle composed of multiple dilated, tortuous vessels (*arrow, D*).

very rare in females over 40.[2] YSTs have a poor prognosis compared with other OMGCTs because they grow rapidly and are prone to rupture. Cases have been described with normal examinations weeks before large tumors were detected. YSTs are a common component of mixed GCTs, usually associated with significant serum AFP elevation.

Imaging

YSTs are typically large, encapsulated masses with septated cystic regions. They are highly vascular with large, tortuous vascular pedicles and avid enhancement of the peripheral solid components (**Fig. 5**). They often show the "bright dot sign" on CT or MR: enhancing foci in the wall of the solid components representing hypervascularity with associated aneurysms. YSTs tend to have expansive growth, causing mass effect and displacement of surrounding structures, rather than infiltration/invasion.[6]

MR shows variable signal intensity in the cystic components of the mass, which may have T1 hyperintense hemorrhage, and large T2 hypointense flow voids.[7]

Tumor rupture with capsular tears is present in ~1/4 of cases, thus peritoneal spread, ascites, and lymphadenopathy are common. Peritoneal metastases are usually hypervascular, similar to the primary tumor.

Since YSTs are often cystic, they show imaging overlap with epithelial neoplasms. YSTs are bilateral in only 8% of cases, so the presence of bilateral adnexal involvement is more suggestive of an epithelial tumor. YSTs have mature teratoma in the contralateral ovary in 10% of cases, which may be a helpful distinguishing feature.[2]

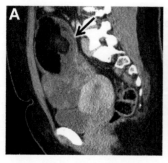
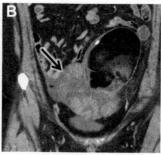

Fig. 4. Dysgerminoma associated with mature teratoma. Sagittal and coronal CECT shows an adnexal mass with a mature teratoma component (*arrow, A*) containing layering macroscopic fat and calcification, and a solid, heterogeneously enhancing dysgerminoma component (*arrow, B*).

MIXED GERM CELL TUMORS

MGCTs contain more than one germ cell element, most commonly dysgerminoma, YST, and immature teratoma (IT) (**Box 4**). They may contain other less common elements that are rarely present in isolation, including embryonal carcinoma, polyembryoma, and choriocarcinoma.[8] These components are usually intimately mixed, but can also be present in separate areas of the mass. MGCTs are often highly malignant, and may show local aggressive behavior.

MGCTs are most common in young females in the second to third decades, with a median age of 15. Approximately two-thirds of patients present with hormonal manifestations, including precocious pseudo-puberty (if the mass contains choriocarcinoma or embryonal carcinoma) and abnormal uterine bleeding. Elevation of serum tumor markers is common, and varies depending on the tumor components.[2]

Imaging

MGCTs are usually predominantly solid masses with regions of hemorrhage and/or necrosis, but may also be a multiloculated cystic lesion with avidly enhancing solid components. Teratomatous elements may produce macroscopic fat or calcifications (**Fig. 6**).

Ultrasound usually shows a heterogeneous solid mass with cystic components and marked color Doppler flow. There are no characteristic ultrasound features distinguishing MGCTs or its rare components, including choriocarcinoma and embryonal carcinoma.[8]

NONGESTATIONAL CHORIOCARCINOMA

Nongestational choriocarcinomas, which are not associated with gestation near the time of diagnosis, are very rare; pure choriocarcinomas constitute up to 3.4% of OMGCTs (**Box 5**).[2] Nongestational choriocarcinoma is an OMGCT that differentiates toward trophoblastic structures, and has worse prognosis compared with the gestational form. Findings indicating nongestational form include the presence of other neoplastic germ cell elements, and diagnosis in

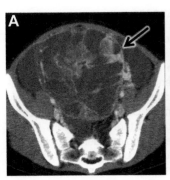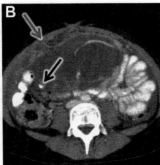

Fig. 5. Yolk sac tumor. Axial CECT at different levels shows a large, multiloculated cystic pelvic mass with avidly enhancing septations/solid components (*arrow, A*). There is associated peritoneal tumor spread with ascites and omental nodularity (*blue arrow, B*). Brightly enhancing foci represent small aneurysms within the wall are known as the "bright dot sign" (*black arrow, B*).

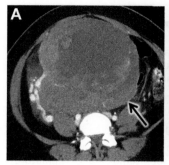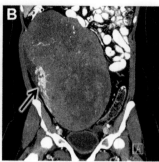

Fig. 6. Mixed germ cell tumor. Axial (*A*) and coronal (*B*) CECT shows a large, right pelvic mass that has features commonly seen with dysgerminomas, including a lobulated, predominantly solid, heterogeneous mass (*arrow, A*) that has a prominent vascular pedicle (*arrow, B*). However, tumor markers were elevated, including AFP, bHCG, and LDH; pathology showed an MGCT that was 59% dysgerminoma, 30% yolk sac tumor, 10% high-grade immature teratoma, and 1% embryonal carcinoma.

the prepubertal or postmenopausal periods. DNA polymorphism analysis helps distinguish gestational and nongestational choriocarcinoma; gestational tumors have both paternal and maternal genomic contributions, whereas nongestational tumors have only maternal genetics.[8] An adnexal mass with elevated serum bHCG may cause clinical confusion for ectopic pregnancy.

Choriocarcinoma is highly malignant and can be locally invasive; hematogenous metastases may be present at diagnosis. Central nervous system metastases occur in 10% to 20% of cases, and are the leading cause of death. Liver and lung metastases are also relatively common. Patients may present with pseudo-precocious puberty, amenorrhea, and symptoms associated with bleeding metastases.[9] Extensive bleeding from hypervascular metastases is known as "choriocarcinoma syndrome," which may be associated with diffuse alveolar hemorrhage, subcapsular hepatic hematomas, and in severe cases, disseminated intravascular coagulation. This is more common in patients with large tumor burden, shortly after beginning chemotherapy.[4]

Imaging

Choriocarcinomas are avidly enhancing solid masses, particularly along the periphery. In contrast to most OMGCTs that are circumscribed, choriocarcinoma may show local invasion of nearby organs (eg, uterus, pelvic sidewall) at the time of diagnosis. Arterial phase imaging often shows enlarged vessels along the periphery of the mass, and delayed post-contrast images are useful to show peritoneal metastases, which can be associated with ascites.[2]

Ultrasound is useful to exclude intrauterine or definite ectopic pregnancy given the elevated serum bHCG. Choriocarcinoma has heterogeneous echogenicity with marked low resistance blood flow in the solid components on color Doppler.

MR shows an avidly enhancing mass that has small T1 hyperintense foci of hemorrhage. The solid components typically have a low T2 signal, with small cystic regions that are T2 hyperintense. Regions of hypervascularity may show T2 hypointense flow voids.

IMMATURE TERATOMA

ITs are the second most common OMGCT, accounting for 36.2% of cases (Box 6).[2] Peak incidence is between 15 and 19 years old, rarely occurring after menopause. Unlike mature teratomas, ITs are malignant and have a relatively poor prognosis among OMGCTs. ITs have components arising from all three germ cells layers, endoderm, mesoderm, and ectoderm. These differ from mature teratoma because they contain immature embryonic elements, most commonly immature neuroepithelium.

Box 5
Nongestational choriocarcinoma pearls

- Typically avidly enhancing solid masses
- US shows heterogeneous masses with marked low-resistance blood flow on color Doppler
- Highly malignant; local invasion and metastases may be present at diagnosis
- Not associated with gestation—a nongestational form reflects a germ cell tumor differentiated toward trophoblastic structures
- Symptomatic bleeding metastases → "Choriocarcinoma syndrome"
- Associated with significantly elevated bHCG → may cause precocious pseudo-puberty
- US useful to evaluate for intrauterine or ectopic pregnancy given elevated bHCG

Box 6
Immature teratoma pearls

- Distinguish from mature teratoma:
  - Larger, more soft-tissue component
  - Smaller fatty foci, fluid rather than fatty attenuation cystic regions
  - Scattered small calcifications instead of "tooth-like" calcifications
- Typically young females
- Grading is based on amount of immature neuroepithelium
- AFP may be mildly elevated
- Peritoneal seeding may cause gliomatosis peritonei
- Likely to develop growing teratoma syndrome after treatment

Most patients present non-acutely with abdominal distention and discomfort, whereas ~10% have acute abdominal pain from mass rupture/hemorrhage or adnexal torsion. Serum markers may show nonspecific elevation of LDH, and sometimes mildly elevated AFP.

Imaging

When macroscopic fat and calcifications are present within an ovarian mass, the knee-jerk diagnosis is mature teratoma, which is benign. It is imperative to distinguish immature and mature teratomas on imaging because ITs account for 30% of deaths from ovarian cancer in patients under 20.

ITs are usually larger than mature teratomas at the time of diagnosis (>14 cm).[2] In contrast to mature teratomas, which usually have larger regions of macroscopic fat, ITs are predominantly heterogeneous cystic and solid masses with small foci of fat interspersed in the lesion. Cysts within ITs are usually fluid attenuation rather than fat. Calcifications are typically small, irregular, and scattered throughout the mass instead of coarse or tooth-like (**Figs. 7** and **8**)[2,10–12]. Ruptured ITs may seed the peritoneum primarily with glial tissue ("gliomatosis peritonei"; **Fig. 9**).[4]

MALIGNANT TRANSFORMATION OF MATURE TERATOMA

Mature teratomas are the most common benign ovarian neoplasm, most commonly diagnosed between 20 to 40 years of age (**Box 7**).[2] They are composed of well-differentiated tissues arising from all three germ cell layers, including endoderm, mesoderm, and ectoderm.

Malignant transformation of mature teratomas is very rare (<2% of cases), most common in postmenopausal patients. Although it is possible for any tissue within a teratoma to undergo malignant degeneration, squamous cell carcinoma is the most common, accounting for >80% of cases.[2] Transformation to squamous cell carcinoma is associated with ascending high-risk human

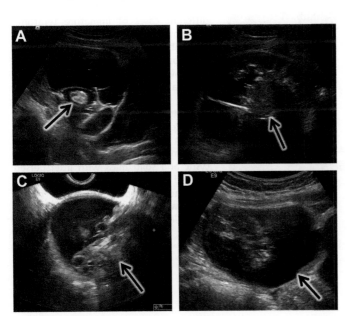

Fig. 7. Immature teratoma. Four different cases of immature teratoma are shown on pelvic ultrasound (*A-D*). These appear as cystic and solid masses with heterogeneous echogenicity. Small foci of fat have increased echogenicity (*arrow, A*).

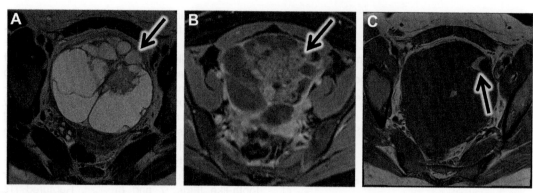

Fig. 8. Immature teratoma. Axial T2 MR (*A*) shows a part cystic and solid pelvic mass (*arrow*). Axial T1 post-contrast MR with fat saturation (*B*) shows heterogeneous enhancement of the solid components (*arrow*), and axial T1 MR (*C*) shows the T1 hyperintense foci of fat within the mass (*arrow*).

papillomavirus infection, and likely arises from squamous metaplasia of the columnar epithelium along the teratoma cyst wall. Serum squamous cell carcinoma antigen levels >2 ng/mL are present in 81.3% of cases.[2]

Imaging

Typical imaging features of mature teratoma include a circumscribed cystic and/or solid adnexal mass with macroscopic fat that may have hair and coarse calcifications/teeth. In cystic lesions, a soft-tissue protuberance from the inner lining of the wall known as the Rokitansky nodule may be present.[10] Malignant transformation with squamous cell carcinoma is most likely to occur along the wall of the cyst or in the Rokitansky

nodule. This typically appears as a heterogeneously enhancing, irregular, solid mass with transmural invasion of the wall. Other findings of malignant behavior include local invasion, lymphadenopathy, and metastases (**Figs. 10** and **11**).

Malignant degeneration of a teratoma should be distinguished from an adnexal collision tumor, such as an epithelial tumor next to a mature teratoma. These often have normal ovarian tissue intervening between the two lesions. Pseudomyxoma peritonei is almost exclusively caused by appendiceal mucinous tumors; however, in extremely rare circumstances a mucinous tumor arising within a mature cystic teratoma may seed the peritoneal cavity, leading to ascites and scalloping of organ surfaces (**Fig. 12**).

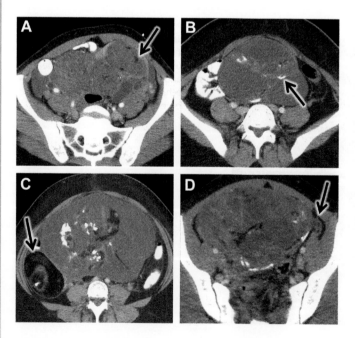

Fig. 9. Immature teratoma. Four different cases of immature teratoma are shown on axial CECT. (*A*) Showing a multilobulated, predominantly solid mass containing small foci of fat (*arrow*). (*B*) Showing a multiloculated cystic mass with calcifications and fat interspersed within the septations (*arrow*). (*C*) Showing a left ovarian cystic and solid mass containing calcifications and fat, and an associated contralateral mature teratoma (*arrow*). (*D*) Showing a mixed cystic and solid mass with interspersed fat and calcification. There is soft-tissue peritoneal stranding in the left pelvis, which was histologically shown to represent gliomatosis peritonei (*arrow*).

MALIGNANT STRUMA OVARII

Although thyroid tissue is present in 5% to 20% of mature teratomas, struma ovarii is defined as a mature teratoma that is composed predominantly of thyroid tissue ("pure") or >50% of the teratoma volume ("impure") (**Box 8**). Despite being the most common monodermal teratoma, struma ovarii is rare, accounting for ~3% of teratomas and ~0.5% of OMGCTs. Median age at diagnosis is 52 years old.[2,13]

Patients occasionally present with a pelvic mass or with hyperthyroidism (~5%). Only 5% of struma ovarii are malignant and are without distinguishing imaging features; typically, small foci of carcinoma found histologically. Treatment includes resection of malignant struma ovarii, with thyroidectomy followed by radio-iodine ablation. Thyroglobulin is a useful tumor marker for surveillance.

Imaging

Struma ovarii is most commonly a circumscribed, multicystic mass with avidly enhancing solid components that are high attenuation on nonenhanced CT (NECT) due to iodinated thyroid hormone and calcification (**Fig. 13**).[13,14] The impure form may have features of mature teratoma, including loculations with fat attenuation or calcifications. They are almost always unilateral, and typically <10 cm in size. Other described patterns include multilocular cystic mass without solid components, unilocular cystic lesion, and a predominantly solid lesion with small, cystic spaces. Besides frank capsular invasion of solid components or metastases, there are no features that distinguish benign and malignant struma ovarii.

The multicystic appearance of struma ovarii has imaging overlap with other malignancies, including mucinous cystic epithelial neoplasms and YSTs. High-density components on NECT can be a key differentiating feature.

On ultrasound, cystic lesions may contain "struma pearls," which are circumscribed, echogenic solid regions with increased vascularity (**Fig. 14**).[11] On MR, the cysts may show areas of T2 hypointensity and T1 hyperintensity corresponding to regions of high CT attenuation. The solid components/septations are usually T2 intermediate to slightly hypointense, T1 intermediate to slightly hyperintense, and show enhancement (**Fig. 15**). T1 may show small foci of hyperintensity in or adjacent to thickened septations/solid components that do not fat suppress.[13]

Struma ovarii is associated with ascites (and sometimes pleural effusion) in up to one-third of cases, known as "pseudo-Meig's syndrome." CA-125 may be elevated, even when benign.[13] Extremely rare cases of metastatic disease are most often associated with peritoneal implantation; hematogenous spread to liver, lungs, bones, and central nervous system may occur, even years after resection of the primary tumor. Struma ovarii may show uptake on I-123 scans if the tumor is hyperfunctioning compared with the orthotopic thyroid gland. In patients with hyperthyroidism, the mass is usually >6 cm in size.[2]

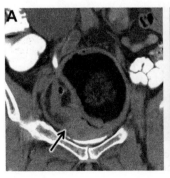
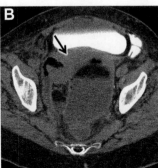

Fig. 10. Malignant transformation of mature teratoma. Coronal (A) and axial (B) CECT show a right adnexal mass composed of soft tissue and fat fluid levels, consistent with a mature teratoma. There is abnormal irregular soft-tissue thickening along the walls (arrows), which represents malignant transformation to squamous cell carcinoma.

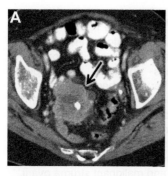 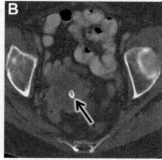

Fig. 11. Malignant transformation of mature teratoma. Axial CECT in soft tissue (*A*) and bone windows (*B*) shows a heterogeneously enhancing, irregular mass in the right adnexa (*arrow, A*) that is engulfing a calcification that resembles a tooth (*arrow, B*). This pathologically represents a squamous cell carcinoma that arose in and engulfed a mature teratoma.

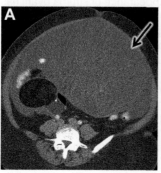 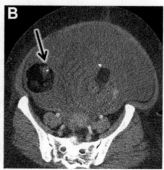

Fig. 12. Mature teratoma containing mucinous tumor. Axial CECT images show a large pelvic lesion with large cystic spaces (*arrow, A*) corresponding to mucinous tumor arising within a mature teratoma, which also contains macroscopic fat and calcifications (*arrow, B*).

Box 8
Struma ovarii pearls

- Typically multicystic mass with avidly enhancing solid components
- Regions of high attenuation due to iodinated thyroid hormone
- "Impure" form may have small foci of fat
- US can show hyperechoic and vascular "struma pearls"
- Typically older females
- Struma ovarii is teratoma with greater than 50% thyroid tissue
- Occasionally causes hyperthyroidism
- Malignancy usually found incidentally histologically; follicular carcinoma is most common
- May cause pseudo-Meig's syndrome, even when benign

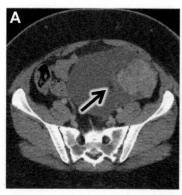 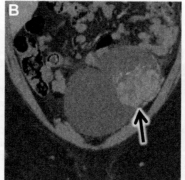 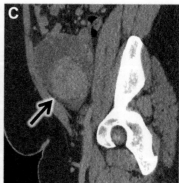

Fig. 13. Struma ovarii on non-enhanced CT. Axial, coronal, and sagittal NECT shows a cystic left adnexal mass with small foci of fat (*arrow, A*), and a larger, high-attenuation mural solid component (*arrow, B and C*). Histologic evaluation incidentally showed follicular carcinoma contained within struma ovarii.

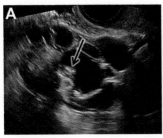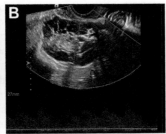

Fig. 14. Struma ovarii. Transvaginal ultrasound shows a multicystic left adnexal mass with echogenic foci along the cyst walls, known as "struma pearls" (*arrow, A*). Color Doppler shows increased vascularity within these regions (*B*).

Carcinoid tumor

Ovarian teratomas may rarely show predominant monodermal differentiation toward argentaffin cells (**Box 9**). These account for <0.5% of all carcinoid tumors, and 0.1% of ovarian tumors.[2] Unlike most OMGCTs, carcinoids are more common in post-menopausal patients (average age 53 years, ranging 23 to 87 years). Although they have malignant potential, most show benign clinical behavior.

Approximately one-third of ovarian carcinoid tumors present with carcinoid syndrome because they release serotonin directly into the systemic circulation, bypassing the liver. Symptoms may include flushing, diarrhea, dyspnea, abdominal pain, and carcinoid heart disease. Carcinoid tumors associated with ovarian stromal luteinization may cause symptoms of estrogen or androgen excess, such as abnormal uterine bleeding or virilization.[15,16]

Imaging

Patterns of ovarian carcinoid tumors include a solid nodule along the wall of a mature teratoma (60% to 80%), a solid ovarian mass, and a multilocular cystic mass with an avidly enhancing solid component (**Fig. 16**).[2] It may be difficult to determine if a carcinoid is primarily ovarian or a metastasis without the presence of other teratomatous elements, such as macroscopic fat. Approximately 15% of cases will have a mature teratoma or mucinous tumor in the contralateral ovary. Carcinoids will typically have increased uptake on octreotide scans and Ga-68 DOTATATE PET/CT due to the presence of somatostatin receptors.

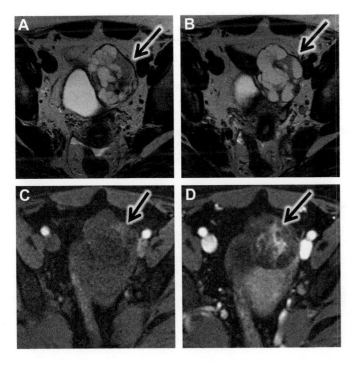

Fig. 15. Struma ovarii. Axial T2 MR at different slices (*A,B*) shows a multiloculated left adnexal mass composed of cystic components with variable signal intensities, and relatively T2 hypointense septations (*arrows*). Axial T1 pre and post-contrast MR with fat saturation shows avid enhancement of the septations/solid components (*arrows, C,D*).

> **Box 9**
> **Ovarian carcinoid pearls**
>
> - Most commonly presents with an avidly enhancing solid component along the wall of a mature teratoma
> - Older females
> - Monodermal differentiation of teratoma toward argentaffin cells
> - Usually benign behavior, but has malignant potential
> - Can cause carcinoid syndrome without liver metastases
> - Ovarian stromal luteinization may cause virilization or abnormal uterine bleeding
> - "Strumal carcinoid" is composed of admixed thyroid and carcinoid cells

On MR, the carcinoid tumor components are usually T1 intermediate to hypointense with intermediate to hypointense T2 signal, although mucinous subtypes will be more T2 hyperintense. The solid component avidly enhances with marked diffusion restriction. Sometimes the solid component may appear "sponge-like," and septal calcifications may be present (**Fig. 17**).[2] Mucinous ovarian carcinoid tumors are more aggressive than other subtypes, behaving similar to mucinous carcinoid tumors originating in the appendix. If metastases do occur, they may present >10 years after the initial diagnosis.

STAGING

Complete clinical staging of OMGCTs requires exploratory surgery, with evaluation of the peritoneal cavity, including the diaphragm, paracolic gutters, omentum, and contralateral ovary. Para-aortic and ipsilateral pelvic lymph nodes may be sampled if they appear suspicious on preoperative imaging, and cytology of ascitic fluid and/or peritoneal washings are obtained before tumor manipulation. Serum tumor markers are measured at the time of diagnosis because persistent elevation after resection indicates residual tumor.

Factors associated with a poorer prognosis include higher International Federation of Gynecology and Obstetrics (FIGO) stage (**Table 2**), higher tumor marker levels, cellular subtype (eg, YST, embryonal carcinoma, and choriocarcinoma), higher grade, increased age, and residual tumor after debulking surgery.[2,17]

Compared with epithelial carcinomas, OMGCTs are more likely to spread to abdominal lymph nodes. Peritoneal spread relatively common, particularly with YSTs, which are prone to rupture. Peritoneal metastases may appear as soft-tissue nodules or peritoneal thickening; ascites or enlarged cardio-phrenic lymph nodes should also raise suspicion. Hepatic capsular or falciform ligament involvement due to peritoneal spread (stage 3) should be distinguished from parenchymal hematogenous metastases (stage 4).[2]

Distant parenchymal metastases are uncommon at presentation, but most often affect the liver and lungs, followed by the central nervous system, bones, and adrenal glands. The most common site of distant spread is to the pleural space, often diagnosed with cytologic analysis/thoracentesis.

TREATMENT

Treatment of OMGCTs is significantly guided by the fact that they are almost always unilateral, commonly affect young females who want to preserve fertility, and are very responsive to chemotherapy with a high cure rate even with incompletely resected disease.[18] Conservative surgical debulking followed by adjuvant chemotherapy (typically platinum-based regimens) is the mainstay of therapy, with survival rates nearing 100% for early-stage disease, and >75% for advanced-stage disease.

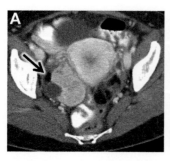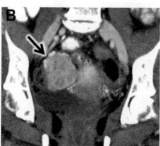

Fig. 16. Ovarian carcinoid tumor. Axial and coronal contrast-enhanced CT shows a right adnexal mass containing macroscopic fat (*arrow, A*) and a larger, avidly enhancing solid component (*arrow, B*) which represents a carcinoid tumor as the predominant component of a mature teratoma.

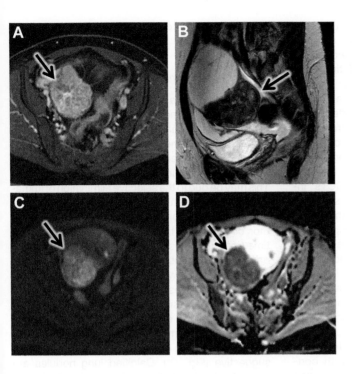

Fig. 17. Ovarian strumal carcinoid tumor. Axial T1 post-contrast MR with fat saturation shows a solid, avidly enhancing right ovarian mass (*arrow, A*). Sagittal T2, shows the solid component is relatively T2 hypointense (*arrow, B*), and is a component of a larger mixed cystic and solid lesion. Axial DWI (*C*) and ADC map (*D*) show the solid component is avidly enhancing (*arrow*). This is a strumal carcinoid arising within a mature cystic teratoma; the solid component represents admixed thyroid and well-differentiated neuroendocrine tumor.

Table 2
International Federation of Gynecology and Obstetrics staging of ovarian malignant germ cell tumors[a]

Stage I	Tumor Confined to Ovaries or Fallopian Tubes.
IA	Tumor limited to one ovary (with intact capsule) or fallopian tube. No tumor on ovarian or fallopian tube surface, or malignant cells in ascites/peritoneal washings.
IB	Tumor limited to both ovaries (with intact capsule) or fallopian tubes. No tumor on ovarian or fallopian tube surface, or malignant cells in ascites/peritoneal washings.
IC	Tumor limited to one or both ovaries or fallopian tubes with: Surgical spill, capsular rupture before surgery, tumor on ovary/fallopian tube surface, or malignant cells in ascites/peritoneal washings.
Stage II	Tumor with pelvic extension below the pelvic brim or peritoneal involvement.
IIA	Extension or implants on uterus, fallopian tubes, and/or ovaries.
IIB	Extension to other pelvic intraperitoneal tissues.
Stage III	Cytologically or histologically confirmed tumor spread to peritoneum outside the pelvis, or metastases to retroperitoneal lymph nodes.
IIIA1	Positive retroperitoneal lymph nodes.
IIIA2	Microscopic extra-pelvic peritoneal involvement.
IIIB	Macroscopic peritoneal metastases beyond the pelvis <2 cm in size.
IIIC	Macroscopic peritoneal metastases beyond the pelvis >2 cm in size, including liver/splenic capsular involvement.
Stage IV	Distant metastasis excluding peritoneal involvement.
IVA	Pleural effusion with positive cytology.
IVB	Parenchymal metastases and metastases to extra-abdominal organs (including lymph nodes outside abdominal cavity)

[a] Note: this does not include staging for malignant struma ovarii; if stuma ovarii is > 2 cm or has extraovarian involvement, total thyroidectomy and I-131 ablation are recommended. Subsequent follow-up is with serum thyroglobulin levels, with I-131 scintigraphy and FDG PET-CT, if necessary.

Treatment of early-stage OMGCT is unilateral salpingo-oophorectomy, followed by adjuvant chemotherapy.[19] Current first-line chemotherapy is bleomycin, etoposide, and cisplatin (BEP) because it is highly effective and does not preclude subsequent pregnancy.[17,20] Patients with Stage I pure dysgerminoma or low-grade IT may undergo resection without adjuvant therapy, followed by surveillance. Although relapse occurs in 15% to 25% of cases, they are almost always successfully salvaged with chemotherapy.[3]

Treatment of advanced-stage OMGCTs includes nonaggressive tumor debulking; standard adjuvant chemotherapy is with BEP, with vincristine, dactinomycin, and cyclophosphamide (VAC) as second-line for nonresponders.[21] Neoadjuvant chemotherapy may be considered in cases where the intra-abdominal tumor is extensive, and the patients are poor surgical candidates. Patients with recurrent or progressive disease (which are usually detected within 2 years by rising serum tumor markers) have worse prognosis compared with their testicular counterparts. These may be treated with conventional dose chemotherapy regimens, which include paclitaxel, ifosfamide, and cisplatin (TIP), or gemcitabine + TIP.[22] Alternative treatment regimens involve high-dose chemotherapy with autologous marrow transplantation rescue, which may be associated with improved long-term survival compared with conventional doses.[3,18]

Growing Teratoma Syndrome

"Growing teratoma syndrome" is an outcome of chemotherapy for nondysgerminoma GCT (particularly IT or MGCT) that occurs in up to 40% of cases, leading to enlargement of metastases that pathologically are composed of only mature teratoma elements after the tumor markers have normalized. This may be due to the selective elimination of immature tumor elements which are chemo-sensitive, and/or the induction of maturation of immature tumor components by chemotherapy. The median time from diagnosis of IT to growing teratoma syndrome is 20 months (range 8 to 42 months).[2,4]

On imaging, growing masses appear at potential sites of metastases, such as the peritoneal cavity or liver. These lesions range from soft tissue to predominantly fat, and may contain calcifications. The presence of macroscopic fat within new lesions in the setting of a recently treated IT is highly suggestive (Fig. 18). Calcified lung nodules are very often benign; however, "ossified metastases" are one of the causes of malignant calcified lung nodules.[4] Surgical resection of growing metastases composed of mature teratoma is usually necessary because these mature tissues are not sensitive to chemotherapy.

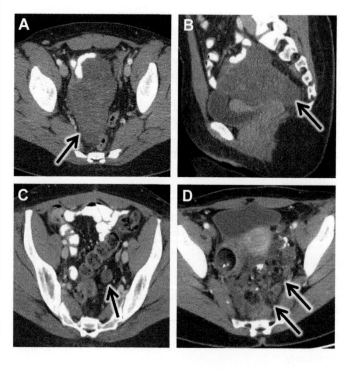

Fig. 18. Growing teratoma syndrome. Axial and coronal CECT (*A,B*) show a solid, right pelvic mass which was resected, showing immature teratoma (*arrows*). Following adjuvant chemotherapy, tumor markers normalized, but the patient developed a solid nodule in the left pelvis 10 months later (*arrow, C*), and extensive tumor within the pelvis with foci of macroscopic fat and calcification 18 months later (*arrow, D*). This pathologically represented mature teratoma, which is resistant to chemotherapy.

SUMMARY

OMGCTs are a diverse set of masses originating from the primitive gonadal germ cells, often in young females. They have useful imaging and clinical features, including serum tumor marker elevation, that may aid the radiologist at the time of diagnosis, and also during follow-up. Accurate and timely diagnosis is essential, as standard-of-care therapies lead to a high rate of cancer remission.

CLINICS CARE POINTS

Bulleted list of evidence-based pearls and pitfalls relevant to the point of care

- An adnexal mass in younger females should raise suspicion for ovarian malignant germ cell tumors (OMGCTs)

- Evaluation of serum tumor markers (particularly alpha fetoprotein, beta-human chorionic gonadotropin, and lactate dehydrogenase) can virtually clinch the diagnosis

- OMGCTs may be associated with carcinoid syndrome, hyperthyroidism, choriocarcinoma syndrome, virilization, precocious pseudo-puberty, and pseudo-Meig's syndrome

- Macroscopic fat in an ovarian mass is not pathognomonic for mature teratoma; recognize the distinguishing features between mature and immature teratoma

- OMGCTs are extremely sensitive to chemotherapy, allowing for fertility-sparing surgeries and conservative debulking with high remission rates

- Growing teratoma syndrome may occur when metastases are growing despite adequate chemotherapy and normalization of tumor markers—mature teratoma is not responsive to chemotherapy

DISCLOSURE

Drs Rogers, Menias, and Shaaban receive royalties from Elsevier for unrelated work. This manuscript did not receive funding.

REFERENCES

1. Crum CP, Drapkin R, Kindelberger D, et al. Lessons from BRCA: the tubal fimbria emerges as an origin for pelvic serous cancer. Clin Med Res 2007;5(1): 35–44.

2. Shaaban AM, Rezvani M, Elsayes KM, et al. Ovarian malignant germ cell tumors: cellular classification and clinical and imaging features. Radiographics 2014;34(3):777–801.

3. Smith HO, Berwick M, Verschraegen CF, et al. Incidence and survival rates for female malignant germ cell tumors. Obstet Gynecol 2006;107(5): 1075–85.

4. Magudia K, Menias CO, Bhalla S, et al. Unusual Imaging Findings Associated with Germ Cell Tumors. Radiographics 2019;39(4):1019–35.

5. Zhao S, Sun F, Chu C, et al. Pure dysgerminoma of the ovary: CT and MRI features with pathological correlation in 13 tumors. J Ovarian Res 2020;13(1):71.

6. Li YK, Zheng Y, Lin JB, et al. CT imaging of ovarian yolk sac tumor with emphasis on differential diagnosis. Sci Rep 2015;5:11000.

7. Yamaoka T, Togashi K, Koyama T, et al. Immature teratoma of the ovary: correlation of MR imaging and pathologic findings. Eur Radiol 2003;13(2): 313–9.

8. Moro F, Castellan LM, Franchi D, et al. Imaging in gynecological disease (22): clinical and ultrasound characteristics of ovarian embryonal carcinomas, nongestational choriocarcinomas and malignant mixed germ cell tumors. Ultrasound Obstet Gynecol 2021;57(6):987–94.

9. Corakci A, Ozeren S, Ozkan S, et al. Pure nongestational choriocarcinoma of the ovary. Arch Gynecol Obstet 2005;271(2):176–7.

10. Saleh M, Bhosale P, Menias CO, et al. Ovarian teratomas: clinical features, imaging findings and management. Abdom Radiol (NY) 2021;46(6):2293–307.

11. Taylor EC, Irshaid L, Mathur M, et al. Multimodality Imaging Approach to Ovarian Neoplasms with Pathologic Correlation. Radiographics 2021;41(1): 289–315.

12. Saba L, Guerriero S, Sulcis R, et al. Mature and immature ovarian teratomas CT, US, and MR imaging characteristics. Eur J Radiol 2009;72(3):454–63.

13. Dujardin MI, Sekhri P, Turnbull LW. Struma ovarii: role of imaging? Insights Imaging 2014;5(1):41–51.

14. Ikeuchi T, Koyama T, Tamai K, et al. CT and MR features of struma ovarii. Abdom Imaging 2012;37(5): 904–10.

15. Zhai LR, Zhang XW, Yu T, et al. Primary ovarian carcinoid : Two cases report and review of literature. Medicine (Baltim) 2020;99(40):e21109.

16. Robboy SJ, Scully RE. Strumal carcinoid of the ovary: an analysis of 50 cases of a distinctive tumor composed of thyroid tissue and carcinoid. Cancer 1980;46(9):2019–34.

17. Guo H, Chen H, Wang W, et al. Clinicopathological Features, Prognostic Factors, Survival Trends, and Treatment of Malignant Ovarian Germ Cell Tumors: A SEER Database Analysis. Oncol Res Treat 2021; 44(4):145–53.

18. Simone CG, Markham MJ, Dizon DS. Chemotherapy in ovarian germ cell tumors: A systematic review. Gynecol Oncol 2016;141(3):602–7.

19. Uccello M, Boussios S, Samartzis EP, et al. Systemic anti-cancer treatment in malignant ovarian germ cell tumours (MOGCTs): current management and promising approaches. Ann Transl Med 2020;8(24):1713.

20. Williams S, Blessing JA, Liao SY, et al. Adjuvant therapy of ovarian germ cell tumors with cisplatin, etoposide, and bleomycin: a trial of the Gynecologic Oncology Group. J Clin Oncol 1994 Apr;12(4): 701–6.

21. Low JJ, Perrin LC, Crandon AJ, et al. Conservative surgery to preserve ovarian function in patients with malignant ovarian germ cell tumors. A review of 74 cases. Cancer 2000;89(2):391–8.

22. Ray-Coquard I, Morice P, Lorusso D, et al. Non-epithelial ovarian cancer: ESMO Clinical Practice Guidelines for diagnosis, treatment and follow-up. Ann Oncol 2018;29(Suppl 4):iv1–18.

Sex Cord-Stromal Tumors of the Ovary

Madeleine Sertic, MBBCh, BAO[a,b,*], Kyle M. Devins, MD[b,c], Esther Oliva, MD[b,c], Susanna I. Lee, MD, PhD[a,b], Aoife Kilcoyne, MBBCh, BAO[a,b]

KEYWORDS

- Female pelvic imaging • Gynecologic oncology • Sex cord-stromal tumors
- Adult granulosa cell tumors • Juvenile granulosa cell tumors • MR imaging • Ultrasound

KEY POINTS

- Ovarian sex cord-stromal tumors (OSCST) are a group of rare tumors, with a broad spectrum of clinical and imaging presentations. It can be challenging to distinguish the tumor subtypes and identify malignant lesions on imaging alone.
- The majority of OSCSTs are benign, and malignant subtypes generally carry a more favorable prognosis than the more common ovarian epithelial malignancies.
- Benign subtypes of OSCSTs can present with aggressive imaging features and mimic malignancies.

Declarations: Funding: Not applicable.

INTRODUCTION

Ovarian sex cord-stromal tumors (OSCST) are a group of rare benign and malignant ovarian neoplasms. As the name suggests, these tumors can arise purely from stromal cells, purely from primitive sex cord cells, or arise from mixed stromal cell and sex cord origin.

OSCSTs account for approximately 7% of primary ovarian neoplasms[1]; benign OSCSTs make up less than 4% of all ovarian benign neoplasms, and malignant OSCSTs account for less than 8% of all malignant ovarian neoplasms.[2] The majority present in the first two to three decades of life.[2] The exception is adult granulosa cell tumors, which have a peak incidence at ages 50 to 55.[3]

OSCSTs typically present with non-specific symptoms of adnexal masses, including abdominal pain, distention, and, rarely, ovarian torsion.[3] However, OSCSTs can be clinically distinguished from the more common ovarian epithelial and germ-cell tumors when they present with signs of hormone production. Tumors originating from ovarian cell types, such as granulosa cells and theca cells, are often hyper-estrogenic, and can present with abnormal uterine bleeding, endometrial hyperplasia, or carcinoma, and isosexual precocious puberty in children.[1] In contrast, tumors composed of cells of testicular cell origin, such as Sertoli cells and Leydig cells, can present with signs of virilization, including hirsutism, acne, male-pattern baldness, voice changes, and irregular menses.[1]

OSCSTs have favorable prognoses. Unlike epithelial ovarian malignancies, of which up to 75% of cases present at Stage III or Stage IV,[4] the majority of patients with OSCSTs present early, at Stage I, and surgery is often curative.[3]

Classification

According to the 2014 WHO Classification of Female Genital Tumors, OSCSTs can be classified into pure stromal tumors, pure sex cord tumors, and mixed sex cord-stromal tumors (Table 1).[5] Within these

[a] Department of Radiology, Massachusetts General Hospital, 55 Fruit Street, Boston, MA, USA; [b] Harvard Medical School, Boston, MA, USA; [c] Department of Pathology, Massachusetts General Hospital, 55 Fruit Street, Boston, MA, USA
* Corresponding author. Division of Abdominal Imaging, Department of Radiology, White 270, Massachusetts General Hospital, 55 Fruit Street, Boston, MA 02114.
E-mail address: msertic@mgh.harvard.edu

Radiol Clin N Am 61 (2023) 595–608
https://doi.org/10.1016/j.rcl.2023.02.005

Table 1
2014 WHO classification of ovarian sex cord-stromal tumors[5]

Pure stromal tumors	Fibroma	Benign
	Cellular fibroma	Benign
	Thecoma	Benign
	Luteinized thecoma associated with sclerosing peritonitis	Benign
	Fibrosarcoma	Malignant
	Sclerosing stromal tumor	Benign
	Microcystic stromal tumor	Benign
	Signet ring stromal tumor	Benign
	Leydig cell tumor	Benign or malignant
	Steroid cell tumor, NOS	Benign
	Malignant steroid cell tumor	Malignant
Pure sex cord tumors	Adult granulosa cell tumor	Malignant
	Juvenile granulosa cell tumor	Malignant
	Sertoli cell tumor, NOS	Benign or malignant
	Sex cord tumor with annular tubules	Benign or malignant
Mixed sex cord-stromal tumors	Sertoli-Leydig cell tumor	Benign or malignant
	Well differentiated	Benign or malignant
	Moderately differentiated	Benign or malignant
	With heterologous elements	Benign or malignant
	Poorly differentiated	Benign or malignant
	With heterologous elements	Benign or malignant
	Retiform	Benign or malignant
	With heterologous elements	Benign or malignant
	Sex cord-stromal tumor, NOS	Benign or malignant
	Gynandroblastoma	Benign or malignant

subtypes, there are benign, borderline, and malignant tumors. Moreover, several benign OSCSTs may be benign in histology but may mimic malignant tumors and present with aggressive clinical and imaging features, as will be discussed below.

IMAGING TECHNIQUES/PROTOCOLS
Computed Tomography

Like most gynecologic pathologies, OSCSTs are incompletely assessed by computed tomography (CT). However, CT is the preferred technique in the pre-treatment evaluation of ovarian malignancy to assess for metastatic disease.[6] CT of the abdomen and pelvis is performed in the axial plane following the administration of intravenous iodinated contrast in the portal venous phase, with coronal and sagittal reformats.

Ultrasound

Ultrasound (US) is a widely available and portable modality that is often performed in the initial assessment of known or suspected ovarian neoplasms. Transvaginal US is preferred, as it permits high-quality imaging of higher resolution than transabdominal ultrasound with a decreased risk of beam attenuation due to overlying structures.[7] Frequencies of common transvaginal US probes range between 5 and 7.5 MHz.[7] The bladder should be emptied, and transvaginal US performed with the patient positioned in a manner that facilitates comfortable probe insertion and caudal positioning. Images of the uterus, ovaries, and adnexa should be acquired in the coronal and sagittal plane. Doppler imaging can be employed to further evaluate focal lesions. At our institution, cine clips of uterus, ovaries, and any focal lesions are also routinely acquired to enable volumetric image review post-exam.

Many OSCSTs present in pediatric patients, with transabdominal US often preferred as a non-invasive imaging technique in this age group. With transabdominal US, the bladder should be filled to displace bowel loops and provide an acoustic window. Probe frequency should be selected based on patient age and size, ranging from 5 to 7.5 MHz curvilinear probes in smaller/younger patients, to 3.5 to 5 MHz curvilinear probes in larger patients/adolescents. As with transvaginal US, coronal and sagittal gray-scale images should be acquired, and Doppler imaging can be applied to further investigate ovarian lesions.

MR Imaging

In the assessment of indeterminate ovarian masses, MR imaging with intravenous gadolinium contrast provides the highest post-test probability of ovarian cancer when compared with CT, Doppler US, or MR imaging without contrast.[6] MR imaging can be performed on a 1.5 T or 3.0 T magnet using a surface-phased array coil. The field of view should be confined to the soft tissues of the central pelvis, and include the uterus, adnexa, vagina, rectum, and bladder. Routine sequences include Fast spin echo (FSE) T2-weighted sequences in the axial, coronal, and sagittal planes, which provide high soft tissue contrast, allowing for both anatomic localization and tissue characterization.[8] At our institution, we also routinely acquire axial T1-weighted sequences with and without fat saturation, and axial diffusion-weighted imaging (DWI). DWI images are acquired in the axial plane with fat-suppressed, single-shot echo-planar images, with tri-directional diffusion gradients with b values between 0 and 1000 s/mm^2. Optimal maximum b values range between 800 to 1000 s/mm^2 and vary based on background tissue and tumor type.[9]

Following injection of intravenous gadolinium contrast, dynamic contrast-enhanced images are typically acquired in the sagittal plane during the arterial (20 second), venous (70 second), and delayed (>3 minute) phases. Further delayed phase post-contrast images are then acquired in the axial and coronal planes. Subtraction images can aid in the detection of lesion enhancement,[8] particularly in the setting of intrinsic hyperintense signal on T1-weighted sequences, such as lesions with internal hemorrhage.

DISCUSSION

OSCSTs are a large group of tumors, with varying clinical presentations and imaging appearances. We will discuss several of the more common malignant tumors, as well as benign tumors that can present aggressively and mimic malignancy. This discussion is by no means exhaustive, but rather an attempt to provide an overview of the more common malignant and clinically aggressive tumors.

OSCSTs are usually large, unilateral, and solid tumors.[3] Larger tumors more often contain hemorrhage or necrosis, occasionally due to torsion. Overall, imaging features vary considerably.

Certain imaging features are seen more commonly in malignant than benign OSCSTs. On MR imaging, the intrinsic T2 signal intensity of solid components is higher in malignant tumors.[10] Very low T2 signal is almost exclusively seen in benign lesions, with the exception of the extremely rare fibrosarcoma.[11] Benign lesions tend to demonstrate mild or hypoenhancement. Excluding fibromas, apparent diffusion coefficient (ADC) values are lower in malignant OSCTs than in benign tumors.[10] However, the accuracy of each of these features in isolation is relatively low. It is the combination of imaging features, in addition to the clinical presentation, that is most useful in evaluating OSCSTs.

Pure Stromal Tumors

Fibroma

Fibromas are benign tumors and are the most common OSCSTs. They are the most common solid ovarian tumors, accounting for 4% of all ovarian neoplasms.[12] Fibromas are hormonally inactive; as their name suggests, they are primarily comprised of fibrous contents, which accounts for their typical imaging findings.

On US, fibromas are solid, hypoechoic masses, with posterior acoustic shadowing. When large, they can be difficult to distinguish from pedunculated subserosal uterine leiomyomas. On CT, fibromas are solid, hypoattenuating masses that demonstrate delayed hypoenhancement following contrast administration.[4] Calcifications may be present.[1]

On MR imaging, fibromas demonstrate intrinsic, homogenous, hypointense signals on T1-weighted sequences and very low intrinsic signals on T2-weighted sequences.[12] Some lesions may contain internal edema or cystic degeneration, which appear hyperintense on T2.[4] Many lesions demonstrate a T2 hypointense capsule that separates the fibroma from the uterus, which can be a helpful feature in distinguishing the lesion from a pedunculated uterine leiomyoma. There is typically no significant diffusion restriction. Fibromas demonstrate poor, heterogeneous, gradual enhancement that is less than the adjacent ovarian stroma and significantly less than the uterine myometrium. This enhancement can also be useful in distinguishing fibromas from uterine leiomyomas, which enhance more avidly than fibromas in all phases.[12]

Although benign, fibromas can mimic malignant tumors at presentation due to their association with Meigs' syndrome (**Fig. 1**). Although less than 1% of ovarian tumors present with Meigs' syndrome, 80% to 90% of cases of Meigs' syndrome are associated with ovarian fibromas.[13] Meigs' syndrome is defined as the triad of ascites, pleural effusion, and a benign ovarian tumor. Lack of peritoneal nodularity, omental caking, or lymphadenopathy can help distinguish Meigs' syndrome from metastatic ovarian cancer. The pathophysiology of Meigs' syndrome is unknown, and hypotheses include the exudative effects of fibroblast growth factors and cytokines released by the ovarian tumor as well as lymphatic congestion secondary to mass effect.[13] Most pleural effusions in

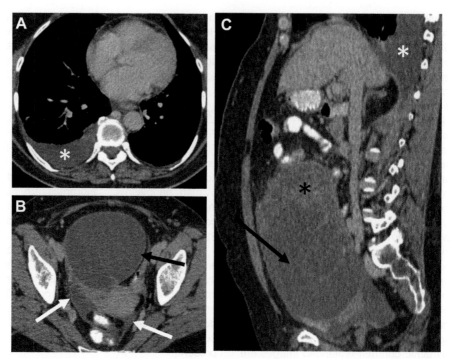

Fig. 1. Fibroma with Meigs' syndrome in a 67-year-old woman presenting with right lower quadrant pain. Axial (*A* and *B*) and sagittal (*C*) contrast-enhanced CT images of the abdomen and pelvis demonstrate the triad of pleural effusion (*asterisk* in *A*), ascites (*white arrows* in *B*), and benign ovarian tumor (*black arrow* in *B*). The tumor is a 24 × 14 × 13 cm heterogeneous mass arising from the right ovary, associated with solid components (*asterisk* in *C*) and hypodense fluid-density regions (*black arrow* in *C*). Following total abdominal hysterectomy and bilateral salpingo-oophorectomy, pathology revealed a cellular focally mitotically active fibroma.

Meigs' syndrome are right-sided, and pleural effusions are thought to be secondary to transdiaphragmatic extension of ascites. This condition is benign, and the ascites and pleural effusion resolve upon resection of the primary tumor.[13]

Thecoma

Thecomas are also benign tumors, though much rarer than fibromas. Although fibromas typically arise in non-functioning ovarian cortex, thecomas and fibrothecomas originate from the ovarian medulla, and can demonstrate estrogenic activity.[4]

Due to their low prevalence, the imaging characteristics of thecomas have not been completely described. Thecomas are predominantly solid, though can contain cystic components, and are most often unilateral.[14]

On CT, thecomas are large, heterogenous masses with internal hypoattenuating regions. The masses demonstrate mild heterogeneous enhancement. Calcifications may be present.[14] On MR imaging, thecomas demonstrate intermediate to mildly hyperintense signal on T2-weighted sequences, and mild heterogeneous enhancement, with multiple non-enhancing regions that correspond to cystic components.[14]

Luteinized thecoma associated with sclerosing peritonitis

As per the 2014 WHO Classification, luteinized thecomas in isolation are not recognized as a distinct subtype of ovarian thecomas. Histologically, they are characterized by spindle cells with scattered luteinized cells.[15] They occur in younger women and can be androgenic. In contrast to typical ovarian thecomas, luteinized thecomas are more likely to be bilateral, and are more often associated with ascites.[15]

Patients present with sudden-onset peritoneal fibrosis, which can cause bowel obstruction.[15] Patients may require surgical intervention, which could precipitate perioperative morbidity such as the development of adhesions, recurrent small bowel obstructions, multiple bowel resections, fistulae, short gut syndrome, and malnutrition.[15]

On imaging, there is diffuse, smooth peritoneal thickening and enhancement, with associated circumferential bowel mural thickening (**Fig. 2**).[15]

Fibrosarcoma

Fibrosarcomas are extremely rare, malignant ovarian tumors. Fewer than one hundred cases have been reported.[11] They may arise de novo,

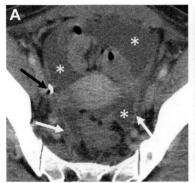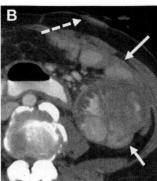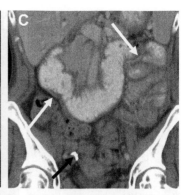

Fig. 2. Sclerosing peritonitis in a 38-year-old woman patient status post right salpingo-oophorectomy for luteinizing thecoma. Contrast-enhanced CT 1-year after resection (*A*) shows clips in the right adnexa (*black arrow*), ascites (*asterisk*), and diffuse peritoneal thickening and enhancement (*white arrows*). Axial (*B*) and coronal (*C*) CT images 7 years later demonstrate sequela of sclerosing peritonitis including multiple small bowel resections, left lower quadrant ileostomy (*dashed arrow*), and diffuse peritoneal and bowel mural thickening (*white arrows*). Multiple dilated loops of the bowel indicate chronic obstruction.

or due to malignant degeneration of an existing ovarian fibroma.

Due to the rarity of these tumors, imaging features are not well described. Histologic diagnosis requires four or more mitotic figures per 10 high-power fields.[16] On imaging, fibrosarcomas are unilateral, solid, heterogeneous ovarian lesions. Intrinsic tumor and enhancement characteristics are similar to fibromas, though they may be more likely to demonstrate internal hemorrhage or necrosis.[11]

Malignant steroid cell tumor

Steroid cell tumors are extremely rare, accounting for less than 0.1% of all ovarian neoplasms.[17] Approximately one-third of all steroid cell tumors are malignant, and up to 43% of the not otherwise specified (NOS) subtype are malignant.[4,17]

On imaging, steroid cell tumors are usually small, less than 3 cm, and almost always unilateral.[4] On US, they are solid masses that may be hyperechoic due to internal lipid content (**Fig. 3**). CT appearance is of a solid, hyperenhancing mass.[17] On MR imaging, they demonstrate intrinsic T1-hyperintense signal on non-fat-saturated sequences, due to the high lipid content. Accordingly, they will demonstrate signal drop on opposed-phase sequences. However, imaging features are variable based on the amount of lipid and fibrous content. Steroid cell tumors are highly vascular and will demonstrate avid enhancement following contrast administration.

As imaging features are variable, steroid cell tumors are more often suspected based on their clinical presentation. The androgenic effects of the tumor cause patients to present with virilization.

In addition, there are reports of cortisol release by these tumors, resulting in a presentation similar to Cushing's syndrome.[17]

Pure Sex Cord Tumors

Granulosa Cell tumors are the most common malignant OSCST, though they account for less than 5% of all ovarian malignant neoplasms and 2% of all ovarian tumors.[4,18] They can be further classified into two subtypes.

Adult granulosa cell tumor

Adult granulosa cell tumors (AGCT) account for up to 95% of all granulosa cell tumors.[2] These malignant tumors typically present in post-menopausal women; the average age of incidence is 50 to 55 years old.[3] Considered low-grade, the clinical course is often indolent, and the 10-year survival rate is greater than 90%.[2]

AGCTs are the most common hormone-secreting ovarian malignancies,[2] and are associated with clinical features of estrogen excess, including abnormal uterine bleeding, endometrial hyperplasia, and endometrial carcinoma.[1]

AGCTs demonstrate a broad spectrum of imaging appearances. They are typically large masses, with average diameters ranging from 9 to 14.5 cm.[18,19] Tumors fall on the solid/cystic spectrum; they can appear primarily solid, contain multiple cystic lesions, or be entirely cystic. The most common forms are multiseptated cystic masses (**Fig. 4**), and solid masses with internal cystic portions (**Fig. 5**).[18] Unilocular cystic masses and homogeneous solid masses are less common.[19] On US, they are well-defined, heterogeneous solid/cystic masses, with echogenic solid components.[18]

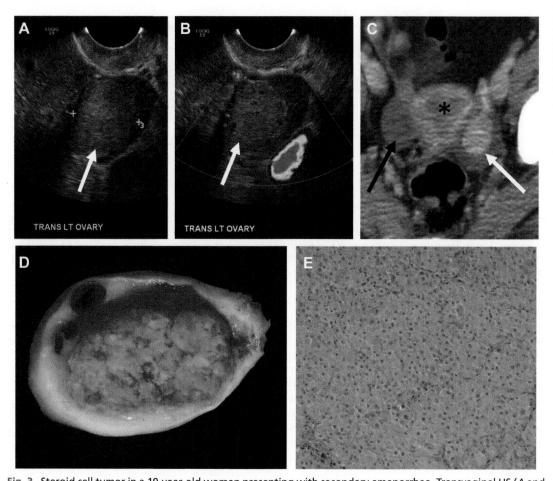

Fig. 3. Steroid cell tumor in a 19-year-old woman presenting with secondary amenorrhea. Transvaginal US (*A* and *B*) reveals a homogeneous hyperechoic solid lesion with peripheral vascularity (*white arrow*). Increased echogenicity is due to intracellular lipid. Axial contrast-enhanced CT (*C*) demonstrates an avidly enhancing left ovarian mass (*white arrow*), normal uterus (*asterisk*), and normal right ovary (*black arrow*). Gross pathology specimen (*D*) demonstrates a well-circumscribed, solid, golden yellow ovarian mass, with histopathology (*E*) confirming the presence of polygonal cells with abundant granular eosinophilic cytoplasm and round nuclei consistent with steroid cell tumor, NOS.

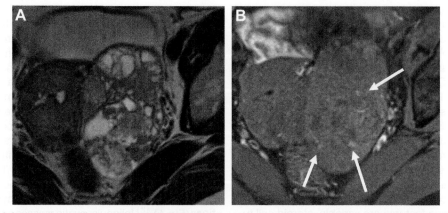

Fig. 4. Adult granulosa cell tumor in a 52-year-old woman. Non-contrast axial T2-weighted MR imaging (*A*) reveals a large mixed solid and cystic left ovarian mass with a "sponge-like" appearance, composed of solid components with intermediate T2 signal, and multiple hyperintense cystic spaces. Axial T1-weighted image with fat saturation (*B*) reveals multiple hyperintense foci (*white arrows*), consistent with internal hemorrhage.

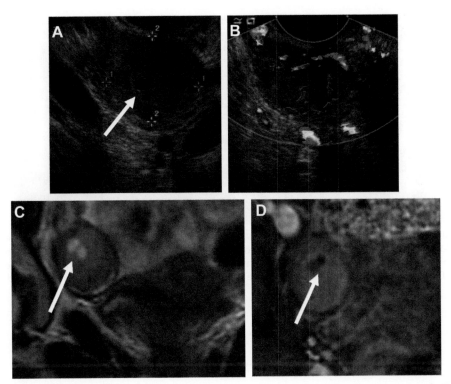

Fig. 5. Adult granulosa cell tumor in a 35-year-old woman presenting with infertility. Transvaginal US grayscale (*A*) and color Doppler images (*B*) demonstrate a solid right ovarian mass with internal vascularity and small anechoic cystic spaces (*arrow* in *A*). Axial T2-weighted (*C*) and T1 with fat saturation post-contrast (*D*) MR images demonstrate a solid mass with intermediate T2 signal, mild enhancement, and non-enhancing, T2 hyperintense cystic foci (*arrows* in *C, D*).

MR imaging appearances vary depending on composition. As with the juvenile granulosa cell tumors (JGCT) described below, AGCTs can demonstrate a "sponge-like" appearance, with multiple small cystic spaces (see **Fig. 4**). On T2-weighted sequences, solid components demonstrate intermediate intensity, while the cystic components are hyperintense. On unenhanced T1-weighted sequences, the solid components also demonstrate intermediate signal, whereas the cystic components range from hypointense to hyperintense, depending on the amount of internal hemorrhage and necrosis. Fluid/fluid levels may be seen.[19] The cystic components typically do not feature papillary projections (**Fig. 6**).[1] The solid components demonstrate heterogeneous

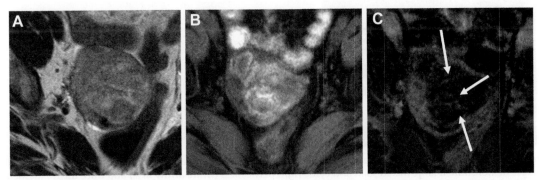

Fig. 6. Adult granulosa cell tumor in a 44-year-old woman. Axial T2-weighted (*A*), T1-weighted contrast-enhanced fat-saturated (*B*), and T1-weighted contrast-enhanced fat-saturated subtraction (*C*) MR images show a solid and cystic right ovarian mass that demonstrates intermediate signal on T2-weighted imaging and hyperintense signal on T1-weighted imaging, consistent with hemorrhage. Subtraction post-contrast images (*C*) reveal mild heterogeneous enhancement of internal septations (*arrows*).

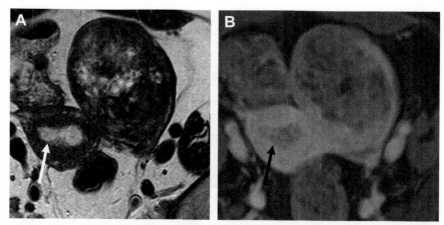

Fig. 7. Adult granulosa cell tumor and endometrial hyperplasia in a 62-year-old woman with post-menopausal bleeding. Axial T2-weighted (*A*) and T1-weighted contrast-enhanced fat-saturated (*B*) MR images show a large left ovarian mass that is predominantly solid and hypoenhancing relative to myometrium, with internal non-enhancing T2-hyperintense cystic foci. There is thickening and heterogeneous enhancement of the endometrium (*arrow*).

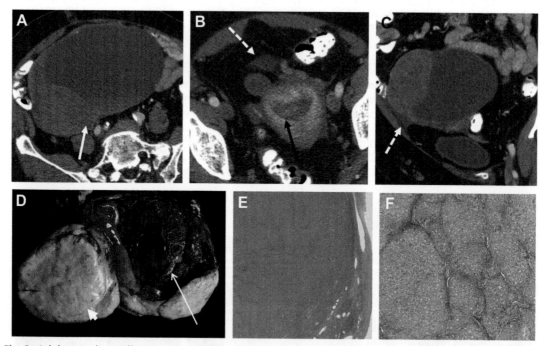

Fig. 8. Adult granulosa cell tumor in a 75-year-old woman. Axial (*A* and *B*) and coronal (*C*) contrast-enhanced CT images demonstrate a large mixed solid and cystic right pelvic mass (*white arrow* in *A*) and trace ascites (*dashed arrow* in *B*). The endometrium is thickened and heterogeneously enhancing (*black arrow* in *B*); this was histopathologically confirmed to reflect endometrial adenocarcinoma. The initial diagnosis was primary ovarian epithelial neoplasm. Gross pathologic specimen of the mass (*D*) demonstrates a solid yellow cut surface (*arrow-head*) with hemorrhage and cystic degeneration (*arrow*). Histopathology revealed both diffuse (*E*) and nested (*F*) patterns of neoplastic granulosa cells, consistent with AGCT.

enhancement, due to internal degeneration, hemorrhage, or infarction.[19]

The estrogenic effects of these tumors, manifest by uterine enlargement and endometrial thickening, are often better assessed on MR imaging, however, endometrial thickening can also be appreciated on CT and US (**Fig. 7**). Endometrial carcinoma can occur secondary to hormonal stimulation (**Fig. 8**), though is rare and typically low-grade and low-stage adenocarcinoma.[1]

Although commonly presenting at a low stage with a favorable prognosis, AGCTs do harbor a risk of late recurrence, up to 10 to 20 years after initial diagnosis.[4] Recurrence often manifests as peritoneal carcinomatosis.[19] However, in contrast to ovarian epithelial malignancies, peritoneal carcinomatosis is rare at the time of initial diagnosis.[18]

Juvenile granulosa cell tumor

JGCT account for only 5% of all granulosa cell tumors, however, they account for 70% of all OSCSTs in women under the age of 20.[20] These malignant neoplasms typically present before age 30; the mean age of diagnosis is 13 years.[2] Clinical presentation is related to the hormonal effects, and children often present with isosexual precocity.

Approximately 10% of JGCTs present during pregnancy (**Fig. 9**).[21] It has been hypothesized that the increased levels of human chorionic

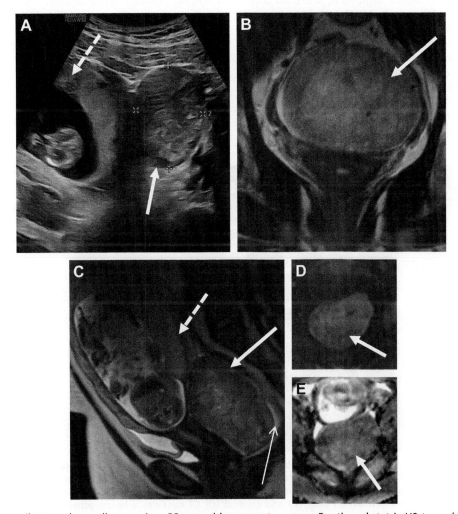

Fig. 9. Juvenile granulosa cell tumor in a 28-year-old pregnant woman. Routine obstetric US to evaluate fetal anatomy (*A*) reveals a heterogeneously hyperechoic solid left adnexal mass (*solid arrow*), adjacent to a gravid uterus (*dashed arrow*). Axial (*B*) and sagittal (*C*) T2-weighted MR images demonstrate a heterogeneous intermediate signal mass (*thick arrows*) arising from the left ovary, with trace ascites (*thin arrow*). There is mild diffusion restriction; axial DWI (*D*) and ADC (*E*) images show hyper- and hypointense signal, respectively, relative to the myometrium.

gonadotropin can stimulate growth of small granulosa cell tumors, which may not have been detected on pre-conception USs.[21] These tumors are often diagnosed incidentally, as estrogenic manifestations are not recognized during pregnancy.[22]

In contrast to AGCTs, recurrence for JGCTs following surgery happens early, within the first 3 years.[21] However, in most cases, JGCT is confined to the ovary and has an excellent prognosis.

Despite differences in clinical presentation and histology, JGCTs and AGCTs demonstrate a similar range of imaging appearances.[19] Although tumors may be entirely solid or entirely cystic, the majority are mixed solid and cystic.[20] They are typically large, unilateral, multilocular cystic masses, with irregular septations, and solid components. On US, as with AGCTs, the solid component of JGCTs is often echogenic (**Fig. 10**). The MR imaging appearance is also similar to that of AGCTs, with a distinctive "sponge-like" appearance. Solid components demonstrate intermediate signal on T1- and T2-weighted sequences, contain multiple small T2-hyperintense cystic components, and hemorrhagic foci that are hyperintense on T1-weighted sequences.[20]

Sertoli cell tumor, not otherwise specified

Sertoli cell tumors are extremely rare OSCTs and can be benign or malignant. They were once considered a subtype of granulosa cell tumor but are now recognized as a distinct sex cord tumor composed of pure Sertoli cells. They are estrogenic and are associated with menstrual irregularity, post-menopausal bleeding, and precocious puberty, depending on the age of the patient.

Classically, Sertoli cell tumors are unilateral solid masses.[19] However, the imaging appearances are variable, and they are primarily cystic lesions with small solid components (**Fig. 11**). The solid components are echogenic on US and demonstrate intrinsic intermediate signal on T1- and T2-weighted sequences, with enhancement following contrast administration. The predominantly cystic tumors can be difficult to distinguish from ovarian epithelial neoplasms on imaging, though Sertoli cell tumors have excellent prognoses and rarely recur.[19]

Mixed Sex Cord-Stromal Tumors

Sertoli-Leydig cell tumor

Previously considered a subtype of the Sertoli stromal tumor, the WHO now classifies

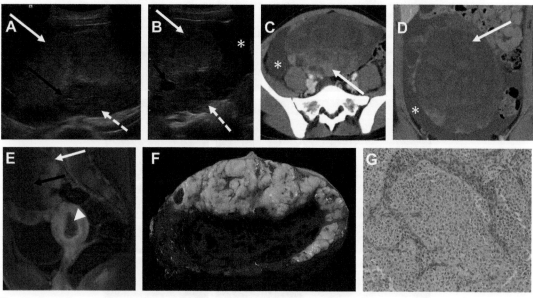

Fig. 10. Juvenile granulosa cell tumor in a 15-year-old woman with right lower quadrant pain. Transabdominal US (*A* and *B*) reveals a heterogeneous, hyperechoic mass (*white arrows*) arising from the right ovary (*dashed arrows*), with ascites (*asterisk* in *B*). Multiple small internal cystic spaces are demonstrated within the mass (*black arrow* in *A, B*). Contrast-enhanced axial (*C*) and coronal (*D*) CT confirms a heterogeneously enhancing solid and cystic mass (*arrows*) and moderate ascites (*asterisk* in *C, D*). Sagittal T1-weighted contrast-enhanced fat-saturated MR imaging (*E*) demonstrates a heterogeneously enhancing mass, with a large non-enhancing central component (*black arrow*), and endometrial thickening (*arrowhead*). Gross pathologic specimen of the tumor (*F*) demonstrates a mass with a nodular, fleshy tan-yellow appearance, with hemorrhage and secondary cystic degeneration. Histopathologic assessment (*G*) confirmed irregular nests of neoplastic granulosa cells with abundant eosinophilic cytoplasm in a collagenous background, consistent with JGCT.

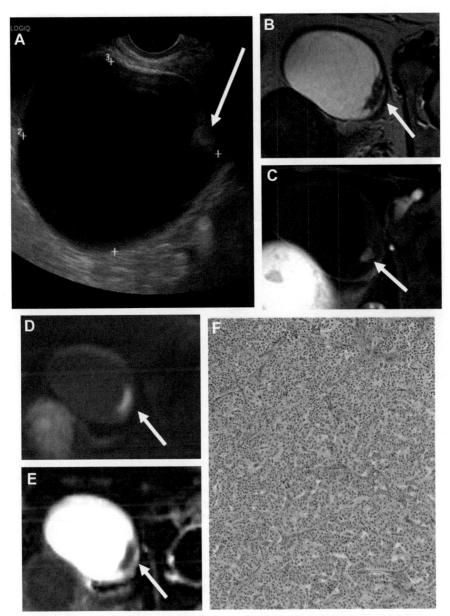

Fig. 11. Sertoli cell tumor in a 51-year-old woman with post-menopausal bleeding. Transvaginal US (*A*) shows a cystic left ovarian lesion with a mural nodule (*arrow*). T2-weighted MR imaging (*B*) demonstrates a cystic mass with a mural nodule (*arrow*), that enhances post-contrast (*C*). The nodule restricts diffusion; it is hyperintense on DWI (*D*) and hypointense on ADC (*E*). Following left salpingo-oophorectomy, histopathologic assessment (*F*) demonstrated trabeculae, solid and hollow tubules of neoplastic cells consistent with Sertoli cell tumor.

Sertoli-Leydig cell tumors as mixed sex cord-stromal tumors. These tumors can be benign or malignant, and are sub-classified based on their pathologic differentiation (see **Table 1**). Sertoli-Leydig cell tumors are the most common androgenic ovarian tumors; approximately 30% of cases are associated with androgenic activity.[4,20] Tumors occur in patients younger than 30 years, with a mean age of incidence of 14 years.[20]

Due to their androgenic effects, presentation is often related to clinical signs of virilization, such as acne, hirsutism, and irregular menstruation. However, some tumors demonstrate estrogenic activity.[1] Heterologous tumor components can undergo hepatic differentiation and cause elevated serum Alpha Fetoprotein (AFP) levels, though this is extremely rare.[1,20]

On imaging, these tumors are almost always unilateral; 80% of tumors are confined to the ovary at

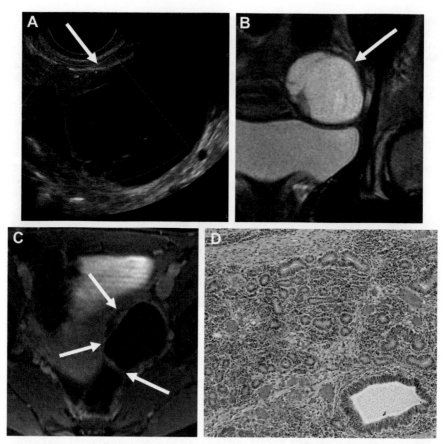

Fig. 12. Sertoli-Leydig cell tumor in a 21-year-old woman. Transvaginal US with color Doppler (*A*) demonstrates a large, predominantly cystic left ovarian mass (*arrow*) containing thick, vascular septations. Coronal T2-weighted (*B*) and contrast-enhanced T1-weighted axial MR imaging (*C*) reveal a predominantly cystic left ovarian mass with enhancing septations and mural nodularity (*arrows*). Following cystectomy, histopathology (*D*) revealed neoplastic Sertoli cells forming irregular aggregates and tubules, with scattered admixed Leydig cells, consistent with Sertoli-Leydig cell tumor of intermediate differentiation. Based on this diagnosis, the patient underwent left salpingo-oophorectomy with diagnostic laparoscopy, partial omentectomy, and pelvic washings, all of which were negative.

diagnosis.[1] Appearances are variable; tumors can be entirely solid, solid and cystic, primarily cystic (**Fig. 12**), or papillary.[4] On US, the tumors may appear as hypoechoic solid masses or mixed solid and cystic masses.[1] On MR imaging, the classic appearance is that of a well-circumscribed mass, containing multiple T2-hyperintense cystic regions.[10] The signal intensity of the solid components varies depending on the fibrous content of the stroma, however, there is typically avid contrast enhancement.[1]

Sex cord-stromal tumor, not otherwise specified

This is a poorly defined group of tumors that can be benign or malignant, and account for less than 10% of all OSCSTs.[22] These neoplasms do not demonstrate a recognizable pattern of predominant differentiation; the radiologic appearance of these tumors is also variable (**Fig. 13**). Like most OSCSTs, tumors are typically mixed solid and cystic. Solid components will enhance following contrast administration, and cystic components may contain internal hemorrhage.

SUMMARY

OSCST represent a broad class of primary ovarian neoplasms. Although some tumors have distinct imaging features, the majority have variable appearances, and it is the combination of imaging and clinical features that is most useful in distinguishing tumor subtypes. It is important to be aware of the imaging features that raise concern for malignant lesions, as well as distinguishing aggressive benign presentations that may mimic metastatic disease. These tumors are rare, and an understanding of their imaging appearances is

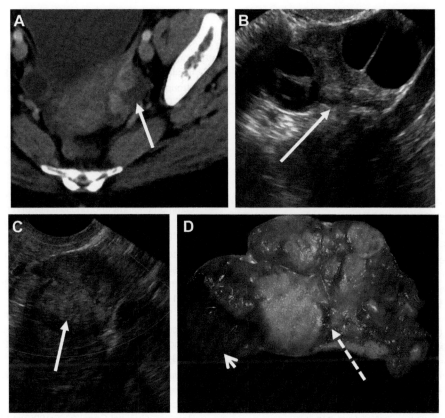

Fig. 13. Mixed sex cord-stromal tumor in a 58-year-old woman with abdominal pain. Contrast-enhanced axial CT (*A*) shows a mixed solid and cystic left ovarian mass. Transvaginal US (*B, C*) confirms the mixed solid and cystic mass (*solid arrows*). The solid components on US are heterogeneously hyperechoic with mild internal vascularity. The patient underwent hysterectomy, bilateral salpingo-oophorectomy, and peritoneal biopsies. Gross pathology (*D*) of the ovarian mass demonstrates yellow nodules embedded in a white background (*dashed arrow*) and tan/hemorrhagic cystic areas (*arrowhead*). A diagnosis of mixed sex cord-stromal tumor was rendered, with roughly equal amounts of Sertoli-Leydig (well to moderately differentiated), JGCT and AGCT components.

essential for the radiologist to raise the possibility of OSCST at presentation.

CLINICS CARE POINTS

- OSCST are a group of rare tumors, with a broad spectrum of clinical and imaging presentations. It can be difficult to distinguish the tumor subtypes and identify malignant lesions on imaging alone.

- The majority of OSCSTs are benign, and malignant subtypes generally carry a more favorable prognosis than the more common ovarian epithelial malignancies.

- Benign subtypes of OSCSTs can present aggressively, and mimic malignancies.

CONFLICTS OF INTEREST

Not applicable.

REFERENCES

1. Horta M, Cunha TM. Sex cord-stromal tumors of the ovary: a comprehensive review and update for radiologists. Diagn Interv Radiol 2015;21(4): 277–86.
2. Al Harbi R, McNeish IA, El-Bahrawy M. Ovarian sex cord-stromal tumors: an update on clinical features, molecular changes, and management. Int J Gynecol Cancer 2021;31(2):161–8.
3. Schultz KA, Harris AK, Schneider DT, et al. Ovarian Sex Cord-Stromal Tumors. J Oncol Pract 2016; 12(10):940–6.
4. Jung SE, Rha SE, Lee JM, et al. CT and MRI findings of sex cord-stromal tumor of the ovary. AJR Am J Roentgenol 2005;185(1):207–15.

5. Sisodia RC, Del Carmen MG. Lesions of the Ovary and Fallopian Tube. N Engl J Med 2022 Aug 25; 387(8):727–36.

6. Iyer VR, Lee SI. MRI, CT, and PET/CT for ovarian cancer detection and adnexal lesion characterization. AJR Am J Roentgenol 2010;194(2):311–21.

7. O'Shea A, Figueiredo G, Lee SI. Imaging Diagnosis of Adenomyosis. Semin Reprod Med 2020;38(2–03): 119–28.

8. Masch WR, Daye D, Lee SI. MR Imaging for Incidental Adnexal Mass Characterization. Magn Reson Imaging Clin N Am 2017;25(3):521–43.

9. Sertic M, Kilcoyne A, Catalano OA, et al. Quantitative imaging of uterine cancers with diffusion-weighted MRI and 18-fluorodeoxyglucose PET/CT. Abdom Radiol (NY) 2022;47(9):3174–88.

10. Zhao S-H, Li H-M, Qiang J-W, et al. The value of MRI for differentiating benign from malignant sex cord-stromal tumors of the ovary: emphasis on diffusion-weighted MR imaging. J Ovarian Res 2018;11(1):73.

11. Ray S, Biswas BK, Mukhopadhyay S. Giant primary ovarian fibrosarcoma: Case report and review of pitfalls. J Cytol 2012;29(4):255–7.

12. Shinagare AB, Meylaerts LJ, Laury AR, et al. MRI features of ovarian fibroma and fibrothecoma with histopathologic correlation. AJR Am J Roentgenol 2012;198(3):W296–303.

13. Vijayaraghavan GR, Levine D. Case 109: Meigs syndrome. Radiology 2007;242(3):940–4.

14. Li X, Zhang W, Zhu G, et al. Imaging features and pathologic characteristics of ovarian thecoma. J Comput Assist Tomogr 2012;36(1):46–53.

15. Altman AD, Bentley JR, Rittenberg PV, et al. Luteinized Thecomas ("Thecomatosis") with Sclerosing Peritonitis (LTSP): Report of 2 Cases and Review of an Enigmatic Syndrome Associated with a Peritoneal Proliferation of Specialized (vimentin+/keratin+/CD34+) Submesothelial Fibroblasts. J Obstet Gynaecol Can 2016;38(1):41–50.

16. Young RH. Ovarian Sex Cord-Stromal Tumors: Reflections on a 40-Year Experience With a Fascinating Group of Tumors, Including Comments on the Seminal Observations of Robert E. Scully, MD. Arch Pathol Lab Med 2018;142(12):1459–84.

17. Lee J, John VS, Liang SX, et al. Metastatic Malignant Ovarian Steroid Cell Tumor: A Case Report and Review of the Literature. Case Rep Obstet Gynecol 2016;2016:6184573.

18. Kim SH, Kim SH. Granulosa cell tumor of the ovary: common findings and unusual appearances on CT and MR. J Comput Assist Tomogr 2002;26(5): 756–61.

19. Javadi S, Ganeshan DM, Jensen CT, et al. Comprehensive review of imaging features of sex cord-stromal tumors of the ovary. Abdom Radiol (NY) 2021;46(4):1519–29.

20. Heo SH, Kim JW, Shin SS, et al. Review of ovarian tumors in children and adolescents: radiologic-pathologic correlation. Radiographics 2014;34(7): 2039–55.

21. Hasiakos D, Papakonstantinou K, Goula K, et al. Juvenile granulosa cell tumor associated with pregnancy: Report of a case and review of the literature. Gynecol Oncol 2006;100(2):426–9.

22. Staats PN, Young RH. Sex Cord-Stromal, Steroid Cell, and Other Ovarian Tumors with Endocrine, Paraendocrine, and Paraneoplastic Manifestations. In: Kurman RJ, Hedrick Ellenson L, Ronnett BM, editors. Blaustein's pathology of the female genital tract. Cham: Springer International Publishing; 2019. p. 967–1045.

Imaging of Endometrial Cancer

Martina Sbarra, MD[a],*, Michela Lupinelli, MD[b], Olga R. Brook, MD[c],
Aradhana M. Venkatesan, MD[d], Stephanie Nougaret, MD, PhD[e,f]

KEYWORDS

- Endometrial cancer • MR imaging • Staging • Personalized management

KEY POINTS

- Although endometrial cancer is a surgically staged disease, preoperative MR imaging helps in the selection of the most appropriate initial therapy.
- The high soft-tissue contrast resolution provided by MR imaging, compared with other imaging modalities, enables optimal evaluation of deep myometrial invasion and local tumor extent compared with other clinical imaging modalities.
- Axial sequences acquired perpendicular to the endometrial cavity are crucial to accurately assess myometrial invasion, which is one of the most important prognostic factors.

INTRODUCTION

Endometrial carcinoma (EC) is the most common gynecologic cancer both in the United States and Europe, with an increasing incidence rate in recent years.[1,2] Risk factors include prolonged exposure to unopposed estrogen (often caused by nulliparity and infertility associated with polycystic ovarian syndrome or tamoxifen use), obesity, and hyperinsulinemia.[3,4] Although most cases of endometrial cancer are sporadic, 5% to 10% are hereditary, usually related to Lynch syndrome.[5]

EC is staged surgically according to the International Federation of Gynecology and Obstetrics (FIGO) system (**Table 1**).[6] Imaging is not a part of the staging system, but it plays an integral role in preoperative assessment, which is crucial to tailor treatment. MR imaging is considered the optimal imaging modality to determine the local extent of the endometrial tumor, due to its excellent soft-tissue contrast resolution.[7] The American College of Radiology (ACR) and the European Society of Urogenital Radiology (ESUR) recommend MR imaging as appropriate for imaging in the preoperative setting.[8,9]

In this article, we emphasize the role of imaging for EC, with a focus on MR imaging. Information about MR imaging protocols, the advantages of MR imaging in the assessment of EC, and the role of MR imaging in endometrial cancer risk stratification and management are illustrated.

MOLECULAR CLASSIFICATION OF ENDOMETRIAL CANCER

According to histopathologic criteria, EC has traditionally been classified into two major types.[10] Type I tumors (>80%) are grade 1 and 2 endometrioid adenocarcinomas. They are estrogen-dependent tumors and associated with a favorable prognosis. Type II tumors (<20%) are grade 3 endometrioid

[a] Unit of Diagnostic Imaging, Fondazione Policlinico Universitario Campus Bio-medico, Via Alvaro Del Portillo 200, 00128 Roma, Italy; [b] Department of Radiology, Morgagni-Pierantoni Hospital, via Carlo Forlanini 34, 47121, Forlì, Italy; [c] Department of Radiology, Beth Israel Deaconess Medical Center, Boston, MA 00215, USA; [d] Department of Abdominal Imaging, Division of Diagnostic Imaging, The University of Texas MD Anderson Cancer Center, Houston, TX 77030, USA; [e] Montpellier Cancer Research Institute, University of Montpellier, INSERM, U1194, Montpellier, France; [f] Department of Radiology, Montpellier Cancer Institute, 208 Avenue des Apothicaires, Montpellier 34295, France
* Corresponding author.
E-mail address: m.sbarra@policlinicocampus.it

Radiol Clin N Am 61 (2023) 609–625
https://doi.org/10.1016/j.rcl.2023.02.007
0033-8389/23/© 2023 Elsevier Inc. All rights reserved.

Table 1
International Federation of Gynecology and Obstetrics staging system and management of endometrial cancer

FIGO Stage	Description	Treatment
IA	Tumor confined to the uterine corpus; < 50% myometrial invasion	Stage I EC: Surgery Hysterectomy and bilateral salpingo-oophorectomy.
IB	Tumor confined to the uterine corpus; > 50% myometrial invasion	• Stage I G1–G2 and G3, minimally invasive surgery; sentinel LNE is recommended.
II	Tumor invades cervical stroma, but does not extend beyond the uterus	• Stage I serous EC or carcinosarcoma, full surgical staging including lymph node staging.
IIIA	Tumor invades uterine serosa and/or adnexa	Stage I–IVA EC: Adjuvant therapy for low- and intermediate-risk patients
IIIB	Tumor invades vagina and/or parametrium	Adjuvant therapy is not recommended Low-Risk:
IIIC1	Positive pelvic lymph nodes	• Stage IA G1–G2 EEC (MMRd or NSMP) and no or focal LVSI
IIIC2	Positive para-aortic lymph nodes with or without positive pelvic lymph nodes	• Stage I–II POLEmut cancers Intermediate-Risk:
IVA	Tumor invades bladder and/or bowel mucosa	• Stage IA p53-abn tumors not infiltrating the myometrium Adjuvant VBT is recommended
IVB	Distant metastases, including intra-abdominal metastases and/or inguinal lymph nodes	Intermediate-Risk: • Stage IA G3 EEC (MMRd or NSMP) and no or focal LVSI • Stage IB G1–G2 EEC (MMRd or NSMP) and no or focal LVSI • Stage II G1 EEC (MMRd or NSMP) and no or focal LVSI Stage I–IVA EC: Adjuvant therapy for high-intermediate and high-risk patients Adjuvant therapy is recommended (EBRT/ChT) High-Intermediate Risk: • Stage IA–IB with substantial LVSI • Stage IB G3 • Stage II G1 with substantial LVSI • Stage II G2–G3 (MMRd or NSMP) High-risk: • All stages and all histologies with p53-abn and myometrial invasion • All stages with serous or undifferentiated carcinoma including carcinosarcoma with myometrial invasion • All Stage III and IVA with no residual tumor, regardless of histologies and molecular subtypes

Abbreviations: ChT, chemotherapy; EBRT, external beam radiotherapy; EC, endometrial cancer; EEC, endometrioid-type endometrial cancer; G, grade; LNE, lymph node evaluation; LVSI, lymphovascular space invasion; MMRd, mismatch repair deficient; NSMP, no specific molecular profile; p53-abn, p53-abnormal; *POLE*mut, polymerase epsilon-ultramutated; VBT, vaginal brachytherapy.

adenocarcinomas and non-endometrioid tumors. Type II tumors are not estrogen-dependent and show a worse prognosis with a higher risk for lymphovascular invasion, intra- or extraperitoneal spread, and relapse.[11] Type I tumors are treated with definitive surgery without lymphadenectomy when sentinel lymph node sampling is negative and in the absence of high-risk histologic features. Conversely, a systematic lymphadenectomy is recommended for type II tumors.[12]

The Cancer Genome Atlas (TCGA) studies have identified four EC molecular subtypes, later updated and incorporated into the ProMisE (Proactive Molecular Risk Classifier for Endometrial Cancer) molecular classifications:[13,14]

- (i) POLE mutation (*POLE*mut group) identified by next-generation sequencing of exons 9 to 14 of *DNA polymerase epsilon (POLE)*;
- (ii) microsatellite instability (mismatch repair deficient [MMRd] group) is defined by loss of expression of one of the mismatch repair proteins (MLH1, PMS2, MSH6, and MSH2) by immunohistochemistry (IHC);
- (iii) high somatic copy-number alterations driven by TP53 mutation (p53abn group);
- (iv) EC without a pathogenic *POLE* variant, with retained MMR protein expression, and wild-type p53 IHC, is classified as "no specific molecular profile" (NSMP) EC (**Fig. 1**).

EC molecular classification has shown improved prognostic relevance and a lack of interobserver variability as compared with the well-established morphological classification.[6] Extensive study of this molecular classification has revealed a good relationship between molecular subgroups and clinical outcome, establishing their prognostic value, particularly in high-risk endometrial cancer. *POLE*-mutated tumors are associated with the most favorable prognosis, whereas p53abn tumors have the poorest clinical outcomes.[15–17] Molecular profiling is encouraged for all ECs, especially in high-grade/high-stage tumors because the molecular results may influence adjuvant treatment recommendations.[12,18]

The molecular EC classification has been implemented in the World Health Organization 2020 classification and the 2021 European treatment guidelines given its prognostic value (see **Table 1**).[12,19] In addition, this molecular classification has resulted in an updated risk classification system for endometrial cancer (**Table 2**).

Prospective studies such as PORTEC-4a, RAINBO, CANSTAMP, NRG-GY018, and GY020 are among the first studies to analyze molecular-based treatments in the primary setting. For example, PORTEC-4a will be the first trial to prospectively investigate the use of adjuvant therapy after combining molecular and clinicopathological features in EC.[20] These clinical trials have the potential to provide key information for tailoring EC treatments based on molecular data, leading to personalized patient management and improved patient outcomes.

MR IMAGING PROTOCOL

MR imaging is the optimal imaging modality to assess deep myometrial invasion and local tumor extent in endometrial cancer. In routine clinical practice, the combination of T2-weighted imaging

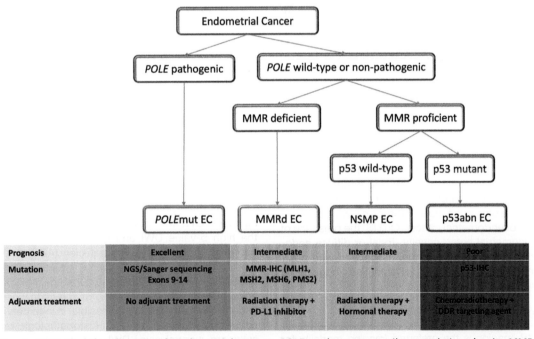

Fig. 1. Molecular classification of endometrial cancer. POLE, polymerase epsilon catalytic subunit; MMR, mismatch repair; POLEmut, polymerase epsilon-ultramutated; MMRd, mismatch repair deficient; NSMP, no specific molecular profile; p53abn, p53-abnormal; NGS, next generation sequencing; IHC, immunohistochemistry; PD-L1, programmed death-ligand 1; DDR, DNA damage repair.

Table 2
Endometrial cancer risk groups including molecular subtypes

Risk Group	
Low risk	• Stage IA (G1–G2) EEC (MMRd or NSMP) and no or focal LVSI • Stage I/II *POLE*mut tumor
Intermediate risk	• Stage IA G3 EEC (MMRd or NSMP) and no or focal LVSI • Stage IA non-endometrioid type and/or p53-abn tumors without myometrial invasion and no or focal LVSI • Stage IB (G1–G2) EEC (MMRd or NSMP) and no or focal LVSI • Stage II G1 EEC (MMRd or NSMP) and no or focal LVSI
High–intermediate risk	• Stage I EEC (MMRd or NSMP) any grade/depth of invasion with substantial LVSI • Stage IB G3 EEC (MMRd or NSMP) regardless of LVSI • Stage II G1 EEC (MMRd or NSMP) with substantial LVSI • Stage II G2–G3 EEC (MMRd or NSMP)
High risk	• All stages and histologies with p53-abn and myometrial invasion • All stages with serous or undifferentiated carcinoma including carcinosarcoma with myometrial invasion • All stage III and IVA with no residual tumor, regardless of histology and regardless of molecular subtypes.

Abbreviations: EEC, endometrioid-type endometrial cancer; LVSI, lymphovascular space invasion; MMRd, mismatch repair deficient; NSMP, no specific molecular profile; *POLE*mut, polymerase epsilon-ultramutated; p53-abn, p53-abnormal.

(T2WI), diffusion-weighted imaging (DWI), and multiphase contrast-enhanced imaging offers a "one-stop shop" approach for the imaging-based evaluation of patients with endometrial cancer.[21]

MR Imaging Protocol

A minimum 1.5 T magnet strength is recommended to ensure adequate image quality. Suggested MR imaging protocols, according to the Society of Abdominal Radiology (SAR) Uterine and Ovarian Cancer (UOC) Diseased Focused Panel (DFP)[22] and the ESUR guidelines,[9] are summarized in **Table 3**.

IMAGING FEATURES
Ultrasonography Imaging Features

Transvaginal ultrasound (TV US) is the first-line imaging technique to evaluate the endometrium in patients presenting with bleeding. Abnormal uterine bleeding is the most common clinical presentation of endometrial cancer. On US, the presence of endometrial heterogeneity, focal or diffuse endometrial thickening (>5 mm) associated with postmenopausal bleeding should be considered suspicious.[23]

MR Imaging Features

MR imaging is the preferred imaging modality for the preoperative assessment of endometrial cancer.[24,25] The European Society for Medical Oncology (ESMO) and National Comprehensive Cancer Network (NCCN) guidelines advise MR imaging as part of the patient's preoperative cancer assessment.[18,26] Preoperative assessment can help to establish a recurrence risk group and to confirm the utility of subsequent surgical management.

Classic MR Imaging Appearance of Endometrial Tumor

The normal zonal anatomy of the uterus is well demonstrated on T2WI and consists of (1) the high-signal intensity (SI) of the endometrium, surrounded by (2) the low-SI of the junctional zone (inner myometrium), which itself is surrounded by (3) the intermediate-SI of the outer myometrium (**Fig. 2**).

Endometrial cancer usually shows intermediate to low-SI compared with the high-SI of normal endometrium, on T2WI (**Fig. 3**). The enhancement of endometrial cancer usually is earlier than normal endometrium but later than the adjacent myometrium, on multi-phase contrast-enhanced MR imaging. On DWI, the tumor generally has high-SI on the high b-value DWI and low-SI on the corresponding apparent diffusion coefficient (ADC) map.

Although endometrial cancer is typically diagnosed by biopsy or dilation and curettage, MR imaging may be very helpful in tumor detection when endometrial sampling is not feasible, due to cervical stenosis, as well as when histopathologic results are inconclusive. DWI can provide useful information in differentiating benign from malignant endometrial lesions. The results of multiple studies have shown that endometrial cancer has

Table 3
Suggested MR imaging protocol for endometrial cancer[9,22]

Patient Preparation
• Fasting and the use of antiperistaltic agent (butylscopolamine bromide or glucagon, if available) to reduce motion artifacts owing to bowel peristalsis • A moderately full bladder to minimize artifacts related to bladder filling • Vaginal distention is optional

Sequences and Imaging Planes	
T2WI	Small FOV high-resolution T2 sequences in sagittal and axial oblique planes. The axial oblique sequences angled perpendicular to the endometrial cavity. Slice thickness ≤4 mm; FOV 20 to 26 cm
Large FOV T2W1/T1WI	Axial T2W sequence of the abdomen and pelvis (ESUR). Coronal T2W sequence to include kidneys and large FOV axial T1WI/T2WI of the pelvis (SAR UOC DFP). Large FOV imaging allows visualization of secondary sign of pelvic mass effect (hydronephrosis) and malignant disease (retroperitoneal lymph nodes or peritoneal carcinosis)
DWI	DWI sequences in at least one plane but preferably two planes (axial oblique along the uterus with the same orientation of axial oblique T2W sequence or sagittal) and with a minimum of 2 b values (0 and 800 to 1000)

Contrast-enhanced T1WI	Contrast-enhanced images acquired at 2 min 30 provide the best contrast between tumor and the myometrium. Suggested contrast-enhanced imaging phases:
	1. A single-phase axial T1WI acquisition at 2 min 30, or
	2. Multi-phase contrast-enhanced MR imaging:
	  • Early phase (30 to 60 s) is optimal to evaluate the sub-endometrial enhancement
	  • Equilibrium phase (120 to 180 s) is optimal to evaluate the depth of myometrial invasion
	  • Delayed phase (4 to 5 min) is helpful for detection of cervical stromal invasion

Abbreviations: DWI, diffusion-weighted imaging; ESUR, European Society of Urogenital Radiology; FOV, field of view; SAR UOC DFP, Society of Abdominal Radiology Uterine and Ovarian Cancer Disease-focused Panel.

a significantly lower ADC value than normal endometrium and myometrium[27–31] (**Fig. 4**).

International Federation of Gynecology and Obstetrics Stage IA/IB and Corresponding MR Imaging Findings

Stage I tumors are confined to the uterine corpus and account for 80% of cases. Stage IA is diagnosed if the tumor involves only the endometrium or less than 50% of the myometrium (**Fig. 5**), whereas stage IB is present if the tumor invades 50% or more of the myometrial thickness (**Fig. 6**). Depth of myometrial invasion can be used as a surrogate imaging marker of potential lymphovascular space invasion (LVSI) and therefore likelihood of nodal metastases and relapse.[6,32] The depth of

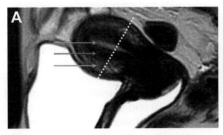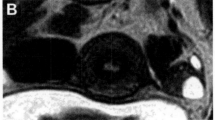

Fig. 2. Sagittal T2WI (*A*) shows the hyperintensity of the endometrium (*blue arrow*), the hypointense junctional zone (*orange arrow*), and the intermediate-signal intensity outer myometrium (*green arrow*). Angling the axis perpendicular to the endometrial cavity (*dashed line, A*) enables a true axial sequence (*B*) providing a plane for the accurate evaluation of the depth of tumor myometrial invasion.

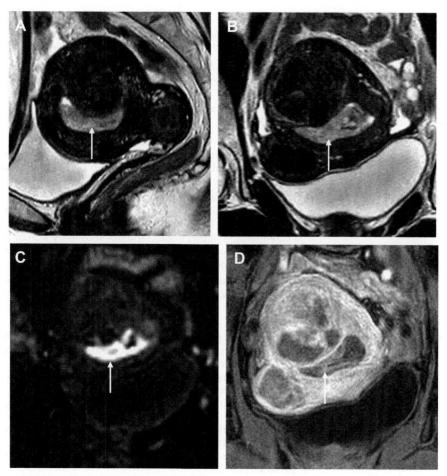

Fig. 3. Sagittal (*A*) and axial-oblique (*B*) T2WI show distension of the endometrial cavity by an intermediate-SI tumor (*arrows*), with no deep myometrial invasion (FIGO stage IA). Endometrial cancer is hyperintense on DWI (*C, arrow*), and shows hypoenhancement on contrast-enhanced imaging (*D, arrow*) with a maximal tumor-to-myometrial contrast on equilibrium phase.

myometrial invasion is best measured on the axial oblique images acquired perpendicular to the endometrial cavity. A line must be drawn parallel to the expected inner edge of the myometrium, then, two orthogonal measurements must be made, one reflecting the maximum tumor extent within the myometrium and one representing the whole thickness of the myometrium. The ratio of these two lengths represents the percentage of the myometrial invasion (see **Fig. 5**).[9,21]

Myometrial invasion is almost completely excluded if an intact low SI junctional zone on T2WI is present and if uninterrupted sub-endometrial early phase enhancement is demonstrated on contrast-enhanced MR imaging (**Fig. 7**).

Pitfalls

- When the zonal anatomy of the uterus is not well defined, as is often in post-menopausal patients or when tumor is isointense to the myometrium on T2WI, tumor margins may not be clearly evaluated on T2WI. Contrast-enhanced imaging and DWI can help to improve the delineation of tumor margins and tumor depth within the myometrium.
- Large tumors can distend the endometrial cavity and compress the surrounding myometrium; the depth of myometrial invasion may be overestimated in these cases. Presence of an intact low SI junctional zone on T2WI and uninterrupted sub-endometrial enhancement on early contrast-enhanced MR imaging are helpful to exclude myometrial invasion (**Figs. 8** and **9**).
- In the cornual regions, the myometrium is physiologically thinner than the other parts of the uterus. Thus, the tumor located in the cornua makes it difficult to estimate the percentage of myometrial invasion. The addition

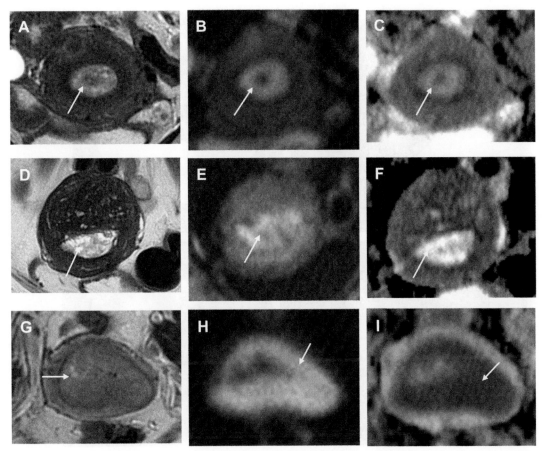

Fig. 4. Endometrial polyp (*A–C, arrows*) shows high-SI on T2WI with a central hypointense fibrous stalk (*A*), high-SI on DWI as T2 shine-through effect (*B*), and high-SI on ADC map (*C*). Endometrial hyperplasia (*D–F, arrows*) shows high-SI on T2WI (*D*) and does not show diffusion restriction with high-SI on DWI (*E*) and ADC map (*F*). Endometrial cancer (*arrows in G–I*) has intermediate-SI on T2-WI (*G*) and shows diffusion restriction with high-SI on DWI (*H*) and low-SI on ADC map (*I*).

of contrast-enhanced imaging and DWI to the axial oblique T2WI acquired perpendicular to the endometrial cavity can improve tumor delineation.

- The normal zonal anatomy of the uterus can be irregular or distorted due to the presence of leiomyomas. Contrast-enhanced imaging and DWI can help to delineate tumor margins and distinguish tumors from leiomyoma.
- Adenomyosis may be responsible for a pseudo-widening of the junctional zone being mistaken for myometrial invasion. Furthermore, the true degree of myometrial invasion may be difficult to evaluate in the setting of concomitant adenomyosis because endometrial cancer frequently extends into the ectopic endometrial tissue in adenomyosis. In these cases, review of the DWI findings is helpful, as adenomyosis will not show diffusion restriction whereas endometrial cancer will **(Fig. 10)**.[33]

International Federation of Gynecology and Obstetrics Stage II and Corresponding MR Imaging Findings

Stage II tumors invade the cervical stroma, but do not extend beyond the uterus. Stage II has a different prognosis compared with stage I. Invasion of the cervical stroma is associated with a higher risk of LVSI, directly correlating with the risk of lymph node metastases, and increased risk of recurrence.[6,34] Cervical stromal invasion is best evaluated on sagittal and axial oblique images. Cervical stromal invasion is diagnosed when (1) on T2WI, the intermediate-SI tumor disrupts the normal low-SI cervical stroma, (2) on contrast-enhanced imaging, the hypoenhancing tumor disrupts the normal enhancement of cervical stroma, and (3) on DWI, the tumor with high-SI on high b value DWI disrupts the low-SI cervical stroma **(Fig. 11)**.

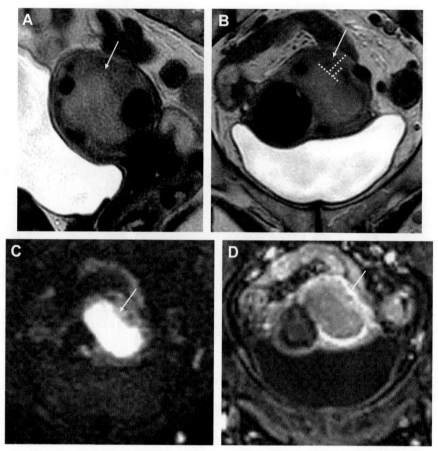

Fig. 5. Sagittal (*A*) and axial oblique (*B*) T2WI show distention of the endometrial cavity by an intermediate-SI tumor (*arrows*) within the fundus; the dashed lines (*B*) confirm the absence of deep myometrial invasion. Axial oblique DWI (*C*) shows a mass associated with hyperintense DWI signal at the level of the endometrial cavity (*arrow*) and axial oblique contrast-enhanced imaging (*D*) shows a hypoenhancing area within the endometrial cavity (*arrow*) in keeping with stage IA tumor, invading less than 50% of the myometrium.

Pitfalls

- Tumor extending into the endocervical canal without the disruption of the normal low-SI cervical stroma is not diagnostic of cervical stromal invasion. Distension of the cervical canal by tumor (see **Fig. 6**) should not be mistaken for true cervical stromal invasion (see **Fig. 11**).
- Cervical stromal invasion may occur without the involvement of the endocervical mucosa when the tumor invades the cervical stroma via adjacent contiguous myometrial invasion (see **Fig. 11**).

International Federation of Gynecology and Obstetrics Stage III and Corresponding MR Imaging Findings

Stage III tumors are those demonstrating spread beyond the uterus but not outside the true pelvis.

Stage IIIA tumors invade the uterine serosa. Uterine serosal invasion is diagnosed when (1) on T2WI, the intermediate to high-SI tumor disrupts both the normal low-SI serosa and the normal smooth outer contour of the uterus, and (2) on contrast-enhanced imaging, the normal rim enhancement of the outer myometrium is disrupted. When the tumor is isointense to the myometrium, the evaluation on T2WI may be limited. Contrast-enhanced imaging and DWI can help to overcome this pitfall, improving tumor delineation.

Stage IIIA tumors also include direct tumor spread to the adnexa or ovarian metastasis. Adnexal involvement by endometrial cancer is a significant parameter in FIGO staging and has an impact on the overall survival rate.[35] It is important to be aware that synchronous ovarian tumors can occur in conjunction with endometrial cancer.[36] Although not always possible on imaging, it is crucial to differentiate synchronous ovarian cancer

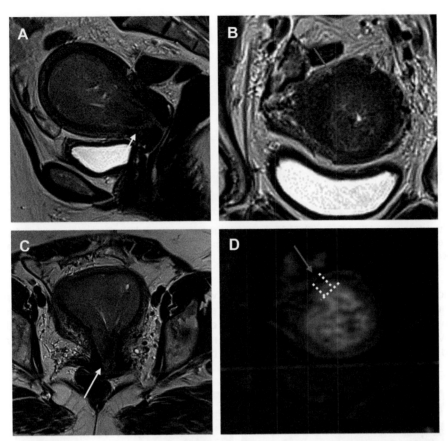

Fig. 6. Sagittal (*A*), axial oblique (*B*), and coronal oblique (*C*) T2WI show an intermediate-SI tumor involving the endometrial cavity with disruption of junctional zone (*A,B, orange arrows*) and prolapsing into the endocervical canal (*A,C,* white arrows) with no stromal invasion (FIGO stage IB). Axial oblique DWI (*D*) helps best delineation of depth of myometrial invasion showing extension of abnormal-SI to greater than 50% of the myometrium (*orange arrow*). The dashed lines (*D*) indicate how the depth of myometrial invasion should be measured on axial oblique sequences.

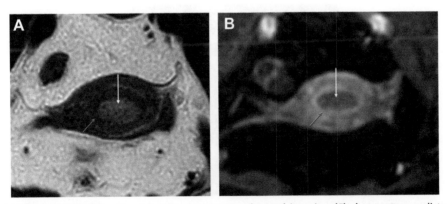

Fig. 7. Axial-oblique T2WI (*A*) and axial oblique contrast-enhanced imaging (*B*) show a tumor distending the endometrial cavity (white arrows); a continuous low signal intensity junctional zone is seen on A (*orange arrow*). A smooth uninterrupted band of early sub-endometrial enhancement on contrast-enhanced MR imaging helps to exclude myometrial invasion (orange arrow, *B*).

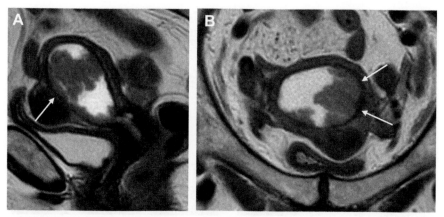

Fig. 8. Sagittal (*A*) and axial oblique (*B*) T2WI show a large tumor distending the endometrial cavity and compressing the surrounding myometrium. The identification of a low-SI junctional zone (*arrows, A,B*) excludes the presence of myometrial invasion.

from endometrial cancer ovarian metastasis because they have different prognoses.[37] Secondary ovarian metastases are more likely when there is a large volume endometrial tumor, high tumor grade, and deep myometrial invasion associated with a small ovarian lesion, or when there is bilateral ovarian involvement. Synchronous ovarian cancers are more frequent in patients with simultaneous involvement of the endometrium and ovary by low-grade endometrioid carcinoma.

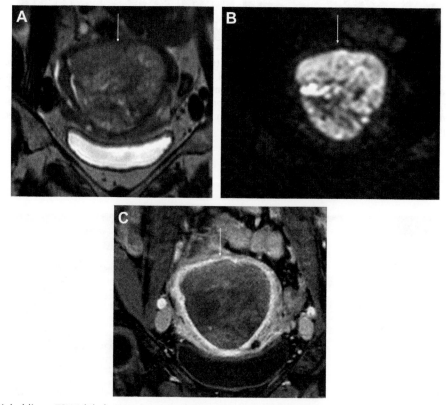

Fig. 9. Axial oblique T2WI (*A*) shows a large endometrial tumor compressing the myometrium associated with a superficial interruption of the low-SI junctional zone (*arrow*). The superficial invasion of the inner myometrium is confirmed on DWI (*B*) and on contrast-enhanced MR imaging (*C*) as shown by the irregular tumor margins (*B, arrow*) and by interrupted sub-endometrial enhancement (*C, arrow*).

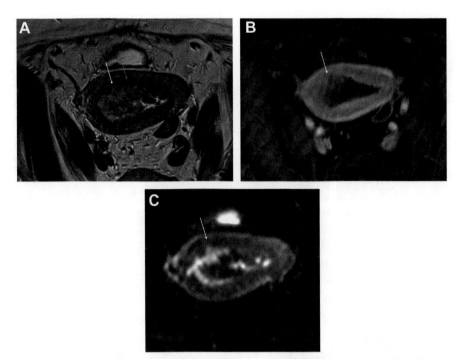

Fig. 10. Axial oblique T2WI (*A*) shows a thick junctional zone (*orange arrow*) and a poorly delineated tumor to myometrium interface (*white arrow*). The tumor margins are difficult to assess on T2WI. Contrast-enhanced imaging (*B*) shows an ill-defined hypoenhancing area (*arrow*). On ADC map (*C*), the myometrial invasion appears superficial (*arrow*) consistent with FIGO IA disease. DWI helps tumor staging in case of adenomyosis.

Stage IIIB tumors involve the parametria and the vagina by either direct invasion or metastatic spread. Parametrial involvement occurs in the context of cervical invasion and is diagnosed on T2WI when there is intermediate-SI tumor extension occupying the full thickness of the cervical stroma, with an irregular interface at the adjacent parametrial fat or frank tumor extension into the parametrial fat. Vaginal involvement—indicated by segmental loss of the low-SI of vaginal wall on T2WI—is very rare at the time of the initial diagnosis and is usually due to the presence of "drop metastases". Although vaginal involvement can be readily apparent on clinical examination, its evaluation can be difficult on MR imaging especially when the drop metastasis is small, and the vaginal vault is collapsed. DWI can improve the depiction of small metastatic deposits at the level of the parametrium or vagina.[38]

Stage IIIC is characterized by the presence of positive lymph nodes and is further subdivided into stage IIIC1 (positive pelvic lymph nodes) (**Fig. 12**) and stage IIIC2 (positive para-aortic lymph nodes). Risk factors for lymph node metastases include high-risk tumor histology, LVSI, deep myometrial invasion, and cervical stromal invasion.[39]

MR imaging evaluation of pelvic and para-aortic lymph nodes can be performed in the preoperative

setting with accuracy comparable to computed tomography (CT), associated with a sensitivity of 44% to 66% and specificity of 73% to 98%.[40] The detection of lymph nodes metastases according to size criteria (short axis >10 mm) has been reported to have high specificity (93% to 100%), low sensitivity (17% to 80%), and moderate accuracy (83% to 90%).[40–42] Morphologic criteria (ie, nodal shape and margins) have not been shown to improve the prediction of nodal metastases.[21] DWI has been studied in lymph node metastases because nodes can be easily detected owing to their high-SI on high b value DWI.[43] However, there is a significant overlap between the ADC value of benign and malignant nodes; therefore, DWI cannot be used to reliably identify lymph node metastases, particularly in normal-sized lymph nodes.[41]

International Federation of Gynecology and Obstetrics Stage IV and Corresponding MR Imaging Findings

Stage IV tumors directly invade the bladder or rectal mucosa (stage IVA) or manifest with distant metastases (stage IVB).

The loss of low T2 SI of the bladder or rectal wall and direct mucosal invasion by a tumor with

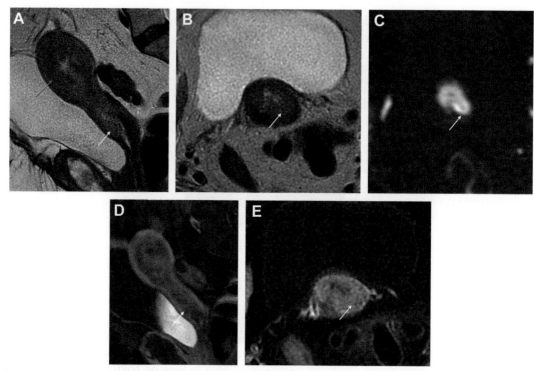

Fig. 11. Sagittal (*A*) and axial oblique (*B*) T2WI show endometrial cancer with deep myometrial invasion (*orange arrow, A*) and cervical stromal invasion (*white arrows, A,B*). Note the interruption of the hypointense cervical stromal signal intensity (*white arrows, A,B*), and the cervical stromal invasion from adjacent myometrium (FIGO stage II). The cervical stromal invasion is confirmed on DWI (*C*) and on sagittal (*D*) and axial oblique (*E*) contrast-enhanced imaging (arrows).

intermediate-SI are suggestive of stage IVA disease; this is often best delineated on sagittal T2-weighted MR imaging. Preservation of the fat planes between the tumor and the bladder or rectal wall excludes stage IVA with high accuracy.[9] However, in inconclusive cases, cystoscopy or rectosigmoidoscopy is recommended.

In stage IVB tumors, distant metastases (including para-aortic lymph nodes above the renal vessels and inguinal lymph nodes), and malignant ascites or peritoneal implants can be demonstrated. Peritoneal disease is more common in patients with non-endometrioid endometrial cancer (ie, serous and undifferentiated carcinomas or uterine carcinosarcoma), who should undergo omentectomy during staging surgery because of the higher risk of microscopic omental metastases.[12] On MR imaging, DWI can improve the detection of small peritoneal implants.[44]

Computed Tomography Imaging Features

CT imaging has a limited role in the local assessment of endometrial cancer. CT has a low sensitivity (83%) and specificity (42%) in evaluating myometrial invasion, as well as in assessing cervical stromal invasion.[45]

Contrast-enhanced CT of the chest, abdomen, and pelvis is appropriate for the assessment of lymph node and distant metastases for high-grade tumor in the initial evaluation of endometrial

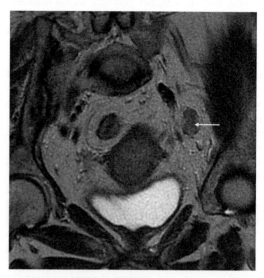

Fig. 12. Axial oblique T2WI shows an intermediate-SI endometrial tumor and positive pelvic lymphadenopathy (*arrow*), in keeping with FIGO stage IIIC1.

cancer.[8] Furthermore, CT of the chest, abdomen, and pelvis with intravenous contrast may be appropriate both for the surveillance of asymptomatic patients with high-risk endometrial cancer and for the post-treatment evaluation of clinically suspected recurrence of known endometrial cancer.[8]

PET-Computed Tomography and PET-MR Imaging Features

[18]F-fluoro-2-deoxy-D-glucose PET-CT (FDG PET/CT) is the best imaging method to evaluate lymph node and distant metastases in endometrial cancer and may be used in high-risk or advanced-stage disease (Fig.13).[6] The yield of FDG PET/CT is low in early-stage disease because of the low prevalence of lymph node metastases. FDG PET/CT has an excellent specificity (94%) and moderate sensitivity (72%) for the assessment of lymph node metastases; the moderate sensitivity probably reflects the need for enough tumoral cells to induce ^{18}F-fluoro-2-deoxy-D-glucose hypermetabolism.[46]

PET-MR imaging is an emergent hybrid imaging modality that may improve endometrial cancer assessment by combining the functional capacity of PET with the high soft-tissue contrast provided by MR imaging. A recent meta-analysis showed an excellent diagnostic performance of FDG-PET-MR imaging to evaluate primary tumor, nodal staging and recurrence in patients with gynecological malignancies, including endometrial cancer.[47] There are known technical and operational challenges associated with PET/MR imaging that have limited its widespread adoption compared with PET/CT.[24]

Nevertheless, PET/MR imaging has the potential to provide a "one-stop shop" imaging modality to evaluate both local and distant extent of disease, with specific practical value in overcoming the limitations of size-based criteria on MR imaging in evaluating nodal involvement.

MR IMAGING FOR ENDOMETRIALCANCER RISK STRATIFICATION AND MANAGEMENT

MR imaging plays an important role in selecting the most appropriate initial therapy for treatment for patients, including those who may be fertility-sparing candidates, those with early and low-intermediate stage disease and patients with advanced and high-risk disease.

Conservative Fertility Sparing Treatment

In premenopausal patients who wish to preserve their fertility, the use of hormonal therapy may be considered as a primary treatment, in lieu of surgery. Fertility-sparing treatment should be considered in patients with atypical hyperplasia/endometrioid intra-epithelial neoplasia, and grade 1 endometrioid carcinoma without myometrial invasion.[48–50] In this setting, it is critical to assess the extent of the disease and to rule out any myometrial invasion (superficial or deep) (Box 1).[51]

Surgical Treatment in Early Stage and Low/Intermediate-Risk Disease

In postmenopausal patients with low- or intermediate-risk disease, lymphadenectomy can safely be avoided when there is no evidence of

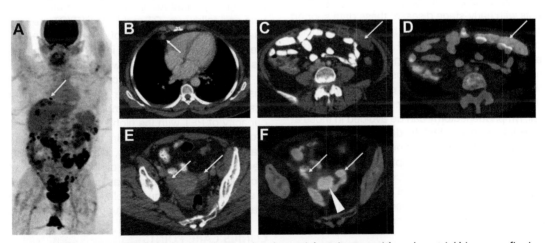

Fig. 13. A 60-year-old woman with newly diagnosed endometrial carcinoma, with endometrial biopsy confirming serous carcinoma. Follow-up 18F-FDG PET/CT, including whole body maximum intensity projection image (A), contrast-enhanced CT (B,C,E) and axial fused PET/CT images (D,F) show multifocal metastatic disease, including anterior diaphragmatic metastatic adenopathy (arrows in A,B), FDG avid omental carcinomatosis (arrows in C,D) and bilateral adnexal metastatic involvement (arrows E,F), as well as focal uptake within the endometrium, consistent with known primary tumor (arrowhead in F).

high-risk features at imaging and no evidence of metastatic disease with sentinel lymph node mapping.[12,26]

In the past, all patients with endometrial cancer had undergone lymphadenectomy as part of staging, along with total hysterectomy, bilateral salpingo-oophorectomy, and careful exploration of the omentum, peritoneum, and intra-abdominal contents.[6] However, performing systematic lymphadenectomy in all patients has been considered controversial, given its association with longer operation time, increased blood loss and subsequent blood transfusions, and the increased risk of long-term complications, such as lymphedema and lymphoceles.[52,53] Moreover, two large clinical trials showed no survival benefit for lymph node dissection in patients with FIGO grade 1 or 2 Stage IA endometrial cancer.[54,55] Sentinel lymph node mapping has been introduced as an alternative to lymph node dissection for lymph node staging. Multiple studies, including prospective cohort ones, confirmed a high degree of sensitivity of sentinel lymph node mapping for lymph node staging in patients with early-stage disease; these data support the positive impact of sentinel lymph node mapping on surgical management and indications for adjuvant treatment.[56-60] According to the ESMO guidelines, sentinel lymph node biopsy can be considered for staging purposes in patients with low/intermediate-risk disease. Per NCCN guidelines as well, lymphadenectomy can be avoided in those at low risk for nodal metastatic disease, with no high-risk features at imaging and no evidence for nodal metastases at sentinel lymph node mapping.[26] Thus, MR imaging plays a crucial role in distinguishing patients who may benefit from this technique from those with more advanced stages who should undergo systematic lymphadenectomy.

Treatment in Advanced and High-Risk Disease

In patients with high-risk endometrial cancer, in whom the extension of disease into adjacent organs is clinically suspected, the role of MR imaging is to assess the presence of extrauterine spread to facilitate treatment planning.[61] In this clinical scenario, a whole-body imaging with CT or PET/CT is recommended to evaluate the presence of lymph nodes and distant metastases.[8]

Endometrial Cancer Radiation Treatment

In patients with localized endometrial cancer, who cannot undergo surgical treatment, radiation therapy is routinely administrated as the definitive treatment. MR imaging helps to determine the local tumor extent and therefore assists in planning the radiation field.[62] Radiation therapy is also administrated in the neoadjuvant or adjuvant setting in patients with high-risk features or advanced disease and in the salvage setting in cases of local recurrence.[12]

SUMMARY

Imaging has become a key tool in the preoperative work-up of endometrial cancer. Although TV US is the first-line imaging technique to evaluate the endometrium in patients presenting with bleeding, MR imaging plays a central role in identifying patients with early-stage disease, including those that may benefit from fertility-sparing therapy, as well as those with high-risk features and evidence of locally advanced or distant disease. Given the controversial role for systemic lymphadenectomy in all patients with endometrial cancer, MR imaging can help surgeons identify those patients with high-risk features who should most likely benefit from systematic lymphadenectomy as part of their definitive management. In those patients triaged for radiation therapy, MR imaging plays an important role in radiation treatment planning and follow-up. CT and FDG PET/CT are also integral to the management of patients with endometrial cancer, particularly in identifying nodal and distant metastases in those with high-risk disease or those at risk for recurrence. PET-MR imaging has the potential to improve endometrial cancer assessment in the future, combining the functional capacity of PET with the high soft-tissue contrast provided by MR imaging. In the contemporary era of personalized medicine, with therapies stratified according to the risk of local and distant recurrence, imaging, particularly with MR imaging, is expected to continue to play a vital role in the management of patients with endometrial cancer.

CLINICS CARE POINTS

- MR imaging plays a vital role in the preoperative work-up of endometrial cancer.

- Imaging findings that can exclude the myometrial invasion are the presence of the continuous hypointense junctional zone on T2-weighted imaging and the presence of uninterrupted sub-endometrial enhancement; deep myometrial invasion represents an imaging marker of potential lymphovascular space invasion and therefore the likelihood of nodal metastases and relapse.
- Lymphadenectomy can be safely avoided in patients with low–intermediate-risk endometrial cancer and without evidence of high-risk features at imaging and no evidence of metastatic disease with sentinel lymph node mapping.
- In patients with high-risk disease or at risk for recurrence, whole-body imaging (computed tomography [CT], PET/CT, PET-MR imaging) is integral to management in identifying nodal and distant metastases.

DISCLOSURE

A.M. Venkatesan receives grant funding from the University of Texas MD Anderson Cancer Center Institutional Research Grant Program, the University of Texas MD Anderson Cancer Center Radiation Oncology Strategic Initiatives Pilot Grant Program, the Oden Institute for Computational Engineering and Sciences, UTMDACC & Texas Advanced Computing Center (TACC) Oncological Data & Computational Sciences Grant Program, and the Department of Defense.

REFERENCES

1. Siegel RL, Miller KD, Fuchs HE, et al. Cancer statistics, 2022. CA Cancer J Clin 2022;72:7–33.
2. World Health Organization. GLOBOCAN 2020: estimated cancer incidence, mortality and prevalence worldwide in 2020. Available at: https://gco.iarc.fr/today/data/factsheets/cancers/24-Corpus-uteri-factsheet.pdf. Accessed September 15, 2022.
3. Karageorgi S, Hankinson SE, Kraft P, et al. Reproductive factors and postmenopausal hormone use in relation to endometrial cancer risk in the Nurses' Health Study cohort 1976-2004. Int J Cancer 2010; 126(1):208–16.
4. Arthur RS, Kabat GC, Kim MY, et al. Metabolic syndrome and risk of endometrial cancer in postmenopausal women: a prospective study. Cancer Causes Control 2019;30(4):355–63.
5. Lynch HT, Snyder CL, Shaw TG, et al. Milestones of Lynch syndrome: 1895–2015. Nat Rev Cancer 2015; 15(3):181–94.
6. Koskas M, Amant F, Mirza MR, et al. Cancer of the corpus uteri: 2021 update. Int J Gynaecol Obstet 2021;155(Suppl 1):45–60.
7. Sala E, Wakely S, Senior E, et al. MRI of malignant neoplasms of the uterine corpus and cervix. AJR Am J Roentgenol 2007 Jun;188(6):1577–87.
8. Expert Panel on GYN and OB Imaging, Reinhold C, Ueno Y, Akin EA, et al. ACR Appropriateness Criteria® Pretreatment Evaluation and Follow-Up of Endometrial Cancer. J Am Coll Radiol 2020; 17(11S):S472–86.
9. Nougaret S, Horta M, Sala E, et al. Endometrial Cancer MRI staging: Updated Guidelines of the European Society of Urogenital Radiology. Eur Radiol 2019;29(2):792–805.
10. Bokhman JV. Two pathogenetic types of endometrial carcinoma. Gynecol Oncol 1983;15(1):10–7.
11. Slomovitz BM, Burke TW, Eifel PJ, et al. Uterine papillary serous carcinoma (UPSC): a single institution review of 129 cases. Gynecol Oncol 2003;91(3): 463–9.
12. Concin N, Matias-Guiu X, Vergote I, et al. ESGO/ESTRO/ESP guidelines for the management of patients with endometrial carcinoma. Int J Gynecol Cancer 2021;31(1):12–39.
13. Cancer Genome Atlas Research Network, Kandoth C, Schultz N, Cherniack AD, et al. Integrated genomic characterization of endometrial carcinoma. Nature 2013;497(7447):67–73.
14. Talhouk A, McConechy MK, Leung S, et al. Confirmation of ProMisE: A simple, genomics-based clinical classifier for endometrial cancer. Cancer 2017; 123:802–13.
15. Kommoss S, McConechy MK, Kommoss F, et al. Final validation of the ProMisE molecular classifier for endometrial carcinoma in a large population-based case series. Ann Oncol 2018;29(5):1180–8.
16. Talhouk A, McConechy MK, Leung S, et al. A clinically applicable molecular-based classification for endometrial cancers. Br J Cancer 2015;113(2):299–310.
17. Leon-Castillo A, de Boer SM, Powell ME, et al. Molecular classification of the PORTEC-3 trial for high-risk endometrial cancer: impact on prognosis and benefit from adjuvant therapy. J Clin Oncol 2020; 38(29):3388–97.
18. Oaknin A, Bosse TJ, Creutzberg CL, et al. Endometrial cancer: ESMO Clinical Practice Guideline for diagnosis, treatment and follow-up. Ann Oncol 2022;33(9):860–77.
19. Herrington CS, WHO Classification of Tumours Editorial Board. WHO classification of tumours female genital tumours. 5th edition. IARC; 2020.
20. van den Heerik ASVM, Horeweg N, Nout RA, et al. PORTEC-4a: International randomized trial of molecular profile-based adjuvant treatment for women with high-intermediate risk endometrial cancer. Int J Gynecol Cancer 2020;30:2002–7.

21. Nougaret S, Lakhman Y, Vargas HA, et al. From Staging to Prognostication: Achievements and Challenges of MR Imaging in the Assessment of Endometrial Cancer. Magn Reson Imaging Clin N Am 2017;25(3):611–33.

22. Society of Abdominal Radiology Uterine and Ovarian Cancer Disease Focused Panel. Endometrial Cancer Example MRI Protocol. Active Panels-Society of Abdominal Radiology. Available at: https://abdominal radiology.org/sar-subpages/dfp-panels/. Accessed November 6, 2022.

23. Lin MY, Dobrotwir A, McNally O, et al. Role of imaging in the routine management of endometrial cancer. Int J Gynaecol Obstet 2018;143(Suppl 2): 109–17.

24. Kinkel K, Kaji Y, Yu KK, et al. Radiologic staging in patients with endometrial cancer: a meta-analysis. Radiology 1999;212(3):711–8.

25. Maheshwari E, Nougaret S, Stein EB, et al. Update on MRI in Evaluation and Treatment of Endometrial Cancer. Radiographics 2022;42(7):2112–30.

26. National Comprehensive Cancer Network. Uterine Neoplasms (version 1.2022). Available at: https:// www.nccn.org/professionals/physician_gls/pdf/ uterine.pdf.

27. Bharwani N, Miquel ME, Sahdev A, et al. Diffusion-weighted imaging in the assessment of tumour grade in endometrial cancer. Br J Radiol 2011; 84(1007):997–1004.

28. Fujii S, Matsusue E, Kigawa J, et al. Diagnostic accuracy of the apparent diffusion coefficient in differentiating benign from malignant uterine endometrial cavity lesions: initial results. Eur Radiol 2008;18(2): 384–9.

29. Inada Y, Matsuki M, Nakai G, et al. Body diffusion-weighted MR imaging of uterine endometrial cancer: is it helpful in the detection of cancer in nonenhanced MR imaging? Eur J Radiol 2009;70(1): 122–7.

30. Rechichi G, Galimberti S, Signorelli M, et al. Endometrial cancer: correlation of apparent diffusion coefficient with tumor grade, depth of myometrial invasion, and presence of lymph node metastases. AJR Am J Roentgenol 2011;197(1):256–62.

31. Tamai K, Koyama T, Saga T, et al. Diffusion-weighted MR imaging of uterine endometrial cancer. J Magn Reson Imaging 2007;26(3):682–7.

32. Larson DM, Connor GP, Broste SK, et al. Prognostic significance of gross myometrial invasion with endometrial cancer. Obstet Gynecol 1996;88(3):394–8.

33. Nougaret S, Sbarra M, Robbins J. Imaging Spectrum of Benign Uterine Disease and Treatment Options. Radiol Clin North Am 2020;58(2):239–56.

34. Sala E, Rockall A, Rangarajan D, et al. The role of dynamic contrast-enhanced and diffusion weighted magnetic resonance imaging in the female pelvis. Eur J Radiol 2010;76(3):367–85.

35. Stewart CJR, Crum CP, McCluggage WG, et al. Guidelines to Aid in the Distinction of Endometrial and Endocervical Carcinomas, and the Distinction of Independent Primary Carcinomas of the Endometrium and Adnexa From Metastatic Spread Between These and Other Sites. Int J Gynecol Pathol 2019; 38(Suppl 1):S75–92.

36. Bese T, Sal V, Kahramanoglu I, et al. Synchronous Primary Cancers of the Endometrium and Ovary With the Same Histopathologic Type Versus Endometrial Cancer With Ovarian Metastasis: A Single Institution Review of 72 Cases. Int J Gynecol Cancer 2016;26(2):394–406.

37. Dokter E, Anderson L, Cho SM, et al. Radiology-pathology correlation of endometrial carcinoma assessment on magnetic resonance imaging. Insights Imaging 2022;13(1):80.

38. Rizzo S, Femia M, Buscarino V, et al. Endometrial cancer: an overview of novelties in treatment and related imaging keypoints for local staging. Cancer Imag 2018;18(1):45.

39. Muallem MZ, Sehouli J, Almuheimid J, et al. Risk Factors of Lymph Nodes Metastases by Endometrial Cancer: A Retrospective One-center Study. Anticancer Res 2016;36(8):4219–25.

40. Rockall AG, Meroni R, Sohaib SA, et al. Evaluation of endometrial carcinoma on magnetic resonance imaging. Int J Gynecol Cancer 2007;17(1):188–96.

41. Kim HJ, Cho A, Yun M, et al. Comparison of FDG PET/CT and MRI in lymph node staging of endometrial cancer. Ann Nucl Med 2016;30(2):104–13.

42. Lin G, Ho KC, Wang JJ, et al. Detection of lymph node metastasis in cervical and uterine cancers by diffusion-weighted magnetic resonance imaging at 3T. J Magn Reson Imaging 2008;28(1):128–35.

43. Shen G, Zhou H, Jia Z, et al. Diagnostic performance of diffusion-weighted MRI for detection of pelvic metastatic lymph nodes in patients with cervical cancer: a systematic review and meta-analysis. Br J Radiol 2015;88(1052):20150063.

44. Fehniger J, Thomas S, Lengyel E, et al. A prospective study evaluating diffusion weighted magnetic resonance imaging (DW-MRI) in the detection of peritoneal carcinomatosis in suspected gynecologic malignancies. Gynecol Oncol 2016; 142(1):169–75.

45. Hardesty LA, Sumkin JH, Hakim C, et al. The ability of helical CT to preoperatively stage endometrial carcinoma. AJR Am J Roentgenol 2001;176(3): 603–6.

46. Bollineni VR, Ytre-Hauge S, Bollineni-Balabay O, et al. High diagnostic value of 18F-FDG PET/CT in endometrial cancer: systematic review and meta-analysis of the literature. J Nucl Med 2016;57:879–85.

47. Nie J, Zhang J, Gao J, et al. Diagnostic role of 18F-FDG PET/MRI in patients with gynecological

malignancies of the pelvis: A systematic review and meta-analysis. PLoS One 2017;12(5):e0175401.

48. Kim SR, van der Zanden C, Ikiz H, et al. Fertility-Sparing Management Using Progestin for Young Women with Endometrial Cancer From a Population-Based Study. J Obstet Gynaecol Can 2018;40(3):328–33.

49. Chae SH, Shim S, Lee SJ, et al. Pregnancy and oncologic outcomes after fertility-sparing management for early stage endometrioid endometrial cancer. International Journal of Gynecologic Cancer 2019;29:77–85.

50. Markowska A, Chudecka-Glaz A, Pitynski K, et al. Endometrial Cancer Management in Young Women. Cancers 2022;14(8):1922.

51. McEvoy SH, Nougaret S, Abu-Rustum NR, et al. Fertility-sparing for young patients with gynecologic cancer: How MRI can guide patient selection prior to conservative management. Abdom Radiol (NY) 2017;42(10):2488–512.

52. Volpi L, Sozzi G, Capozzi VA, et al. Long term complications following pelvic and para-aortic lymphadenectomy for endometrial cancer, incidence and potential risk factors: a single institution experience. Int J Gynecol Cancer 2019;29(2):312–9.

53. Konno Y, Todo Y, Minobe S, et al. A retrospective analysis of postoperative complications with or without para-aortic lymphadenectomy in endometrial cancer. Int J Gynecol Cancer 2011;21(2):385–90.

54. Benedetti Panici P, Basile S, Maneschi F, et al. Systematic pelvic lymphadenectomy vs. no lymphadenectomy in early-stage endometrial carcinoma: randomized clinical trial. J Natl Cancer Inst 2008; 100(23):1707–16.

55. Kitchener H, Swart AM, Qian Q, et al, ASTEC study group. Efficacy of systematic pelvic lymphadenectomy in endometrial cancer (MRC ASTEC trial): a randomised study. Lancet 2009;373(9658):125–36.

56. Backes FJ, Cohen D, Salani R, et al. Prospective clinical trial of robotic sentinel lymph node assessment with isosulfane blue (ISB) and indocyanine green (ICG) in endometrial cancer and the impact of ultrastaging (NCT01818739). Gynecol Oncol 2019; 153(3):496–9.

57. Rajanbabu A, Agarwal R. A prospective evaluation of the sentinel node mapping algorithm in endometrial cancer and correlation of its performance against endometrial cancer risk subtypes. Eur J Obstet Gynecol Reprod Biol 2018;224:77–80.

58. Bodurtha Smith AJ, Fader AN, Tanner EJ. Sentinel lymph node assessment in endometrial cancer: a systematic review and meta-analysis. Am J Obstet Gynecol 2017;216(5):459–76.e10.

59. Bogani G, Murgia F, Ditto A, et al. Sentinel node mapping vs. lymphadenectomy in endometrial cancer: A systematic review and meta-analysis. Gynecol Oncol 2019;153(3):676–83.

60. Accorsi GS, Paiva LL, Schmidt R, et al. Sentinel Lymph Node Mapping vs Systematic Lymphadenectomy for Endometrial Cancer: Surgical Morbidity and Lymphatic Complications. J Minim Invasive Gynecol 2020;27(4):938–45.e2.

61. Silva C, Carneiro C, Cunha TM. Role of Imaging in the Management of High-Risk Endometrial Cancer. Cureus 2021;13(11):e19286.

62. Kidd EA. Imaging to optimize gynecological radiation oncology. Int J Gynecol Cancer 2022;32(3):358–65.

Current Concepts in the Imaging of Uterine Sarcomas

Robert Petrocelli, MD[a],*, Nicole Hindman, MD[b],
Caroline Reinhold, MD, MSc[c,d]

KEYWORDS

- Uterine sarcoma • Leiomyosarcoma • STUMP • Endometrial stromal sarcoma
- Undifferentiated uterine sarcoma • Adenosarcoma

KEY POINTS

- Pelvic MRI with intravenous contrast is the gold standard imaging technique for preoperative identification of uterine sarcomas.
- Leiomyosarcoma is a myometrial-based mass reliably differentiated from benign leiomyoma (and associated variants) based on MR imaging appearance.
- Uterine smooth muscle tumor of uncertain malignant potential is a myometrial-based mass that cannot be reliably differentiated from leiomyosarcoma or leiomyoma.
- Endometrial stromal sarcomas and adenosarcoma are typically endometrial-based masses with differing biologic behavior and typical imaging features.
- Undifferentiated uterine sarcoma is a dedifferentiated sarcoma with nonspecific overtly malignant imaging features.

INTRODUCTION
Discussion of Problem

Background

Uterine sarcomas are a group of rare tumors accounting for approximately 3% of all uterine malignancies.[1] Classified according to World Health Organization (WHO) guidelines, the most common subtypes include leiomyosarcoma (LMS) (63%), endometrial stromal sarcoma (ESS) (21%), adenosarcoma (6%), and undifferentiated uterine sarcoma (UUS) (5%). Additional rarer subtypes exist (5%), with smooth muscle tumor of uncertain malignant potential (STUMP) included among uterine sarcomas.[2]

Leiomyomas are a common indication for medical and surgical intervention. Fertility-sparing minimally invasive procedures associated with reduced surgical morbidity are popular treatment alternatives to hysterectomy for symptomatic leiomyomata. Minimally invasive surgery (including laparoscopic myomectomy with or without morcellation) can lead to piecemeal resection of uterine masses and inadvertent dissemination of tumor which sharply contrasts with the goal of en bloc resection of uterine sarcomas via total abdominal hysterectomy and bilateral salpingoophorectomy (TAH-BSO). When sarcoma is not initially suspected, minimally invasive surgery may compromise oncologic outcomes. Uterine artery embolization of unsuspected sarcoma can delay appropriate surgical management, potentially worsening patient prognosis. Prospective identification and differentiation of uterine sarcomas from benign leiomyomata is thus critical for optimal surgical management and patient outcomes.

a Department of Radiology, New York University Grossman School of Medicine, 660 First Avenue, 3rd Floor, New York, NY 10016, USA; b Department of Radiology, New York University Grossman School of Medicine, 660 First Avenue, 3rd Floor, New York, NY 10016, USA; c Department of Radiology, McGill University Health Center, 1001 Decarie Boulevard, Montréal, QC H4A 3J1, Canada; d Montreal Imaging Experts Inc., Montréal-Nord, QC H1G 2T2, Canada
* Corresponding author.
E-mail address: Robert.Petrocelli@nyulangone.org

Radiol Clin N Am 61 (2023) 627–638
https://doi.org/10.1016/j.rcl.2023.02.008

This article reviews the spectrum of disease in uterine sarcomas with a focus on reviewing the classification of primary sarcoma subtypes and the typical MR appearances at presentation used to inform the staging of these rare tumors.

Leiomyosarcoma

LMS is the most common uterine sarcoma. The incidence of LMS in patients undergoing surgical management for leiomyomata is generally accepted as 1 in 770, supported by expert consensus from the American College of Obstetrics and Gynecology, although published estimates are variable.[3–5] Risk of LMS increases with age. It is estimated to be as high as 1 in 65 patients over 60 undergoing surgical therapy for leiomyomata and is also higher than baseline in patients with symptomatic fibroids.[3] The incidence of LMS is highest in patients of Black race and those with solitary uterine tumors.[3,6]

Pathologic diagnosis of classic spindle cell LMS requires 2 of the following 3 features: mitotic index of $\geq$10 mitotic figures per 10 high-power fields (HPF), moderate to severe cytologic atypia, and presence of tumor necrosis (unique to malignancy and differentiated from ischemic necrosis in leiomyomata).[7] Conventional leiomyomata will display mitotic indices of <5 mitotic figures per HPF, only up to mild cytologic atypia, and no tumor necrosis. A spectrum of pathologic findings exists between LMS and leiomyomata and tumor necrosis remains a challenging feature, with only moderate interobserver agreement among gynecologic pathologists.[8]

A minority of LMSs arise within existing leiomyomas (0.2%). The remainder originates within the myometrium. Sensitivity for detection on endometrial biopsy has been reported as low as 32%, with smaller tumors at earlier disease stages more difficult to detect. Patients presenting with postmenopausal bleeding have higher detection rates, especially when the tumor contacts the endometrium.[9]

Lack of residual tumor following primary resection and initial tumor size are the most important prognostic factors, with 86% 5-year survival for LMS <5 cm versus 18% 5-year survival for LMS >10 cm. Tumor mitotic index > 10 mitosis per 10 HPF confers a worse prognosis.[2] Treatment of LMS is centered on TAH-BSO (en-bloc intact resection). Minimally invasive treatment techniques such as myomectomy, uterine artery embolization, and morcellation should be avoided when there is suspicion of uterine sarcoma due to the risk of disease spread.[10]

Uterine smooth muscle tumor of uncertain malignant potential

Uterine STUMP is a rare uterine mesenchymal tumor subtype existing between leiomyoma and LMS. STUMP is diagnosed when uterine smooth muscle tumors show intermediate histologic characteristics that are subdiagnostic for LMS but more atypical than would be encountered with leiomyoma.[7,11]

STUMPs remain a challenging diagnosis due to rarity, lack of standardized diagnostic criteria, and unclear management strategies. Recurrence risk after myomectomy or hysterectomy varies depending upon histologic features.[12] Heterogeneous recurrence risk is likely a manifestation of the diverse biologic behavior of STUMP that may behave like benign uterine disease or low-grade (LG) malignancy. STUMPs associated with tumor necrosis and low mitotic indices have the highest recurrence risk, whereas STUMPs with high mitotic indices (>15 mitotic figures per 10 HPF) but lacking tumor necrosis or atypia have the lowest recurrence risk based on a small patient cohort.[13] Frequency of imaging surveillance after surgery is guided by recurrence risk.

Endometrial stromal tumors

The WHO classification of uterine sarcomas includes ESS and UUS among the endometrial stromal tumors. The biologic behavior of high-grade (HG) ESS and UUS is far more aggressive than LG-ESS.[14] LG-ESS typically occurs in premenopausal patients (mean age 39 years) with indolent growth rate and favorable prognosis (91% 5-year survival), whereas HG-ESS typically occurs in older patients (mean age 61 years) with aggressive growth rate and poor prognosis (33% 5-year survival).[15,16]

Histologically, endometrial stromal tumors arise from the endometrial stroma and exist on a spectrum from benign endometrial stromal nodules to malignant sarcomas. The malignant ESS include LG-ESS composed of well-differentiated cells with mild atypia showing finger-like projections that display myometrial and often lymphovascular invasion. In contrast, HG-ESS displays higher atypia, higher mitotic count, and more destructive pattern of invasion with necrosis, with ESS subtype genetic alterations having been defined.[16] Morphologically, UUS also differs from HG-ESS in part due to lack of smooth muscle or endometrial stromal differentiation, which remains a diagnosis of exclusion.[17] ESSs are treated with TAH-BSO.

Adenosarcoma

Adenosarcoma accounts for approximately 0.2% of all uterine malignancies and 6% of uterine sarcomas.[2,6] Histologically, these tumors include benign epithelial elements and a malignant mesenchymal component and may arise from both the uterine myometrium and the endometrial stroma. Prognosis is variable and related to the presence of sarcomatous overgrowth. Tumors without sarcomatous overgrowth are considered low grade with a more favorable prognosis (79% 5-year survival for stage I disease) as compared with those with sarcomatous overgrowth. Adenosarcoma is treated with TAH-BSO. After surgery, local recurrence at the vaginal cuff is common.[16]

Clinical presentation

The clinical presentation of uterine sarcoma patients is variable but often nonspecific, mimicking symptoms commonly attributed to leiomyomata. Symptoms encountered include abnormal uterine bleeding, pain, and bulk symptoms including pressure and rapid growth of a palpable mass.[18,19] Symptoms related to metastasis can manifest in advanced disease.[20]

Superficial endometrial biopsy is often negative as many tumors are confined to myometrium, although endometrial biopsy is useful to exclude endometrial malignancy. Additional sampling techniques may yield false-negative diagnoses due to tumor heterogeneity and are not typical in standard clinical practice. Ultimately, final diagnosis of sarcomas is made on surgical specimens.

Typical pattern of disease spread

In early-stage disease confined to the uterus, pelvic lymphadenopathy is generally uncommon in sarcomas. In advanced disease sarcomas may display local invasion beyond uterus into adjacent pelvic structures. Common sites of distant metastatic disease include the peritoneum, lung, liver, and lymph nodes. Nodal drainage from the uterus and cervix occurs predominantly via the obturator, internal and external iliac chains, and para-aortic chains although additional pathways involving inguinal and sacral nodes are possible.

Staging

Malignant uterine sarcomas are staged according to the International Federation of Gynecology and Obstetrics (FIGO) classification. Imaging plays a critical role in preoperative staging and the assessment for recurrence after treatment.

Imaging Technique and Protocols

MR imaging

MR imaging is the imaging modality of choice for the characterization of uterine masses and the local preoperative staging of suspected uterine sarcoma. A representative MR imaging protocol for the assessment of uterine masses including benign leiomyomas and suspected uterine sarcomas is provided in **Box 1**.

> **Box 1**
> **Representative MRI pelvis protocol for uterine sarcomas**
>
> - T2-weighted imaging (axial, coronal, and sagittal)
>   - Small FOV[a]—uterus and pelvic sidewalls
>   - 3 mm slice thickness
> - Diffusion-weighted imaging (axial preferred)
>   - Small FOV[a]—uterus and nodal stations
>   - 5 mm slice thickness
>   - B values—50 and 1000 or 1200 (preferred)
> - Dual echo opposed phase gradient recalled echo imaging (axial)
> - T1-weighted imaging (axial and sagittal), pre/post-contrast fat suppressed
>   - Small FOV[a] sagittal—uterus and pelvic sidewalls (30-, 60-, and 90-s delay)
>   - Large FOV axial (delay)
>   - Generate subtraction for post-contrast sequences
> - T2-weighted imaging (axial or coronal) and diffusion-weighted imaging (axial) of the abdomen may be obtained if locally advanced malignancy is suspected to assess for hydronephrosis and lymphadenopathy.
>
> [a]Small FOV should include the whole uterus and pelvic sidewalls. As a baseline, 25 cm × 25 cm is typically an adequate FOV, although this should be adjusted accordingly to ensure coverage of the whole uterus.

Computed tomography

Computed tomography (CT) is used for preoperative distant staging of suspected or known uterine sarcoma and assessing for recurrence after therapy. A standard protocol intended for general oncology patients performed with oral and IV contrast in the portal venous phase (70 s) can be used. Chest CT is typically obtained concurrently in the venous phase.

PET/CT

Fluorodeoxyglucose (FDG) PET/CT can assist in detecting metastatic disease at initial staging or after therapy. A standard protocol intended for general oncology patients using weight-based FDG administered intravenously 60 min before imaging with the acquisition from the skull base to proximal thighs is used.

Ultrasound

The role of ultrasound in imaging uterine sarcomas is primarily as an initial screening exam to identify

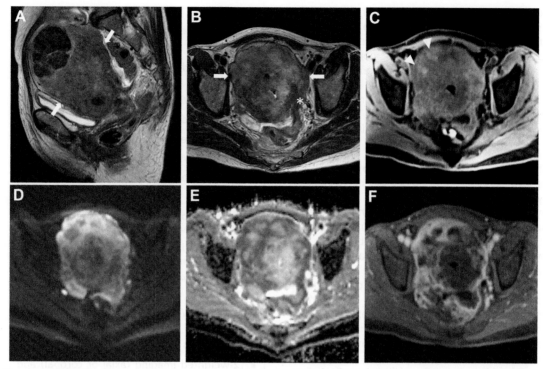

Fig. 1. 57-year-old woman with leiomyomas and LMS. Sagittal (*A*) and axial (*B*) T2-weighted imaging (T2WI) shows an infiltrative heterogeneous myometrial mass with hyperintense and intermediate T2 signal (*arrows*) invading the rectosigmoid colon (*asterisk*). (*C*) Axial T1 fat-suppressed pre-contrast MR imaging shows foci of T1 hyperintensity (*arrowhead*) in nonenhancing necrotic portion reflecting intratumoral hemorrhage, along with restricted diffusion (*D*) with ADC value of 850×10^{-3} mm²/s (*E*). Heterogeneous peripheral enhancement with central necrosis is seen on post-contrast T1WI (*F*).

leiomyomata or other masses. Ultrasound exams performed for uterine mass screening use a standard female pelvis protocol. Omission of transabdominal imaging may reduce sensitivity for detecting large uterine masses that extend beyond the depth of transvaginal ultrasound (TVUS).

Imaging Findings/Diagnostic Criteria/ Differential Diagnosis

Leiomyosarcoma and smooth muscle tumor of uncertain malignant potential

MR imaging has emerged as the gold standard imaging modality for preoperative characterization of uterine sarcomas and the published literature supports the use of MR imaging as a screening tool for LMS in patients presenting for surgical management of fibroids.[21]

The classic MR imaging appearance of LMS is a solitary uterine mass arising from the myometrium with poorly circumscribed or infiltrating/irregular borders.[22] On T2-weighted imaging, tumors often show heterogeneous T2 signal with areas within the solid component showing intermediate or hyperintense T2 signal intensity.[22] On T1-weighted imaging, the solid viable portion of tumor may show early heterogeneous enhancement on dynamic post-contrast imaging with areas of nonenhancing necrotic tumor that may display scattered intrinsic T1 hyperintensity (indicating intratumoral hemorrhage).[22–24] LMS will appear hyperintense on diffusion-weighted imaging (DWI) (similar or greater than the DWI signal of endometrium and lymph nodes) and hypointense on apparent diffusion coefficient (ADC) maps.[25–28] A representative appearance of LMS is illustrated in **Fig. 1**.

However, in clinical practice many of the "classic" LMS features may be absent and some may be present in benign leiomyomas. With the challenge of prospective differentiation in mind, substantial overlap in imaging features between LMS and benign uterine disease is a known confounding factor.

Hemorrhage, as well as T2 hyperintensity and intermediate signal can be seen in leiomyoma

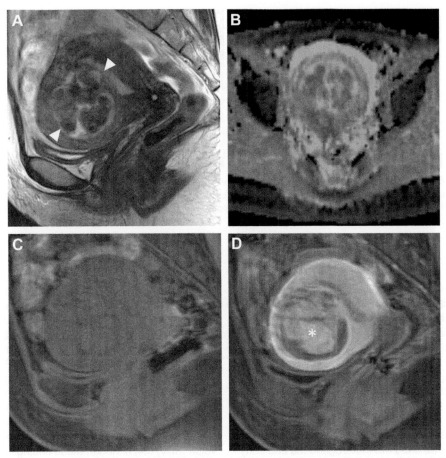

Fig. 2. A 48-year-old woman with STUMP. Sagittal T2WI (*A*) shows lobulated well-circumscribed mildly T2 hypo-intense anterior uterine body mass (*arrowheads*) with ADC value of 1050 × 10-3 mm²/s on ADC map (*B*). No intra-tumoral hemorrhage evident on pre-contrast T1WI (*C*). The mass enhances homogeneously (*asterisk*) on post-contrast T1WI (*D*).

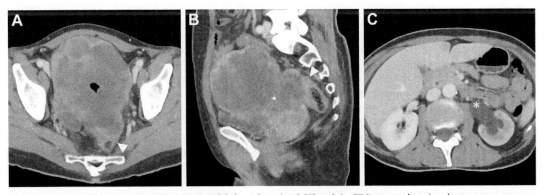

Fig. 3. A 57-year-old woman with LMS. Axial (*A*) and sagittal (*B*) pelvic CT images showing heterogeneous cen-trally necrotic infiltrative myometrial mass with extrauterine extension invading the rectosigmoid colon (*arrow-head*) and ureter (not shown) resulting in obstructive uropathy (*asterisk*) (*C*).

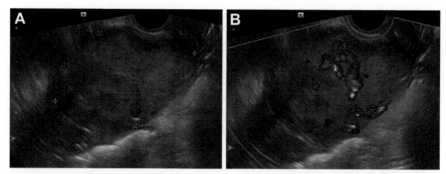

Fig. 4. An 87-year-old woman with malignant spindle cell uterine neoplasm most likely reflecting myxoid leiomyosarcoma. Sagittal TVUS images reveal a large hypoechoic uterine mass with relatively circumscribed borders (calipers) (*A*). Color Doppler assessment of the mass shows an increased central color Doppler signal, beyond that expected for patient's age (*B*).

variants. DWI and ADC values also have several pitfalls. Cellular leiomyomas can display DWI hyperintensity ($\geq$ endometrium and lymph nodes) and low ADC values (1.19 $\pm$ 0.18 [SD] $\times$ 10^{-3}mm^2/s) which overlap with LMS (1.17 $\pm$ 0.15 [SD] $\times$ 10^{-3}mm^2/s).[25] Conventional leiomyomas typically have lower ADC values ranging from 0.88 to 1.40 10^{-3} mm^2/s and overlap with LMS; therefore, DWI must be assessed to confirm true diffusion restriction.[24,25,29,30]

Classic enhancement pattern of leiomyomas (homogeneous, progressive, and delayed enhancement) and LMS (heterogeneous and early enhancement) have been described although significant overlap exists. Presence of necrosis is typical of LMS but can also be observed in STUMP and degenerating leiomyoma. Even a rapidly growing uterus/leiomyoma has not proven specific, with only 1 out of 371 patients in a surgical cohort found to have LMS (0.27%).[31]

Individual imaging features lack the sensitivity and specificity needed for reliable prospective differentiation of LMS from benign uterine disease. As a result, diagnostic algorithms have been developed with the goal of excluding LMS. Wahab and colleagues[32] published an algorithm for differentiation of LMS from atypical benign leiomyomata at MR imaging with reported sensitivity and specificity of 88% and 94%. Features predictive of malignancy included lymphadenopathy and peritoneal metastasis, DWI hyperintensity of the uterine mass (> endometrium or lymph nodes), and ADC value less than 0.905 $\times$ 10^{-3}mm^2/s. Global or focal areas of T2 hypointensity, low to intermediate DWI signal intensity less than endometrium, or absence of pelvic lymphadenopathy were strongly predictive of benign lesions. This lower ADC cutoff may reduce the risk of LMS false positives.[32]

STUMP lacks specific imaging features that would allow prospective diagnosis or reliable differentiation from leiomyoma and LMS.[33] An example of STUMP is illustrated in **Fig. 2**.

Neither CT nor FDG PET plays a significant role in primary diagnosis of LMS or STUMP. CT can identify grossly invasive uterine masses but cannot reliably differentiate LMS from benign masses.[34] An example of LMS on CT is illustrated in **Fig. 3**. On PET, LMS displays moderate to intense FDG uptake (mean standardized uptake value [SUV] 6.4) although these findings can overlap with leiomyoma (mean SUV 2.2) which precludes SUV cutoffs that exclude LMS.[35,36]

Early publications on Doppler characteristics of LMS described increased central or peripheral vascularity, lower resistive index, and higher peak systolic velocity for LMS compared with leiomyoma.[37–39] Grayscale features of LMS which have been described include large size, noncircumscribed borders, cystic changes or areas of necrosis, and heterogeneous echogenicity.[40,41] Later work on the combined diagnostic performance of grayscale and Doppler features reported a positive predictive value of only 60% for LMS and US is considered unreliable for definitive characterization.[34,41,42] An example of LMS on ultrasound is illustrated in **Fig. 4**.

Endometrial stromal sarcomas and adenosarcoma

ESSs, adenosarcoma, and malignant mixed Müllerian tumor (carcinosarcoma) typically present as endometrial-based masses rather than masses arising from the myometrium which may serve as a basis for differentiation from LMS and leiomyomas. However, large endometrial-based stromal

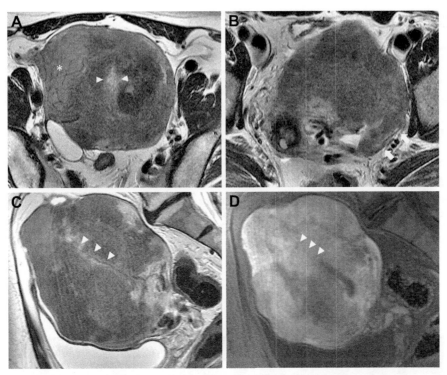

Fig. 5. A 59-year-old woman with LG-ESS. Axial (*A*, *B*) and Sagittal (*C*) T2WI show an infiltrative mass of low to intermediate T2 signal intensity replacing the myometrium. No normal endometrium is identified (*arrowheads A*, *C*, *D*). Characteristic worm-like pattern (*A*, *asterisk*) due to infiltrative/nodular tumor growth interspersed with T2 hypointense bands of preserved myometrium is seen; as well as tumor extension within periuterine vessels and along pelvic ligaments (*B*, *arrows*). On the sagittal post-contrast (*D*), there is heterogeneous enhancement. In addition, the nodular uterine contour further helps to differentiate this low-grade ESS from adenomyosis.

tumors may be difficult to distinguish from other uterine sarcomas.[43–45]

Low-grade endometrial stromal sarcoma LG-ESS typically appears on MR imaging as a polypoid mass based in the endometrial cavity with heterogeneous signal intensity on T1/T2-weighted images. Tumor margins may be circumscribed or show diffuse infiltrative/nodular growth pattern of tumor extension along myometrial lymphatics, interspersed with T2 hypointense bands of preserved myometrial bundles, giving a characteristic "worm-like" appearance. Tumor may also extend beyond the uterus within periuterine vessels or along pelvic ligaments characteristic of ESS.[16,43,46,47] The masses may invade or appear to arise within the myometrium and thus may mimic adenomyosis or other myometrial tumors.[48] Intravenous (IV) leiomyomatosis may mimic LG-ESS with tumor thrombus. The representative appearance of LG-ESS is illustrated in **Fig. 5**. An example of LG-ESS with venous tumor thrombus is illustrated in **Fig. 6**.

High-grade endometrial stromal sarcoma and undifferentiated uterine sarcoma HG-ESS typically presents as a large heterogeneous polypoid mass based in the endometrium with intermediate signal or hyperintensity on T2-weighted images and grossly invasive behavior with infiltrative or nodular contours.[16,43] Alternate appearances of HG-ESS can manifest as a myometrial-based or well-defined mass. Compared with LG-ESS, HG-ESS typically displays greater extent of necrosis and hemorrhage.[49] Feather-like enhancement, defined as fine wispy enhancement interspersed within tumor, is also a characteristic feature that can differentiate HG-ESS from LG-ESS and benign intracavitary leiomyoma.[49] Preserved myometrial bands contributing to a "worm-like" appearance of tumor growth are less common in HG-ESS due to its more invasive nature.[50] A representative appearance of HG-ESS is illustrated in **Fig. 7**.

UUS does not display distinct features allowing for prospective imaging differentiation; it may appear similar to HG-ESS and other uterine

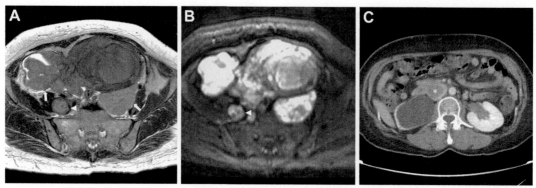

Fig. 6. A 54-year-old woman with LG-ESS with venous tumor thrombus. Axial T2-weighted imaging (*A*) shows bulky heterogeneous T2 intermediate signal mass with diffusion restriction on DWI (*B* = 500) (*B*) (low ADC not shown) with tumor extending into both adnexa (*arrows*). Tumor thrombus extends via the right iliac veins (*arrowhead*) into the inferior vena cava (*asterisk*) (*C*).

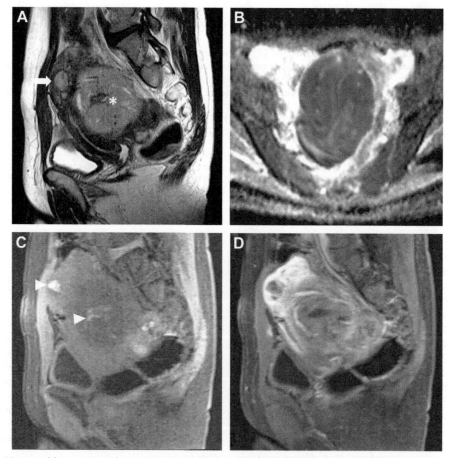

Fig. 7. A 36-year-old woman with HG-ESS. Sagittal T2WI (*A*) shows homogeneous T2 intermediate signal mass with small component arising within endometrium (*arrow*) and large invasive posterior uterine body myometrial component (*asterisk*) with low signal on ADC map (*B*). Intratumoral hemorrhage (*arrowheads*) is evident on pre-contrast T1WI (*C*). Heterogeneous enhancement of tumor on post-contrast T1WI (*D*).

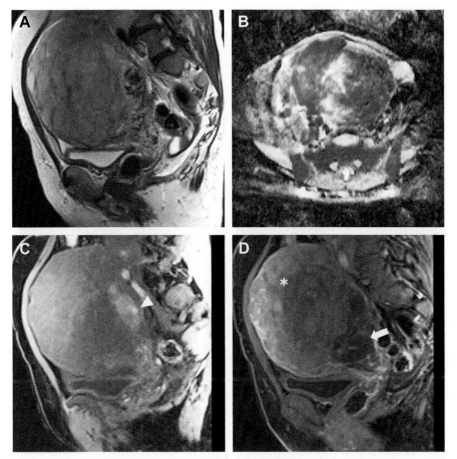

Fig. 8. A 47-year-old woman with UUS. Sagittal T2WI (*A*) shows heterogeneous T2 hyperintense infiltrative uterine mass extending throughout uterus with intense diffusion restriction on ADC map (*B*) (DWI not shown). Mass shows intratumoral hemorrhage posteriorly on sagittal T1-weighted fat suppressed pre-contrast MR imaging (*arrowhead*) (*C*). Enhancement is heterogeneous with hypoenhancing tumor seen superiorly (*asterisk*) and necrotic tumor seen inferiorly (*arrow*) on post-contrast T1WI (*D*).

sarcomas on MR imaging. A representative appearance of UUS is illustrated in Fig. 8.

Adenosarcoma Adenosarcoma is typically an endometrial-based mass with multiple well-defined cystic spaces in additional to T2 hypointense solid areas corresponding to the mesenchymal component. Adenosarcoma may contain hemorrhage and display lattice-like enhancement of the septae separating the cystic spaces. Enhancement within the solid mesenchymal component may be isointense to myometrium (rather than hypointense as seen with LG-ESS).[16,43] ADC values in LG adenosarcoma are reportedly higher than HG uterine sarcomas.[16] Size of solid component is variable and dependent on the presence of sarcomatous overgrowth. Typical LG adenosarcomas appear well defined and can prolapse through the cervix.

Aggressive subtypes can invade adjacent organs beyond the uterus and display vascular invasion with tumor thrombus.[44,51] The representative appearance of adenosarcoma is illustrated in Fig. 9.

CONCLUSION/SUMMARY

Prospective identification of uterine sarcomas and their differentiation from benign uterine disease including leiomyomata and associated variants is an impactful and increasingly required skillset for radiologists. Familiarity with the typical imaging appearances of the most common uterine sarcomas can facilitate differentiation of sarcomas from uterine leiomyomas and direct appropriate patient management in suspected malignancy.

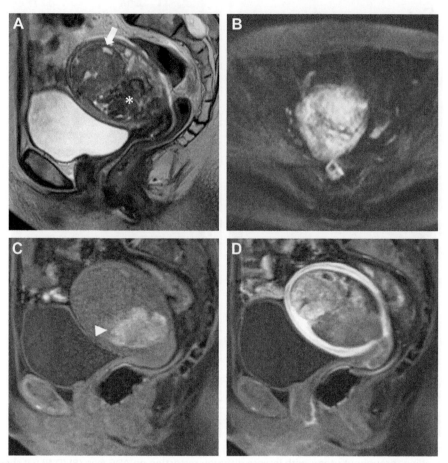

Fig. 9. A 69-year-old woman with low-grade adenosarcoma. Sagittal T2WI (*A*) shows heterogeneous mass based in the endometrial cavity with T2 intermediate to hyperintense component superiorly (*arrow*) and T2 hypointense component inferiorly (*asterisk*). Axial DWI (*B*) shows diffusion restriction (ADC not shown). Intratumoral hemorrhage inferiorly within mass (*arrowhead*) on pre-contrast T1WI (*C*). Heterogeneous enhancement is identified in the superior aspect of this mass on post-contrast T1WI (*D*).

CLINICS CARE POINTS

- Ultrasound does not reliably differentiate leiomyosarcoma from benign uterine disease although is often the initial method of detection of uterine masses.

- Preoperative MRI pelvis with intravenous contrast reliably differentiates uterine sarcomas from conventional fibroids and benign variants. Computed tomography and fluorodeoxyglucose PET facilitate the detection of distant metastasis and recurrence.

- Leiomyosarcoma and smooth muscle tumor of uncertain malignant potential are based in the myometrium. Leiomyosarcoma has specific MRI features that can be prospectively differentiated from benign uterine disease.

- Endometrial stromal sarcomas (endometrial stromal sarcoma, undifferentiated uterine sarcoma, and adenosarcoma) arise from the endometrium although higher grade disease may invade the myometrium.

DISCLOSURE

All authors have no relevant financial disclosures.

REFERENCES

1. Koh WJ, Abu-Rustum NR, Bean S, et al. Uterine neoplasms, Version 1.2018, NCCN clinical practice guidelines in oncology. J Natl Compr Cancer Netw 2018;16(2):170–99.

2. Tropé CG, Abeler VM, Kristensen GB. Diagnosis and treatment of sarcoma of the uterus. A review. Acta Oncologica (Stockholm, Sweden) 2012;51(6): 694–705.

3. Mao J, Pfeifer S, Zheng XE, et al. Population-based estimates of the prevalence of uterine sarcoma among patients with leiomyomata undergoing surgical treatment. JAMA Surgery 2015;150(4):368–70.

4. Wang L, Li S, Zhang Z, et al. Prevalence and occult rates of uterine leiomyosarcoma. Medicine 2020; 99(33):e21766.

5. Uterine Morcellation for presumed leiomyomas: ACOG committee opinion, number 822. Obstet Gynecol 2021;137(3):e63–74.

6. Brooks SE, Zhan M, Cote T, et al. Surveillance, epidemiology, and end results analysis of 2677 cases of uterine sarcoma 1989-1999. Gynecol Oncol 2004;93(1):204–8.

7. Bell SW, Kempson RL, Hendrickson MR. Problematic uterine smooth muscle neoplasms. A clinicopathologic study of 213 cases. Am J Surg Pathol 1994;18(6):535–58.

8. Lim D, Alvarez T, Nucci MR, et al. Interobserver variability in the interpretation of tumor cell necrosis in uterine leiomyosarcoma. Am J Surg Pathol 2013;37(5):650–8.

9. Hinchcliff EM, Esselen KM, Watkins JC, et al. The role of endometrial biopsy in the preoperative detection of uterine leiomyosarcoma. J Minim Invasive Gynecol 2016;23(4):567–72.

10. Laparoscopic Uterine Power Morcellation in Hysterectomy and Myomectomy: FDA Safety Communication. 2014. Available at: https://wayback.archive-it.org/7993/20170404182209/https://www.fda.gov/MedicalDevices/Safety/AlertsandNotices/ucm424443.htm. Accessed June 15, 2022.

11. Travaglino A, Raffone A, Gencarelli A, et al. Stanford parameters stratify the risk of recurrence in gynecologic smooth muscle tumors of uncertain malignant potential. APMIS 2021;129(6):283–90.

12. Şahin H, Karatas F, Coban G, et al. Uterine smooth muscle tumor of uncertain malignant potential: fertility and clinical outcomes. Journal of Gynecologic Oncology 2019;30(4):e54.

13. Stewart E.A., Laughlin-Tommaso S.K. and Schoolmeester J.K., UpToDate and Barbieri R.L., UpToDate, Waltham, MA.

14. Conklin CM, Longacre TA. Endometrial stromal tumors: the new WHO classification. Adv Anat Pathol 2014;21(6):383–93.

15. Seagle B-LL, Shilpi A, Buchanan S, et al. Low-grade and high-grade endometrial stromal sarcoma: a national cancer database study. Gynecol Oncol 2017;146(2):254–62.

16. Sousa FAe, Ferreira J, Cunha TM. MR Imaging of uterine sarcomas: a comprehensive review with radiologic-pathologic correlation. Abdominal Radiology 2021;46(12):5687–706.

17. Isiksacan Özen Ö, Ayhan A. Endometrial stromal neoplasms. Webpage. 2021. Available at: https://www.pathologyoutlines.com/topic/uterusessgeneral.html. Accessed 6/15, 2022.

18. Wu TI, Yen TC, Lai CH. Clinical presentation and diagnosis of uterine sarcoma, including imaging. Best Pract Res Clin Obstet Gynaecol 2011;25(6):681–9.

19. Santos P, Cunha TM. Uterine sarcomas: clinical presentation and MRI features. Diagn Interventional Radiol 2015;21(1):4–9.

20. D'Angelo E, Prat J. Uterine sarcomas: a review. Gynecol Oncol 2010;116(1):131–9.

21. Tong A, Kang SK, Huang C, et al. MRI screening for uterine leiomyosarcoma. J Magn Reson Imag 2019; 49(7):e282–94.

22. Rio G, Lima M, Gil R, et al. T2 hyperintense myometrial tumors: can MRI features differentiate leiomyomas from leiomyosarcomas? Abdominal Radiology (New York) 2019;44(10):3388–97.

23. Goto A, Takeuchi S, Sugimura K, et al. Usefulness of Gd-DTPA contrast-enhanced dynamic MRI and serum determination of LDH and its isozymes in the differential diagnosis of leiomyosarcoma from degenerated leiomyoma of the uterus. Int J Gynecol Cancer 2002;12(4):354–61.

24. Lin G, Yang LY, Huang YT, et al. Comparison of the diagnostic accuracy of contrast-enhanced MRI and diffusion-weighted MRI in the differentiation between uterine leiomyosarcoma/smooth muscle tumor with uncertain malignant potential and benign leiomyoma. J Magn Reson Imag 2016;43(2):333–42.

25. Tamai K, Koyama T, Saga T, et al. The utility of diffusion-weighted MR imaging for differentiating uterine sarcomas from benign leiomyomas. Eur Radiol 2008;18(4):723–30.

26. Valdes-Devesa V, Jimenez MDM, Sanz-Rosa D, et al. Preoperative diagnosis of atypical pelvic leiomyoma and sarcoma: the potential role of diffusion-weighted imaging. J Obstet Gynaecol 2019;39(1):98–104.

27. Sato K, Yuasa N, Fujita M, et al. Clinical application of diffusion-weighted imaging for preoperative differentiation between uterine leiomyoma and leiomyosarcoma. Am J Obstet Gynecol 2014;210(4):368.e1–8.

28. Tasaki A, Asatani MO, Umezu H, et al. Differential diagnosis of uterine smooth muscle tumors using diffusion-weighted imaging: correlations with the apparent diffusion coefficient and cell density. Abdom Imag 2015;40(6):1742–52.

29. Namimoto T, Yamashita Y, Awai K, et al. Combined use of T2-weighted and diffusion-weighted 3-T MR imaging for differentiating uterine sarcomas from benign leiomyomas. Eur Radiol 2009;19(11):2756.

30. Barral M, Placé V, Dautry R, et al. Magnetic resonance imaging features of uterine sarcoma and mimickers. Abdominal Radiology 2017;42(6):1762–72.

31. Parker WH, Fu YS, Berek JS. Uterine sarcoma in patients operated on for presumed leiomyoma and

rapidly growing leiomyoma. Obstet Gynecol 1994; 83(3):414–8.

32. Abdel Wahab C, Jannot AS, Bonaffini PA, et al. Diagnostic algorithm to differentiate benign atypical leiomyomas from malignant uterine sarcomas with diffusion-weighted MRI. Radiology 2020;297(2): 361–71.

33. Tanaka YO, Nishida M, Tsunoda H, et al. Smooth muscle tumors of uncertain malignant potential and leiomyosarcomas of the uterus: MR findings. J Magn Reson Imaging 2004;20(6):998–1007.

34. Gaetke-Udager K, McLean K, Sciallis AP, et al. Diagnostic accuracy of ultrasound, contrast-enhanced CT, and conventional MRI for differentiating leiomyoma from leiomyosarcoma. Acad Radiol 2016; 23(10):1290–7.

35. Kitajima K, Murakami K, Yamasaki E, et al. Standardized uptake values of uterine leiomyoma with 18F-FDG PET/CT: variation with age, size, degeneration, and contrast enhancement on MRI. Ann Nucl Med 2008;22(6):505–12.

36. Tsujikawa T, Yoshida Y, Mori T, et al. Uterine tumors: pathophysiologic imaging with 16alpha-[18F]fluoro-17beta-estradiol and 18F fluorodeoxyglucose PET–initial experience. Radiology 2008;248(2):599–605.

37. Kurjak A, Kupesic S, Shalan H, et al. Uterine sarcoma: a report of 10 cases studied by transvaginal color and pulsed Doppler sonography. Gynecol Oncol 1995;59(3):342–6.

38. Szabó I, Szánthó A, Csabay L, et al. Color Doppler ultrasonography in the differentiation of uterine sarcomas from uterine leiomyomas. Eur J Gynaecol Oncol 2002;23(1):29–34.

39. Hata K, Hata T, Maruyama R, et al. Uterine sarcoma: can it be differentiated from uterine leiomyoma with Doppler ultrasonography? A preliminary report. Ultrasound Obstet Gynecol 1997;9(2):101–4.

40. Ludovisi M, Moro F, Pasciuto T, et al. Imaging in gynecological disease (15): clinical and ultrasound characteristics of uterine sarcoma. Ultrasound Obstet Gynecol 2019;54(5):676–87.

41. Exacoustos C, Romanini ME, Amadio A, et al. Can gray-scale and color Doppler sonography differentiate between uterine leiomyosarcoma and leiomyoma? J Clin Ultrasound 2007;35(8):449–57.

42. Aviram R, Ochshorn Y, Markovitch O, et al. Uterine sarcomas versus leiomyomas: gray-scale and Doppler sonographic findings. J Clin Ultrasound 2005;33(1):10–3.

43. Tirumani SH, Ojili V, Shanbhogue AK, et al. Current concepts in the imaging of uterine sarcoma. Abdom Imag 2013;38(2):397–411.

44. Szklaruk J, Tamm EP, Choi H, et al. MR imaging of common and uncommon large pelvic masses. Radiographics 2003;23(2):403–24.

45. Hélage S, Vandeventer S, Buy JN, et al. Uterine sarcomas: are there MRI signs predictive of histopathological diagnosis? A 50-patient case series with pathological correlation. Sarcoma 2021;2021: 8880080.

46. Koyama T, Togashi K, Konishi I, et al. MR imaging of endometrial stromal sarcoma: correlation with pathologic findings. AJR Am J Roentgenol 1999;173(3): 767–72.

47. Gandolfo N, Gandolfo NG, Serafini G, et al. Endometrial stromal sarcoma of the uterus: MR and US findings. Eur Radiol 2000;10(5):776–9.

48. Furukawa R, Akahane M, Yamada H, et al. Endometrial stromal sarcoma located in the myometrium with a low-intensity rim on T2-weighted images: report of three cases and literature review. J Magn Reson Imag 2010;31(4):975–9.

49. Huang Y-L, Ueng S-H, Chen K, et al. Utility of diffusion-weighted and contrast-enhanced magnetic resonance imaging in diagnosing and differentiating between high- and low-grade uterine endometrial stromal sarcoma. Cancer Imag 2019; 19(1):63.

50. Lucas R. and Cunha T.M., Uterine sarcomas, In: Forstner R., Cunha T.M. and Hamm B., *MRI and CT of the female pelvis*, 2019, Springer International Publishing, New York, NY, 209–224.

51. Kim SA, Jung JS, Ju SJ, et al. Mullerian adenosarcoma with sarcomatous overgrowth in the pelvic cavity extending into the inferior vena cava and the right atrium. Pathol Int 2011;61(7):445–8.

MR Imaging in Cervical Cancer
Initial Staging and Treatment

Taemee Pak, MD[a],*, Elizabeth A. Sadowski, MD[b,c],
Krupa Patel-Lippmann, MD[d]

KEYWORDS

• Cervical cancer • FIGO • MR imaging • Staging

KEY POINTS

- Cervical cancer is the fourth most common cause of cancer-related death for women worldwide.
- The 2018 iteration of the International Federation of Gynecology and Obstetrics classification system allows for advanced imaging modalities to have a significant impact on the staging of cervical cancer, when available while still allowing for clinical staging.
- MR imaging is used for assessment of local disease extent and is highly accurate for locoregional staging of cervical cancer.

INTRODUCTION

Cervical cancer is the 4th most common cancer in women worldwide, with 604,000 new cases diagnosed and 342,000 deaths attributed to cervical cancer in 2020.[1,2] Ninety percent of cervical cancers are squamous cell carcinoma, and the remaining subtypes include adenocarcinoma, clear cell, neuroendocrine tumors, adenosarcomas, carcinosarcomas, and germ cell tumors. Nearly all cases of squamous cell carcinoma are associated with the human papillomavirus (HPV) infection, specifically the HPV-16 and HPV-18 subtypes, and these subtypes are the primary targets of the HPV vaccine.[3–7] Vaccine development, in conjunction with the relative availability of HPV and Pap smear screening, has significantly decreased the incidence of cervical cancer in most developed countries.[8] Unfortunately, health care disparities exist, even in the United States, with nearly 14,100 new cases projected in 2022 of which approximately 35% of those women will die from the disease.[2,9]

Before 2018, the initial staging of cervical cancer by the International Federation of Gynecology and Obstetrics (FIGO) was based primarily on clinical examination, cystoscopy, and sigmoidoscopy.[10,11] This staging schema was used because those areas with limited imaging resources had the highest number of women with cervical cancer. However, in more developed countries, imaging has been routinely used to assess the disease burden before therapy because while clinical staging is relatively accurate in early-stage disease, its accuracy significantly decreases in later-stage disease.[12–16] In 2018, the FIGO organization revised the cervical cancer staging system to incorporate imaging into the disease stage, with further subdivision of tumor size in early-stage disease and inclusion of suspected nodal metastatic disease (Table 1).[17] These revisions were based on data showing that these key factors allow for better prognostic risk stratification in patients and help guide treatment planning.[18–20]

[a] Department of Radiology, UT Southwestern Medical Center, 5323 Harry Hines Boulevard, Dallas, TX 75390, USA; [b] Department of Radiology, University of Wisconsin Hospital and Clinics, 600 Highland Avenue, Madison, WI 53792, USA; [c] Department of Obstetrics and Gynecology, University of Wisconsin Hospital and Clinics, 600 Highland Avenue, Madison, WI 53792, USA; [d] Department of Radiology and Radiological Sciences, Vanderbilt University, Medical Center North, 1161 21st Avenue South, Nashville, TN 37232, USA
* Corresponding author.
E-mail address: taemee.pak@gmail.com
Twitter: @TaemeePakMD (T.P.); @LizSadowski (E.A.S.); @KPatelLippmann (K.P.-L.)

Radiol Clin N Am 61 (2023) 639–649
https://doi.org/10.1016/j.rcl.2023.02.009
0033-8389/23/Published by Elsevier Inc.

Table 1
2018 International Federation of Gynecology and Obstetrics staging classification of cervical cancer

Stage	Description
I	Carcinoma is strictly confined to the cervix (extension to uterine corpus should be disregarded)
IA	Invasive carcinoma that can be diagnosed only by microscopy with a maximum depth of invasion <5 mm
IA1	Measured stromal invasion ≤3 mm in depth
IA2	Measured stromal invasion >3 and ≤5 mm in depth
IB	Invasive carcinoma with measured deepest invasion >5 mm; lesion limited to the cervix uteri with size measured by maximum tumor diameter
IB1	Invasive carcinoma >5 mm depth of stromal invasion and ≤2 cm in greatest dimension
IB2	Invasive carcinoma >2 and ≤ 4 cm in greatest dimension
IB3	Invasive carcinoma >4 cm in greatest dimension
II	The carcinoma invades beyond the uterus, but has not extended into the lower third of the vagina or to the pelvic wall
IIA	Involvement limited to the upper two-thirds of the vagina without parametrial involvement
IIA1	Invasive carcinoma ≤4 cm in greatest dimension
IIA2	Invasive carcinoma >4 cm in greatest dimension
IIB	With parametrial involvement but not up to the pelvic wall
III	The carcinoma involves the lower third of the vagina and/or extends to the pelvic wall and/or causes hydronephrosis or nonfunctioning kidney and/or involves pelvic and/or para-aortic lymph nodes
IIIA	The carcinoma involves the lower third of the vagina, with no extension to the pelvic wall
IIIB	Extension to the pelvic wall and/or hydronephrosis or nonfunctioning kidney (unless known to be due to another cause)
IIIC	Involvement of pelvic and/or para-aortic lymph nodes (including micrometastases), irrespective or tumor size and extent
IIIC1	Pelvic lymph node metastasis only
IIIC2	Para-aortic lymph node metastasis
IV	The carcinoma has extended beyond the true pelvis or has involved (biopsy proven) the mucosa of the bladder or rectum.
IVA	Spread to adjacent pelvic organs
IVB	Spread to distant organs

Currently, the initial workup of cervical cancer includes a multiparametric pelvic MR imaging to assess for local disease and a PET/computed tomography (CT) or PET/MR imaging for assessment of metastatic disease, although a CT of the chest, abdomen, and pelvis is a viable alternative to PET imaging.[12,16,21–26] This monograph will focus on MR imaging of cervical cancer for the assessment of local disease extent, including current imaging protocols, imaging interpretation, and local staging.

NORMAL ANATOMY
Cervical Anatomy and Histopathology

The cervix is a cylindrical structure that links the uterus to the vagina and is composed of stroma, glandular elements, and epithelium. The cervix is covered by both nonkeratinized squamous and glandular epithelium, the latter of which lines the endocervical canal to form the mucosa. Where the two epithelial layers meet is the transformation zone that changes location as a woman ages and is the origin of most cervical cancers.[3,27] The stroma is the outer layer of the cervix that contacts the parametrium. The lower cervix projects into the vagina that in turn surrounds it, forming the anterior, posterior, and lateral vaginal fornices. The donut-shaped cervix seen on speculum examination is the external os. The internal os, which is located at the uterocervical junction, cannot be seen on physical examination. The

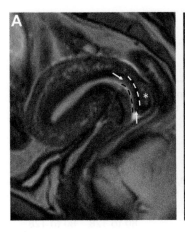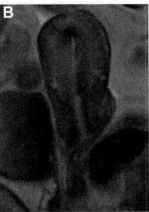

Fig. 1. Normal anatomy. (*A*) Sagittal T2WI of the normal premenopausal cervix delineating the cervical zonal anatomy: intermediate signal endocervical mucosa (*white arrow*), hypointense signal fibromuscular stroma (*white dashed line*), and outer intermediate SI loose glandular stroma (*asterisk*). The center of the cervix is filled with mucus that appears hyperintense (black dashed line) between the mucosa of the anterior and posterior cervix. (*B*) Sagittal T2WI of the normal postmenopausal cervix shows less delineation between the different zones of the cervical anatomy compared with the premenopausal cervix. (Courtesy of D Pinho, MD, Fort Worth, TX.)

endocervical canal extends from the internal os to the external os.

Imaging Appearance of Normal Cervical Anatomy

Normal cervical anatomy is best delineated on standard fast spin echo nonfat-saturated T2-weighted image (WI). The normal premenopausal cervix spans 3 to 4 cm in length with a trilaminar appearance consisting of the inner hyperintense endocervical mucosa, a middle layer of hypointense dense cervical fibromuscular stroma, and an outer layer of intermediate signal intensity (SI) loose stroma (**Fig. 1**A). In contrast, the normal postmenopausal cervix has less prominent endocervical mucosa, whereas the middle and outer layers are more homogeneously hypointense (**Fig. 1**B).

MR IMAGING PROTOCOL

A sample MR imaging protocol adapted from the Society of Abdominal Radiology (SAR) is detailed in **Table 2** and is similar to the protocol guidelines published by the European Society of Urogenital Radiology (ESUR).[28,29] Recommended patient preparation includes patient voiding 30 min before scanning to allow for moderate bladder distension and optimal positioning of the uterus. To reduce artifacts from bowel motion, administration of an anti-peristaltic agent can be helpful. The administration of vaginal gel is optional but can be helpful in delineation of exophytic tumors and detection of vaginal invasion.

MR imaging should be performed with the patient supine on a 1.5 or 3 Tesla magnet with a phased array body/torso coil. Sagittal non-fat-saturated T2-weighted image (T2WI) through the uterus is performed first, and helps with the

prescribing of axial oblique nonfat-saturated T2WI and diffusion-weighted images (DWI) with similar slice thickness oriented perpendicular to the long axis of the cervix. These T2WI and DWI are key to depicting tumor size, parametrial invasion, and vaginal involvement.

Axial non-fat-saturated T1-weighted image (T1WI) through the pelvis can help with identifying lymph nodes and a coronal T2WI including the kidneys should be performed to assess for hydronephrosis. Axial fat-saturated T2WI are optional and can be helpful for bone lesions, stress fractures, lymph nodes, edema, and fluid.

Post-contrast T1WI is helpful in identifying the extent of tumor, particularly in smaller tumors when fertility-sparing surgery is being considered or if recurrence is suspected. Post-contrast imaging should be performed in the sagittal plane with dynamic imaging at 40 and 90 s post-contrast injection followed by acquisition in the axial plane at 180 s.

MR IMAGING INTERPRETATION
Imaging Appearance of Cervical Cancer

Tumors typically show intermediate to high SI on nonfat-saturated T2WI (**Fig. 2**). On DWI, tumor is intermediate to high SI on low B-value images but becomes higher in signal on high B-value images with corresponding low signal on apparent diffusion coefficient (ADC) images, reflecting the tumor's dense cellularity.[30] DWI can provide better contrast between the tumor and adjacent tissue and can be particularly helpful for small lesions or those difficult to visualize on T2WI.[29] On early phase contrast-enhanced images, small tumors may be hyperenhancing to the cervical stroma, appearing hypoenhancing on delayed images (**Fig. 3**). Larger tumors have a more variable

Table 2
Example MR imaging protocol scanning parameters for initial staging of cervical cancer[28]

	Orientation or Region	Dimension	FOV	Slice/Skip	Frequency	Phase
Coronal T2WI without fat saturation	Include kidneys	2D	36 to 40	6 mm; skip 0.5 to 1 mm	256	192 to 256
Sagittal T2WI without fat saturation	Acetabulum to acetabulum	2D	24 to 26	4 mm	256	192 to 256
Axial oblique T2WI without fat saturation	Perpendicular to long axis of cervix/tumor	2D	24 to 26	3 to 4 mm; skip 0.5 mm	256 to 320	256 to 320
Axial oblique DWI	Perpendicular to long axis of cervix/tumor	2D	28 to 32	4 mm	80 to 128	80 to 128
Axial T1WI without fat saturation	Perineum through top of L5	2D	30 to 34	5 mm; skip 1 mm	256 to 320	256 to 320
Sagittal pre-contrast, 40 s, 90 s T1WI	OPTIONAL Acetabulum to acetabulum	3D	28	4 mm	256 to 320	192
Axial 180 s T1WI	OPTIONAL Perineum through top of L5	3D	28	4 mm	256 to 320	192 to 224
Axial T2WI with fat saturation	OPTIONAL Perineum through top of L5	2D	24 to 26	4 mm; skip 0.5 mm	256 to 320	256 to 320

enhancement pattern due to their heterogeneity and may contain necrotic areas.

Lymph Node Evaluation

Lymph node evaluation is important on MR imaging and understanding the common drainage pathways and specific imaging features may aid in discerning normal from abnormal nodes. There are three lymphatic pathways by which cervical cancer disseminates after it has spread to the parametrial nodes: the lateral pelvic route to the external iliac nodes, the hypogastric route to the internal iliac and junctional nodes, and the presacral route along the uterosacral ligaments. All routes ultimately ascend to the common iliac and para-aortic nodes.[31–33] With regards to imaging features, normal lymph nodes tend to be randomly distributed, reniform in shape, contain hila with bulk fat, and show smooth margins. Abnormal nodes are rounder, lose their fatty hila, may show heterogeneity on T2WI including central necrosis, and may cluster together.[34–37]

In addition to appearance, pelvic nodes greater than 8 mm in the short axis and abdominal nodes

greater than 10 mm in the short axis are considered suspicious.[38] Although DWI can be helpful to identify lymph nodes, diffusion restriction is not specific for metastatic disease and should be used in the context of size and other imaging features.[39]

LOCAL STAGING BY MR IMAGING TO GUIDE TREATMENT
MR Imaging in the Management of International Federation of Gynecology and Obstetrics Stage I and II

Stage I disease includes tumors limited to the cervix without evidence of regional or distant disease. Stage IA disease is diagnosed microscopically and is not visible on imaging. Stage IB disease is a measurable disease visible on clinical and imaging evaluation. In 2018, Stage IB was divided into three substages based on maximum tumor size: Stage IB1 (smaller than 2 cm), Stage IB2 (greater than 2 but less than 4 cm), and Stage IB3 (greater than 4 cm).

The new substages within Stage IB in the 2018 FIGO system were prompted by differential

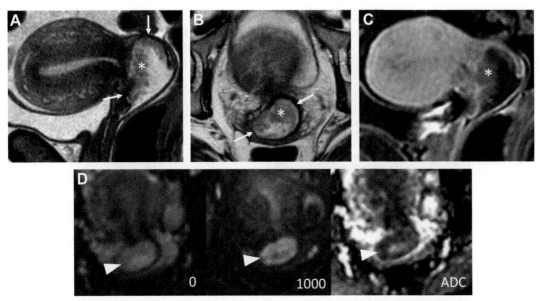

Fig. 2. Tumor appearance. A 41-year-old woman with Stage IB2 squamous cell carcinoma. (*A*) Sagittal T2WI with vaginal gel shows a T2 intermediate signal tumor that measured 3.7 cm (white *asterisk*) which expands the endocervical canal (*arrows*) without extension beyond the cervix. (*B*) Axial T2W images with vaginal gel show a T2 intermediate signal tumor that expands the endocervical canal (*arrows*) but does not invade beyond the T2 hypointense stroma (*arrows*). (*C*) Sagittal fat suppressed post-contrast T1WI at 180 s shows the tumor (*asterisks*) is hypoenhancing relative to the myometrium. (*D*) Diffusion-weighted imaging with B0, B1000 and corresponding ADC map show increasing SI on higher B value with corresponding decreased SI on ADC confirming restricted diffusion (*arrowheads*).

prognostic outcomes based on tumor size and optimal eligibility for consideration of fertility-sparing treatment. A large retrospective cohort study by Matsuo and colleagues[19] reported that patients with tumors less than 2 cm (Stage IB1) had a twofold increase in survival compared with patients with tumors greater than 2 cm but less than 4 cm (Stage IB2). An additional large multi-center retrospective study found that patients with tumors less than 2 cm had a lower risk of parametrial involvement and more favorable 5-year overall survival compared with those with tumors greater than 2 cm.[40] Horn and colleagues[41] reported that patients with tumors less than 2 cm had a significantly lower frequency of pelvic lymph node involvement (13.3%) compared with larger tumors (23.4% for IB2 and 43.5% for IB3). These studies support the division between Stage IB1 (<2 cm) and IB2 (2 to 4 cm) tumors and allow patients with tumors less than 2 cm to be considered for fertility-sparing surgery if they so desire. Fertility-sparing alternatives to hysterectomy in early-stage cancer include cone resection, loop electrosurgical excision procedure, and trachelectomy.[42]

Stage II disease includes tumors that have spread beyond the uterus, including spread to the upper 2/3 of the vagina (Stage IIA) or the parametrium (Stage IIB), but do not involve the lower 1/3 of the vagina or the pelvic sidewall. Stage IIA disease is further divided into substages, with IIA1 describing tumors less than or equal to 4 cm and IIA2 describing tumors greater than 4 cm. For the assessment of vaginal invasion, vaginal gel is helpful in distending the vagina and determining if the intermediate signal of the tumor has invaded the normal hypointense signal of the vaginal wall on T2WI (**Fig. 4**).[43,44]

In the treatment planning of both Stage I and II tumor, the treating physician will take into account the size of the tumor, parametrial extension, and extrauterine spread. It is important to accurately assess and report these findings on MR imaging. Tumor size is measured as the maximum cross-sectional diameter in any plane. Parametrial invasion is best seen on nonfat-saturated T2WI as full-thickness disruption of the markedly T2 hypointense cervical fibromuscular stromal ring with extension of tumor signal into the parametrium (**Fig. 5**). The parametrium refers to the fatty tissue surrounding the uterus and cervix between the uterine corpus and the pelvic sidewall. This encapsulates the uterine vascular pedicles and their lymphatics, as well as the cardinal and uterosacral ligaments. Additional imaging features, such as an irregular tumor-parametrial interface or tumoral

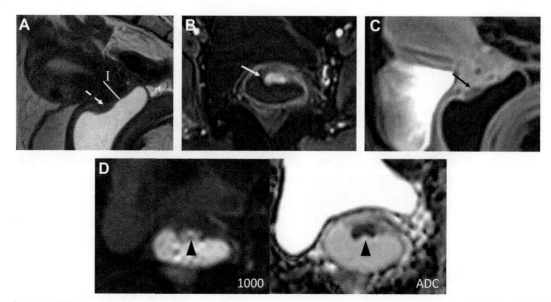

Fig. 3. Small tumor appearance. A 43-year-old woman with Stage IB1 squamous cell carcinoma. (*A*) Sagittal T2WI shows a small 1.2 cm T2 intermediate signal-enhancing tumor (dashed *white arrow*) at the anterior lip of the external os of the cervix. Note that this tumor is somewhat difficult to delineate on T2W image alone. The line shows how to measure the distance from the tumor to the internal os (I), which is nearly 2 cm in this patient. (*B*) Axial oblique fat suppressed post-contrast T1WI at 40 s shows early hyperenhancement of the tumor (*white arrow*). (*C*) Sagittal fat-suppressed post-contrast T1W images at 180 s show hypoenhancement of the tumor relative to the adjacent normal cervix (*black arrow*). (*D*) Diffusion-weighted imaging with B1000 and corresponding ADC map shows tumor with restricted diffusion (*black arrowhead*) with tumor margins well demarcated on the ADC map.

encasement of periuterine vessels, allow for confident diagnosis of parametrial invasion, with a sensitivity of 76% and specificity of 94%.[24] On the other hand, preservation of the hypointense stromal ring has a high negative predictive value of 94% to 100% for invasion.[15,45] The axial oblique nonfat-saturated T2WI is helpful in the assessment of parametrial invasion, as this eliminates blurring of the cervical fibromuscular stroma seen on straight axials that could be misinterpreted as parametrial invasion.[46] Larger tumors may compress the cervical stroma and cause peritumoral edema, also mimicking stromal disruption and parametrial invasion. In these cases, co-interpretation of DWI and T2-weighted sequences compared with T2WI alone significantly increases sensitivity

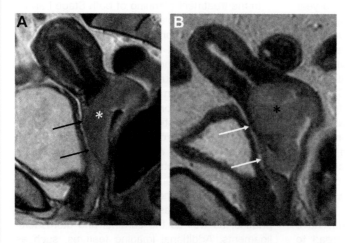

Fig. 4. Vaginal invasion versus vaginal protrusion in two different patients. (*A*) Sagittal T2WI in a 40-year-old woman with Stage IIIA squamous cell carcinoma shows a large cervical tumor (*white asterisk*) extending into the posterior vaginal fornix and inferiorly into the lower 1/3 of the vagina with loss of the normal T2 hypointense anterior vaginal wall consistent with lower 1/3 vaginal wall invasion. (*B*) Sagittal T2W images through the cervix in a 50-year-old woman with Stage IIB squamous cell carcinoma show a large tumor (*black asterisk*) extending posteriorly from the cervix into the posterior vaginal fornix and protruding inferiorly in the vagina. There is preservation of the normal wall signal along the inferior anterior vaginal wall (*white arrows*) suggesting no lower 1/3 vaginal invasion.

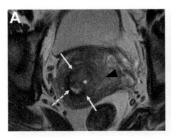
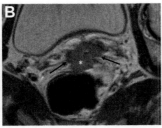

Fig. 5. Parametrial invasion in two different patients. (*A*) Axial T2W image in a 47-year-old woman with Stage IIB squamous cell carcinoma shows tumor (*white asterisk*) obliterating the hypointense cervical fibromuscular stroma from the 10 o'clock to 5 o'clock axis (*white arrows*) with ill-defined extension into the left parametrium (*black arrowhead*). Note the normal preserved T2 hypointense fibromuscular stroma on the right (*dashed white arrow*) (*B*) Axial oblique T2W image in a 53-year-old woman with Stage IIB squamous cell carcinoma shows tumor circumferentially obliterating the cervical fibromuscular stroma with nodular spiculated bilateral parametrial invasion (*black arrows*).

(83% to 92% vs 67% to 75%), specificity (99% vs 85% to 86%), and accuracy (97% to 98% vs 83%) in predicting parametrial invasion.[25]

When the tumor measures less than 2 cm without parametrial invasion, tumoral extension outside of the cervix, or abnormal lymph nodes, the patient can be offered surgery. If the patient is of childbearing age, trachelectomy can be offered if the tumor is more than 0.5 to 1 cm from the internal cervical os, allowing for cerclage to prevent cervical incompetence.[47–51] Reporting cervical length measurement and the distance between the tumor and the internal cervical os are important in these patients and the length of the cervix should be measured on a midline sagittal T2WI (see **Fig. 3**). In patients who do not desire fertility preservation, radical hysterectomy, and pelvic lymphadenectomy can be offered if the tumor measures greater than 2 cm and less than or equal to 4 cm, there is no parametrial invasion,

and the tumor is confined to the cervix (Stages IB1 and IB2) or involves the upper 2/3 of the vagina (Stage IIA1). If the tumor measures greater than 4 cm or if there is parametrial invasion, the patient will proceed with chemoradiation. A tumor of any size with parametrial invasion will be treated with chemoradiation.

MR Imaging in the Management of International Federation of Gynecology and Obstetrics Stage III and IV

Stage III disease includes tumors that involve the lower 1/3 of the vagina, extend to the pelvic wall, cause hydronephrosis, or involve the pelvic and para-aortic lymph nodes. In Stage IIIA, protrusion of tumor into the vagina should be differentiated from true vaginal wall involvement by assessing for disruption of the normal hypointense T2 signal of the lower vaginal wall. In Stage IIIB, invasion of

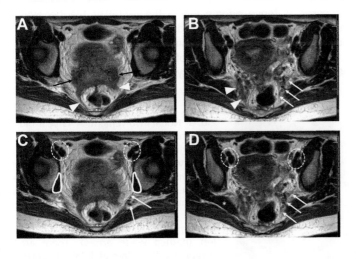

Fig. 6. 43-year-old woman with Stage IIIB squamous cell carcinoma with pelvic sidewall invasion. (*A*) Axial T2WI shows a large cervical tumor with bilateral parametrial invasion (*black arrows*), extending along the uterosacral ligaments right greater than left (*arrowheads*). (*B*) Axial T2WI image slightly cephalad to (*A*) shows the cervical tumor extending to the pelvic sidewall on the right (*arrowheads*) with ill-defined T2 intermediate signal tissue invading the posterior peritoneal lining and abutting the right piriformis muscle (*white arrowheads*). The normal posterior peritoneal lining (*white arrows*) with fat planes around the pelvic sidewall vessels can be seen on the left and used as a comparison. (*C*) Similar axial T2WI as figure component (*A*) illustrating the components of the pelvic sidewall including locations of the obturator internus muscles (white outline), the posterior peritoneal lining and associated vessels/nerves (*white arrows*), and external iliac vessels (*dashed oval*). (*D*) Similar axial T2WI as figure subpart (*B*) illustrating the components of the pelvic sidewall including locations of the posterior peritoneal lining and associated vessels/nerves (*white arrows*), piriformis muscle (*asterisk*), and external iliac vessels (dashed oval). (Courtesy of D Pinho, MD, Fort Worth, TX.)

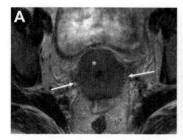
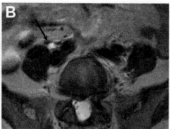
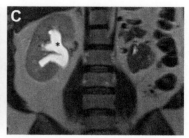

Fig. 7. Cervical mass with hydronephrosis. A 57-year-old woman with Stage IIIB squamous cell carcinoma. (A) Axial T2WI shows a diffuse enlargement of the cervix with loss of the normal T2 hypointense fibromuscular stroma and replacement by intermediate signal tumor (white *asterisk*) with bilateral parametrial invasion (*white arrows*). (B) Axial T2WI in the upper pelvis shows distal right hydroureter (*black arrow*). (C) Axial T2WI at the level of the kidneys shows right hydronephrosis (*black asterisk*).

the pelvic sidewall will be evident by gross tumor extending into the pelvic sidewall that is defined as involvement of the peritoneal lining, the obturator internus, piriformis, and levator ani muscles, and the iliac vessels (Fig. 6).[52] Pelvic sidewall involvement can lead to ureteral obstruction and subsequent hydronephrosis or a nonfunctioning kidney (Fig. 7). This highlights the importance of including at least one sequence with a larger coronal field of view to include the kidneys; otherwise, hydronephrosis may be missed.

New in the 2018 FIGO staging system is Stage IIIC, which incorporates the involvement of pelvic and/or para-aortic lymph nodes irrespective of primary tumor size and extent. Multiple studies have shown nodal disease to be an important prognostic indicator of reduced overall survival and increased disease recurrence (Fig. 8).[18,26,53] Stage IIIC is further subdivided into IIIC1 (pelvic nodes) and IIIC2 (para-aortic nodes) due to the necessity of extended field radiotherapy if para-aortic lymph nodes are involved and because the involvement of the para-aortic nodes increases the risk of recurrence.

Stage IV disease includes tumors that have spread beyond the true pelvis and is divided

into two substages. Stage IVA disease reflects tumor invasion into the mucosa of the bladder or rectum. Stage IVB involves tumor spread to distant organs and to lymph nodes beyond the pelvic and para-aortic regions. For Stage IVA, MR imaging has a sensitivity of 71% to 100% and a specificity of 88% to 91% for bladder and rectal invasion.[54] On imaging, loss of the fat plane between tumor and the bladder or rectal wall and loss of the normal T2 hypointense SI of the bladder or rectal wall with or without an intraluminal mass is needed to report invasion of these structures (Fig. 9). Of note, a preserved fat plane essentially excludes invasion with a negative predictive value of 100%; however, loss of the plane alone does not necessarily indicate invasion.[29,55] A mimic of bladder invasion is bullous edema that appears as a lobulated band of T2 hyperintensity projecting into the bladder lumen. Additionally, mural T2 hyperintense edema within the rectal or bladder wall may also make a definitive evaluation for tumoral invasion challenging and DWI can be helpful to define the extent of tumor. In some cases, further evaluation with cystoscopy may be needed to stage the patient.

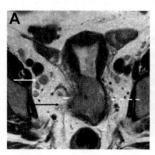
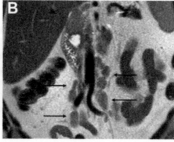

Fig. 8. Nodal involvement. A 49-year-old woman with Stage IIIC2 cervical cancer. (A) Axial T2WI shows T2 intermediate signal tumor (black *asterisk*) obliterating the hypointense cervical fibromuscular stroma on the right with nodular extension into the right parametrium (*black arrow*). Note the normal preserved T2 hypointense fibromuscular stroma on the left (dashed *white arrow*). There are several mildly enlarged bilateral pelvic lymph nodes, largest a rounded right external iliac lymph node (*white arrow*) compatible with pelvic lymph node metastasis. (B) Coronal T2WI demonstrating mildly enlarged lymph nodes tracking along the bilateral iliac chains and leftward aspect of the aorta (*black arrows*) compatible with paraortic lymph node metastases.

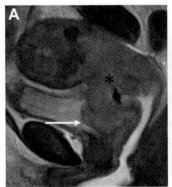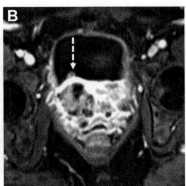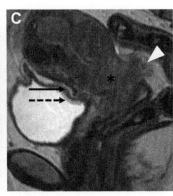

Fig. 9. Bladder invasion versus bullous edema in two different patients: a 44-year-old woman with Stage IVA squamous cell carcinoma of the cervix with bladder wall invasion (*A,B*) and a 42-year-old woman with Stage IIB squamous cell carcinoma of the cervix with bullous edema of the bladder wall (*C*). (*A*). Sagittal T2WI shows a large tumor centered at the cervix (*black asterisks*) with direct nodular extension into the lower uterus, anterior vaginal wall, and posterior bladder wall. The full thickness of the bladder wall shows abnormal T2 signal similar to the primary tumor (*white arrow*). (*B*) Axial T1WI fat suppressed post-contrast image depicts an enhancing tumor nodule protruding into the right posterior bladder wall lumen (*white dashed arrow*). (*C*) Sagittal T2WI shows a large ill-defined cervical mass (*black asterisks*) with preservation of the fat plane between the tumor and the anterior bladder wall superiorly (*black arrow*). Although there is loss of this fat plane more inferiorly, the T2 hypointense bladder wall anteriorly is preserved, and there is only a band of T2 hyperintense signal along the interior bladder wall compatible with bullous edema (*black dashed arrow*), without bladder wall invasion. There is tumor invasion into the fat posterior to the uterus, but no rectal wall invasion (*arrowhead*).

In Stage III and IV disease, chemoradiation is the primary therapy and MR imaging is critical in delineating locoregional spread of tumor to assure that the appropriate radiation field coverage is prescribed. The standard radiation field in early-stage disease includes the primary tumor, parametria, uterosacral ligaments, presacral nodes, and a portion of the vagina measured from the tumor margin. In patients with known common iliac or para-aortic nodal involvement, the radiation field is extended cephalad. In patients with lower 1/3 vaginal involvement, the bilateral groins are included. In patients with bulky pelvic sidewall disease, a parametrial radiation booster dose is often administered after initial whole pelvic radiation.[21]

SUMMARY

Cervical cancer remains a significant cause of morbidity and mortality despite advances in both preventative medicine and treatment. Although clinical staging of cervical cancer can still be performed, the profound role of imaging in prognostication and clinical management is now reflected in the 2018 FIGO staging system. Having a robust understanding of the newest staging iteration, the MR imaging features of cervical cancer, and their impact on treatment pathways will aid the radiologist in generating valuable and practical reports to guide and optimize subsequent treatment strategies.

CLINICS CARE POINTS

- The new subdivisions in Stage IB disease set forth by the 2018 International Federation of Gynecology and Obstetrics system were prognostically driven by tumor size and optimal eligibility for consideration of fertility-sparing treatment.

- Accurate measurement of tumor size is critical in Stages I and II to guide treatment. Tumor size is measured as the maximum cross-sectional diameter in any plane and best practice involves using a combination of multiplanar T2-weighted image and diffusion-weighted images.

- In patients of childbearing age with tumors measuring less than 2 cm, including the length of the cervix and the distance of tumor from the internal cervical os in the sagittal plan is important, as trachelectomy can be offered if the tumor is greater than 0.5 to 1 cm from the internal cervical os.

- In Stage II and III disease with tumors greater than 4 cm and/or when parametrial invasion is present, as well as Stage III and IV disease, chemoradiation is the primary therapy administered and MR imaging is critical in delineating locoregional spread of tumor to ensure that the appropriate radiation field coverage is prescribed.

DISCLOSURE

The Authors have nothing to disclose.

REFERENCES

1. Sung H, Ferlay J, Siegel RL, et al. Global Cancer Statistics 2020: GLOBOCAN Estimates of Incidence and Mortality Worldwide for 36 Cancers in 185 Countries. CA Cancer J Clin 2021;71(3):209–49.
2. American Cancer Society | Cancer Facts & Statistics. American Cancer Society | Cancer Facts & Statistics. Available at: http://cancerstatisticscenter. cancer.org/. Accessed July 14, 2022.
3. Burd EM. Human papillomavirus and cervical cancer. Clin Microbiol Rev 2003;16(1):1–17.
4. Cervical cancer. https://www.who.int/news-room/fact-sheets/detail/cervical-cancer. Accessed June 9, 2022.
5. Walboomers JMM, Jacobs MV, Manos MM, et al. Human papillomavirus is a necessary cause of invasive cervical cancer worldwide. J Pathol 1999;189(1): 12–9.
6. Arbyn M, Xu L, Simoens C, et al. Prophylactic vaccination against human papillomaviruses to prevent cervical cancer and its precursors. Cochrane Database Syst Rev 2018;5:CD009069.
7. Muñoz N, Bosch FX, Castellsagué X, et al. Against which human papillomavirus types shall we vaccinate and screen? the international perspective. Int J Cancer 2004;111(2):278–85.
8. Cervical cancer mortality statistics. Cancer Research UK. 2015. Available at: https://www.cancerresearchuk.org/health-professional/cancer-statistics/statistics-by-cancer-type/cervical-cancer/mortality. Accessed June 12, 2022.
9. Cancer of the Cervix Uteri - Cancer Stat Facts. SEER. Available at: https://seer.cancer.gov/statfacts/html/cervix.html. Accessed July 14, 2022.
10. Pecorelli S, Zigliani L, Odicino F. Revised FIGO staging for carcinoma of the cervix. Int J Gynecol Obstet 2009;105(2):107–8.
11. FIGO staging for carcinoma of the vulva, cervix, and corpus uteri. Int J Gynecol Obstet 2014;125(2):97–8.
12. Hricak H, Gatsonis C, Chi DS, et al. Role of imaging in pretreatment evaluation of early invasive cervical cancer: results of the intergroup study american college of radiology imaging network 6651–gynecologic oncology group 183. J Clin Oncol 2005; 23(36):9329–37.
13. Qin Y, Peng Z, Lou J, et al. Discrepancies between clinical staging and pathological findings of operable cervical carcinoma with stage IB-IIB: a retrospective analysis of 818 patients. Aust N Z J Obstet Gynaecol 2009;49(5):542–4.
14. Zhang W, Chen C, Liu P, et al. Staging early cervical cancer in China: data from a multicenter collaborative. Int J Gynecol Cancer 2019;29(5). https://doi.org/10.1136/ijgc-2019-000263.
15. Balcacer P, Shergill A, Litkouhi B. MRI of cervical cancer with a surgical perspective: staging, prognostic implications and pitfalls. Abdom Radiol 2019;44(7):2557–71.
16. Salvo G, Odetto D, Perrotta MCS, et al. Measurement of tumor size in early cervical cancer: an ever-evolving paradigm. Int J Gynecol Cancer 2020; 30(8). https://doi.org/10.1136/ijgc-2020-001436.
17. Bhatla N, Aoki D, Sharma DN, et al. Cancer of the cervix uteri. Int J Gynaecol Obstet 2018;143(Suppl 2):22–36.
18. Wright JD, Matsuo K, Huang Y, et al. Prognostic performance of the 2018 international federation of gynecology and obstetrics cervical cancer staging guidelines. Obstet Gynecol 2019;134(1):49–57.
19. Matsuo K, Machida H, Mandelbaum RS, et al. Validation of the 2018 FIGO cervical cancer staging system. Gynecol Oncol 2019;152(1):87–93.
20. de Gregorio A, Widschwendter P, Ebner F, et al. Influence of the new FIGO classification for cervical cancer on patient survival: a retrospective analysis of 265 histologically confirmed cases with FIGO stages IA to IIB. Oncology 2020;98(2):91–7.
21. Guidelines Detail. NCCN. Available at: https://www.nccn.org/guidelines/guidelines-detail. Accessed July 14, 2022.
22. Haldorsen IS, Lura N, Blaakær J, et al. What is the role of imaging at primary diagnostic work-up in uterine cervical cancer? Curr Oncol Rep 2019; 21(9):77.
23. Dappa E, Elger T, Hasenburg A, et al. The value of advanced MRI techniques in the assessment of cervical cancer: a review. Insights Imaging 2017;8(5): 471–81.
24. Woo S, Suh CH, Kim SY, et al. Magnetic resonance imaging for detection of parametrial invasion in cervical cancer: An updated systematic review and meta-analysis of the literature between 2012 and 2016. Eur Radiol 2018;28(2):530–41.
25. Qu JR, Qin L, Li X, et al. Predicting Parametrial Invasion in Cervical Carcinoma (Stages IB1, IB2, and IIA): Diagnostic Accuracy of T2-Weighted Imaging Combined With DWI at 3 T. AJR Am J Roentgenol 2018;210(3):677–84.
26. Singh AK, Grigsby PW, Dehdashti F, et al. FDG-PET lymph node staging and survival of patients with FIGO stage IIIb cervical carcinoma. Int J Radiat Oncol 2003;56(2):489–93.
27. Colposcopy and treatment of cervical intraepithelial neoplasia: a beginners' manual. Available at: https://screening.iarc.fr/colpochap.php?lang=1&chap=1. Accessed September 24, 2022.
28. Society of Abdominal Radiology Uterine and Ovarian Cancer Disease Focused Panel. Cervical Cancer Example MRI Protocol. Available at: https://view.

officeapps.live.com/op/view.aspx?src=https%3A%2F%2Fcdn.ymaws.com%2Fabdominalradiology.site-ym.com%2Fresource%2Fresmgr%2Feducation_dfp%2Fuoc%2Fsar_uoc_dfp_cervix_ca_mr_pr.docx&wdOrigin=BROWSELINK. Accessed July 16, 2022.

29. Manganaro L, Lakhman Y, Bharwani N, et al. Staging, recurrence and follow-up of uterine cervical cancer using MRI: Updated Guidelines of the European Society of Urogenital Radiology after revised FIGO staging 2018. Eur Radiol 2021;31(10):7802–16.

30. Fournier LS, Bats AS, Durdux C. Diffusion MRI: technical principles and application to uterine cervical cancer. Cancer Radiother 2020;24(5):368–73.

31. Park JM, Charnsangavej C, Yoshimitsu K, et al. Pathways of nodal metastasis from pelvic tumors: CT demonstration. Radiographics 1994;14(6):1309–21.

32. Sakuragi N. Up-to-date management of lymph node metastasis and the role of tailored lymphadenectomy in cervical cancer. Int J Clin Oncol 2007;12(3):165–75.

33. Buchsbaum HJ. Extrapelvic lymph node metastases in cervical carcinoma. Am J Obstet Gynecol 1979;133(7):814–24.

34. McMahon CJ, Rofsky NM, Pedrosa I. Lymphatic metastases from pelvic tumors: anatomic classification, characterization, and staging. Radiology 2010;254(1):31–46.

35. Fukuya T, Honda H, Hayashi T, et al. Lymph-node metastases: efficacy for detection with helical CT in patients with gastric cancer. Radiology 1995;197(3):705–11.

36. Brown G, Richards CJ, Bourne MW, et al. Morphologic predictors of lymph node status in rectal cancer with use of high-spatial-resolution MR imaging with histopathologic comparison. Radiology 2003;227(2):371–7.

37. Yang WT, Lam WW, Yu MY, et al. Comparison of dynamic helical CT and dynamic MR imaging in the evaluation of pelvic lymph nodes in cervical carcinoma. AJR Am J Roentgenol 2000;175(3):759–66.

38. Koh DM, Hughes M, Husband JE. Cross-sectional imaging of nodal metastases in the abdomen and pelvis. Abdom Imaging 2006;31(6):632–43.

39. Lin G, Ho KC, Wang JJ, et al. Detection of lymph node metastasis in cervical and uterine cancers by diffusion-weighted magnetic resonance imaging at 3T. J Magn Reson Imaging JMRI 2008;28(1):128–35.

40. Kato T, Takashima A, Kasamatsu T, et al. Clinical tumor diameter and prognosis of patients with FIGO stage IB1 cervical cancer (JCOG0806-A). Gynecol Oncol 2015;137(1):34–9.

41. Horn LC, Bilek K, Fischer U, et al. A cut-off value of 2cm in tumor size is of prognostic value in surgically treated FIGO stage IB cervical cancer. Gynecol Oncol 2014;134(1):42–6.

42. Park BK, Kim TJ. Useful MRI findings for minimally invasive surgery for early cervical cancer. Cancers 2021;13(16):4078.

43. Akata D, Kerimoglu U, Hazırolan T, et al. Efficacy of transvaginal contrast-enhanced MRI in the early staging of cervical carcinoma. Eur Radiol 2005;15(8):1727–33.

44. Atcı N, Özgür T, Öztürk F, et al. Utility of intravaginal ultrasound gel for local staging of cervical carcinoma on MRI. Clin Imaging 2016;40(6):1104–7.

45. Kaur H, Silverman PM, Iyer RB, et al. Diagnosis, staging, and surveillance of cervical carcinoma. Am J Roentgenol 2003;180(6):1621–31.

46. Woo S, Moon MH, Cho JY, et al. Diagnostic performance of MRI for assessing parametrial invasion in cervical cancer: a head-to-head comparison between oblique and true axial T2-weighted images. Korean J Radiol 2019;20(3):378–84.

47. McEvoy SH, Nougaret S, Abu-Rustum NR, et al. Fertility-sparing for young patients with gynecologic cancer: how MRI can guide patient selection prior to conservative management. Abdom Radiol N Y 2017;42(10):2488–512.

48. Dargent D, Mathevet P. 4 Schauta's vaginal hysterectomy combined with laparoscopic lymphadenectomy. Baillières Clin Obstet Gynaecol. 1995;9(4):691–705.

49. Rob L, Skapa P, Robova H. Fertility-sparing surgery in patients with cervical cancer. Lancet Oncol 2011;12(2):192–200.

50. Plante M. Evolution in fertility-preserving options for early-stage cervical cancer: radical trachelectomy, simple trachelectomy, neoadjuvant chemotherapy. Int J Gynecol Cancer 2013;23(6):982–9.

51. Lakhman Y, Akin O, Park KJ, et al. Stage IB1 cervical cancer: role of preoperative MR imaging in selection of patients for fertility-sparing radical trachelectomy. Radiology 2013;269(1):149–58.

52. Bourgioti C, Chatoupis K, Moulopoulos LA. Current imaging strategies for the evaluation of uterine cervical cancer. World J Radiol 2016;8(4):342–54.

53. Tomizawa K, Kaminuma T, Murata K, et al. FIGO 2018 staging for cervical cancer: influence on stage distribution and outcomes in the 3D-image-guided brachytherapy era. Cancers 2020;12(7):1770.

54. Sala E, Wakely S, Senior E, et al. MRI of malignant neoplasms of the uterine corpus and cervix. AJR Am J Roentgenol 2007;188(6):1577–87.

55. Rockall AG, Ghosh S, Alexander-Sefre F, et al. Can MRI rule out bladder and rectal invasion in cervical cancer to help select patients for limited EUA? Gynecol Oncol 2006;101(2):244–9.

Imaging of Vaginal and Vulvar Malignancy

Melissa McGettigan, MD[a],*, Maria Zulfiqar, MD[b], Anup S. Shetty, MD[c]

KEYWORDS

- Vaginal cancer • Vulvar cancer • Vagina • Vulva • MRI

KEY POINTS

- Squamous cell carcinoma is the most common type of vaginal and vulvar malignancy and strongly associated with high-risk human papilloma virus infection.
- MRI allows depiction of the tumor and local extent of disease as well as regional lymph nodes.
- MRI features include focal mass or nodular thickening with intermediate T2 signal, enhancement, and restricted diffusion.
- Lymph node drainage can be variable but most commonly involves the iliac lymph nodes for the upper and middle thirds of the vagina and the inguinofemoral lymph nodes for the lower third of the vagina and vulva.

INTRODUCTION

Vaginal and vulvar cancers are rare gynecologic malignancies. Vaginal malignancy accounts for approximately 2% to 3% of cancers in the female genital tract whereas vulvar malignancy accounts for approximately 4% of female genital tract cancers in the United States.[1,2] These diseases share similar epidemiology patterns, predisposing factors, and etiologies. Advances in pathology and genetics have increased knowledge regarding pathogenesis of these malignancies. Cumulative evidence-based data have led to better understanding of prognosis and refinements in staging.

Vaginal and vulvar malignancies can be asymptomatic, particularly in the early stages. Potential signs and symptoms of vaginal malignancy include bleeding, pain, dyspareunia, dysuria, and vaginal mass. The most common presenting symptom of vulvar malignancy is pruritis.[3] Other presentations include a vulvar mass, bleeding, and pain.[1,2]

Although history and physical examination are essential as a means of first-line detection, imaging plays an increasingly important role in diagnosis, staging and management. MRI is valuable in diagnosis, characterization, and localization because of exceptional contrast resolution and tissue-specific imaging capabilities, allowing accurate locoregional staging. Positron emission tomography (PET) and computed tomography (CT) of the chest, abdomen, and pelvis are complementary imaging modalities for assessment of local disease and are indicated for evaluation of regional and distant spread in high-risk patients.

NORMAL ANATOMY AND IMAGING TECHNIQUES

Vaginal Anatomy

The vagina is a distensible midline fibromuscular tubular structure that extends from the uterine cervix to the external vulva. The vagina is divided into 3 anatomic zones: a deep forniceal zone, a central wedge-shaped transition zone, and a superficial sphincteric zone into which the external urethral orifice opens, also known as the vestibule (Fig. 1).[4,5]

[a] Moffitt Cancer Center, University of South Florida College of Medicine, 12902 USF Magnolia Drive, Tampa, FL 33612, USA; [b] Mayo Clinic Arizona, 13400 East Shea Boulevard, Scottsdale, AZ 85259, USA; [c] Mallinckrodt Institute of Radiology, Washington University School of Medicine, 510 South Kingshighway Boulevard, Box 8131, St Louis, MO 63110, USA
* Corresponding author.
E-mail address: melissa.mcgettigan@moffitt.org

Radiol Clin N Am 61 (2023) 651–670
https://doi.org/10.1016/j.rcl.2023.02.010
0033-8389/23/© 2023 Elsevier Inc. All rights reserved.

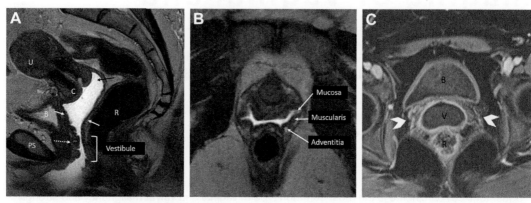

Fig. 1. Anatomy of the vagina. Sagittal T2W MRI (A) shows the vagina distended with aqueous gel, separating the anterior and posterior walls (white arrows). The deep forniceal zone (black arrow) has a dome-shaped configuration around the cervix. The superficial zone is known as the vestibule. Transverse folds (rugae) are prominent in young women (dashed arrow). Axial T2W MRI (B) shows the vaginal wall layers with inner hyperintense mucosa and outer hypointense muscularis layer covered by an outer fibrous layer of adventitia and associated fat. Axial T1W fat-suppressed postcontrast MRI in a different patient (C) demonstrates enhancement of the venous plexus (arrowheads) surrounding the gel-distended vagina. B, bladder; C, cervix; PS, pubic symphysis; R, rectum; U, uterus; V, vagina.

The vaginal wall is composed of 4 histologic layers including an inner layer of stratified squamous epithelium, a connective tissue layer of elastic lamina propria, a fibromuscular layer, and an outer fibrous layer of adventitia. MRI depicts the inner high T2 signal mucosa containing transverse folds (rugae), the low T2 signal muscular layer, and the outer layer of intermediate signal adventitia (see Fig. 1).[5,6] Postcontrast MRI demonstrates diffuse surrounding enhancement of the perivaginal venous plexus (see Fig. 1).[6]

Lymphatic drainage of the vagina is variable, but frequently follows the 3 anatomic zones. The upper one-third drains to the external iliac and para-aortic lymph nodes; the middle one-third drains to the internal and common iliac lymph nodes, and the lower one-third drains to the superficial and deep inguinal lymph nodes.[4–6]

Vulvar Anatomy

The vulva is the region external to the vagina and includes the mons pubis, clitoris, labia, and Bartholin glands in addition to the urethral meatus and vaginal introitus, collectively referred to as the external genitalia. The labia majora are paired folds covered in hair-bearing skin that fuse anteriorly at the mons pubis (anterior prominence of the

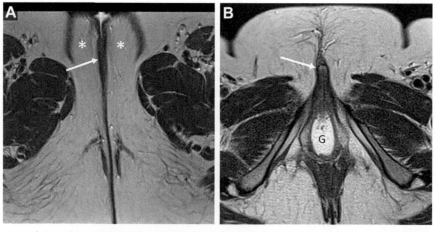

Fig. 2. Anatomy of the vulva on axial T2W MRI. (A) The labia majora (asterisks) are fatty outer folds that lie lateral to the labia minora (arrow). (B) The labia minora fuse anteriorly to form the clitoris (arrow). G, aqueous gel in the vagina.

Table 1
Representative MRI protocol for vaginal and vulvar disease

			MRI Vaginovulvar Protocol						
Sequence Name	Slice Thickness (mm)	Matrix (pixels)	FOV (mm)	TR (ms)	TE (ms)	NSA	Acquisition Time (s)	Notes	
T2W Single Shot FSE Coronal	6	320 × 320	400 × 400	1000	100	1	120 (multi breath-hold)	Whole pelvis coverage	
T1W 3D Spoiled GRE Dixon Axial	3	260 × 320	300 × 380	6.68	2.39	1	14 (single breath-hold)	Acquire in-phase and opposed-phase, reconstruct fat-only and water-only	
T2W FSE Axial	6	260 × 320	300 × 380	4000	98	2	180 (free breathing)	Whole pelvis coverage	
T2W FSE Sagittal	4	320 × 320	300 × 300	4630	96	2	270 (free breathing)	Cover femoral head to femoral head	
T2W FSE Oblique Axial Small FOV	4	320 × 320	240 × 240	4570	108	2	270 (free breathing)	Angle perpendicular to long axis of vagina/vulva; cover from perineum through top of uterus	
T2W FSE Oblique Coronal Small FOV	4	320 × 320	240 × 240	4000	108	2	270 (free breathing)	Angle coronal to the plane of the vagina and vulva	
T2W 3D Oblique Axial	1.5	256 × 256	240 × 240	1600	95	1	300 (free breathing)	Multiplanar reconstructions can be created from 3-dimensional dataset, if necessary	
DWI Single Shot Axial	3	144 × 192	300 × 380	8900	68	2, 4, 8	360 (free breathing)	Obtain b-values of 50, 500, 1000; reconstruct ADC map and calculated b-value of 1400	

(continued on next page)

Table 1
(continued)

MRI Vaginovulvar Protocol

Sequence Name	Slice Thickness (mm)	Matrix (pixels)	FOV (mm)	TR (ms)	TE (ms)	NSA	Acquisition Time (s)	Notes
T1W 3D Spoiled GRE Axial Precontrast	3	260 × 320	300 × 380	5.09	2.33	1	12 (single breath-hold)	
T1W 3D Spoiled GRE Axial Arterial	3	260 × 320	300 × 380	5.09	2.33	1	12 (single breath-hold)	Generate subtraction from precontrast acquisition
T1W 3D Spoiled GRE Axial Venous	3	260 × 320	300 × 380	5.09	2.33	1	12 s (single breath-hold)	Generate subtraction from precontrast acquisition
T1W 3D Spoiled GRE Axial Equilibrium	3	260 × 320	300 × 380	5.09	2.33	1	12 s (single breath-hold)	Generate subtraction from precontrast acquisition
T1W 3D Spoiled GRE Coronal	3	320 × 320	400 × 400	4.67	2.39	1	14 s (single breath-hold)	
T1W 3D Spoiled GRE Sagittal	3	320 × 320	300 × 380	4.67	2.39	1	14 s (single breath-hold)	

Abbreviations: 3D, 3-dimensional; ADC, apparent diffusion coefficient; DWI, diffusion-weighted imaging; FOV, field of view; FSE, fast spin echo; GRE, gradient-recalled echo; NSA, number of signal averages; T1W, T1-weighted; T2W, T2-weighed; TE, echo time; TR, repetition time.

Table 2
Representative positron emission tomography/MRI protocol for vaginal and vulvar disease

			PET/MRI Vaginovulvar Protocol					
Sequence Name	Slice Thickness (mm)	Matrix (pixels)	FOV (mm)	TR (ms)	TE (ms)	NSA	Acquisition Time (s)	Notes
T1W WB Two-Point GRE Dixon Axial	3	312 × 384	400 × 500	3.85	2.46	1	11 s × 6 stations (breath-hold)	Skull vertex to thighs in 6 stations; composed image set, coronal reformat, and MRAC map created from source data for attenuation correction
T2W WB Single-Shot FSE axial	5	240 × 320	400 × 500	3000	116	1	120 s × 6 stations (free breathing)	Skull vertex to thighs in 6 stations; composed image set created from source data
WB PET Acquisition							Acquired simultaneously during whole body T1W MRAC and T2W MRI	PET stations matched to MR stations
T1W pelvis Two-Point GRE Dixon Axial	3	312 × 384	400 × 500	3.85	2.46	1	11 s (breath-hold)	Pelvis only; MRAC map created from source data for attenuation correction
Pelvis PET acquisition							Acquired simultaneously during pelvis T1W MRAC	A separate regional acquisition facilitates fusion with regional MR images
DWI Pelvis Single Shot Axial	5	96 × 128	337 × 450	8100	71	2, 4, 8	180 s (free breathing)	Obtain b-values of 50, 500, 800; reconstruct ADC map
T2W Pelvis FSE Oblique Axial Small FOV	4	280 × 320	227 × 260	4710	102	2	270 s (free breathing)	Angle perpendicular to long axis of vaginal/vulva; cover from

(continued on next page)

Table 2
(continued)

			PET/MRI Vaginovulvar Protocol					
Sequence Name	Slice Thickness (mm)	Matrix (pixels)	FOV (mm)	TR (ms)	TE (ms)	NSA	Acquisition Time (s)	Notes
T2W Pelvis 3D Oblique Axial	1.5	256 × 320	280 × 360	1710	88	2	430 s (free breathing)	perineum through top of uterus; Multiplanar reconstructions can be created from 3D dataset, if necessary; high-resolution images helpful for PET/MR fusion
T1W Pelvis 3D Spoiled GRE Axial Precontrast	3	240 × 320	300 × 400	3.53	1.23	1	18 s (single breath-hold)	
T1W Pelvis 3D Spoiled GRE Axial Arterial	3	240 × 320	300 × 400	3.53	1.23	1	18 s (single breath-hold)	
T1W Pelvis 3D Spoiled GRE Axial Venous	3	240 × 320	300 × 400	3.53	1.23	1	18 s (single breath-hold)	
T1W Pelvis 3D Spoiled GRE Axial Equilibrium	3	240 × 320	300 × 400	3.53	1.23	1	18 s (single breath-hold)	
T1W Pelvis 3D Spoiled GRE Coronal	3	320 × 320	350 × 350	4.11	1.82	1	20 s (single breath-hold)	
T1W Pelvis 3D Spoiled GRE Sagittal	3	320 × 320	350 × 350	4.11	1.82	1	20 s (single breath-hold)	

Abbreviations: 3D, 3-dimensional; ADC, apparent diffusion coefficient; DWI, diffusion-weighted imaging; FOV, field of view; FSE, fast spin echo; GRE, gradient-recalled echo; MRAC, MRI-based attenuation correction; NSA, number of signal averages; T1W, T1-weighted; T2W, T2-weighed; TE, echo time; TR, repetition time; WB, whole body.

Table 3
International Federation of Gynecologic Oncology staging of vaginal cancer

Stage	Description
I	Tumor confined to the vagina
II	Tumor involves paravaginal tissue without extension to the pelvic side wall
III	Tumor extends to the pelvic side wall and/or causes hydronephrosis without or with regional lymph nodes
IV	Tumor extends beyond the true pelvis or involves bladder or rectal mucosa or distant metastases
IVA	Tumor extends beyond true pelvis or involves bladder or rectal mucosa
IVB	Distant metastases

Table 4
International Federation of Gynecologic Oncology staging of vulvar cancer (updated 2021)

Stage	Description
I	Tumor confined to the vulva
IA	Tumor size ≤2 cm and stromal invasion ≤1 mm
IB	Tumor size >2 cm or stromal invasion >1 mm
II	Tumor of any size with extension to lower one-third of the urethra, lower one-third of the vagina, lower one-third of the anus with negative lymph nodes
III	Tumor of any size with extension to upper part of adjacent perineal structures or with any number of nonfixed, nonulcerated lymph nodes
IIIA	Tumor of any size with extension to upper two-thirds of urethra or upper two-thirds of vagina, bladder or rectal mucosa or regional lymph node metastases ≤5 mm
IIIB	Regional lymph node metastases >5 mm
IIIC	Regional lymph node metastases with extracapsular spread
IV	Tumor of any size fixed to bone or fixed, ulcerated lymph node metastases or distant metastases
IVA	Tumor fixed to pelvic bone or fixed or ulcerated regional lymph node metastases
IVB	Distant metastases

symphysis pubis) and posteriorly at the posterior commissure of the perineum. The labia minora are smaller skin folds, medial to the labia majora, and are covered by vaginal mucosa medially. These fuse anteriorly to form the prepuce of the clitoris and posteriorly in the fossa navicularis (**Fig. 2**).

Vulvar lymphatic drainage is via the superficial inguinal lymph nodes, then to the deep inguinal lymph nodes. Deep inguinal lymph nodes drain into iliac and para-aortic lymph nodes.[7,8] Lymphatic vessels can cross midline in lesions associated with median structures such as the clitoris as well as in large paramedian lesions.[8]

MRI offers exquisite anatomic detail and soft tissue contrast in delineating vaginovulvar masses and their anatomic relationship to adjacent structures. Distension of the vaginal vault with a water-soluble gel is achieved either by the technologist/radiologist or the patient at his or her discretion. A torso phased-array receiver coil is used anteriorly in conjunction with the posterior table/spine receiver coil to achieve a high signal-to-noise ratio. An endocavitary coil may obscure a vaginovulvar mass and should be avoided. Small field-of-view, high-resolution axial and coronal imaging should be angled along the plane of the vagina and vulva to minimize off-axis volume averaging. A representative MRI protocol is summarized in **Table 1**.

Hybrid PET/MRI offers the combination of MRI soft tissue detail with metabolic data from PET to overcome potential shortcomings of anatomic imaging such as poor sensitivity in detecting nodal metastases in nonenlarged lymph nodes. Considerations unique to PET/MRI compared with PET/ CT include MR attenuation correction, implant/device safety, gadolinium contrast safety, precertification/billing, and examination length.[9] A lower dose of ionizing radiation from PET/MR as compared to PET/CT may be beneficial for patients in whom cumulative dose exposure is a concern. Conversely, the bore width of 60 cm for hybrid PET/MRI compared with 70 cm for conventional MRI may be a consideration precluding imaging of larger or claustrophobic patients. A representative PET/MRI protocol is summarized in **Table 2**.

PATHOLOGY
Vaginal Cancer

Squamous cell carcinoma (SCC), accounting for approximately 80% to 90% of vaginal malignancies,

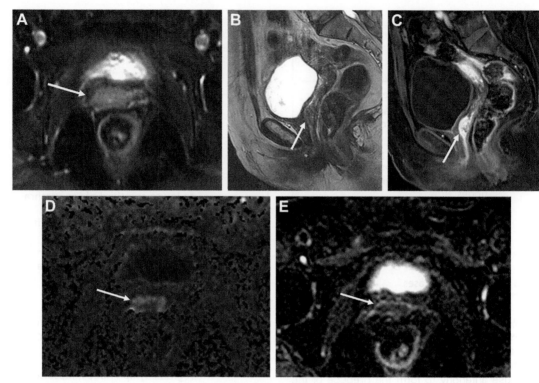

Fig. 3. 78-year-old woman with Stage II invasive SCC of the vagina. Axial T2W fat-suppressed (*A*) and sagittal T2W MRI (*B*) demonstrate a 5 × 3 cm mass in the mid-vagina that has intermediate signal (*arrow*). Sagittal T1W fat-suppressed postcontrast MRI (*C*) demonstrates avid enhancement. Axial DWI (b-1000) (*D*) and ADC map (*E*) show high and low signal, respectively (*arrows*), indicating restricted diffusion in the tumor.

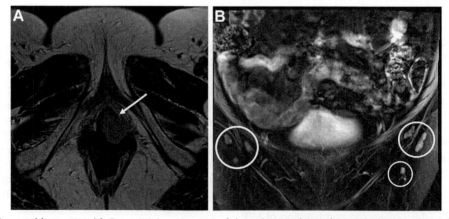

Fig. 4. 66-year-old woman with Stage IIIB invasive SCC of the vulva involving the Bartholin gland. Axial T2W MRI (*A*) demonstrates a 2.6 cm intermediate signal mass extending through the left vaginal wall to involve the urethra (*arrow*). Coronal T1W fat-suppressed postcontrast MRI (*B*) shows small, nonspecific bilateral inguinal lymph nodes (circles) without lymphadenopathy. Pathology from bilateral inguinal lymph node dissection confirmed a 6.5 mm focus of metastatic disease in 1 of 6 nodes on the left without extracapsular spread and negative right inguinal nodes.

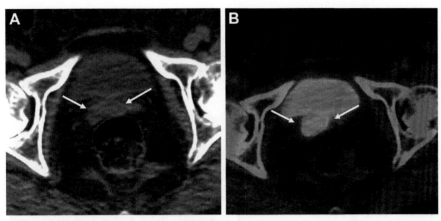

Fig. 5. 78-year-old woman (same as in Fig. 3) with Stage II invasive SCC of the vagina. Axial noncontrast CT (*A*) and axial fused PET/CT (*B*) demonstrate focal nodular thickening in the right and mid-aspects of the vagina with hypermetabolic activity (SUV 10.2), consistent with malignancy (*arrows*).

is frequently found in the upper one-third of the vagina.[10,11] Risk factors for vaginal SCC include infection with high-risk oncogenic strains of human papilloma virus (HPV), particularly HPV 16, with viral DNA detected in more than half (55% to 64%) of invasive vaginal cancers.[12] Thus, risk factors for HPV infection, including initiation of sexual intercourse at a young age and high number of sexual partners, are also risk factors for vaginal SCC.[13]

Few primary vaginal malignancies are non-SCC. These include vaginal adenocarcinoma, accounting for approximately 5-10% of primary malignancies and typically found in younger females (peak age of 19), occasionally arising in foci of adenosis, endometriosis or Wolffian rest remnants.[14,15] Rarer subtypes include small cell carcinoma, melanoma, sarcoma, lymphoma, and carcinoid.[5,10]

Secondary vaginal involvement by malignancy is significantly more common than primary malignancies (accounting for approximately 80% of cases), frequently caused by direct invasion of other genitourinary or rectal tumors.[10,11]

Vulvar Cancer

The majority (>90%) of invasive vulvar cancers are SCC and most commonly involve the labia with about 50% of cases involving the labia majora.[16] Vulvar intraepithelial neoplasias (VIN) are precursor lesions to invasive SCC, characterized by histopathologic atypia. Similar to vaginal cancer, high-risk HPV infection with oncogenic strains, most commonly HPV 16 followed by HPV 11, 18, and 33, is a risk factor for vulvar cancer, with approximately 43% of SCC attributed to

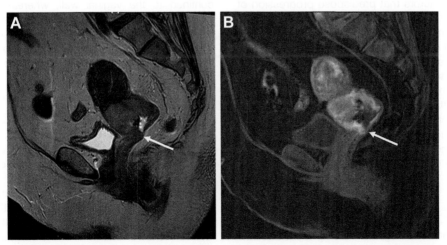

Fig. 6. 55-year-old woman with stage IIIC SCC of the cervix. Sagittal T2W (*A*) and T1W fat-suppressed post-contrast MRI (*B*) show a cervical mass extending into the upper one-third of the vagina (*arrow*).

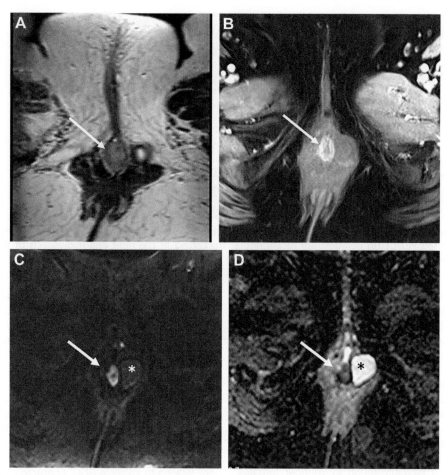

Fig. 7. 62-year-old woman with history of endometrial adenocarcinoma presenting with a vaginal mass. Axial T2W MRI (*A*) shows an intermediate signal mass in the vaginal introitus (*arrow*). Biopsy confirmed disease recurrence. Axial T1W fat-suppressed postcontrast MRI (*B*) shows avid enhancement of the mass. Axial DWI (b-1000) (*C*) and ADC map (*D*) show marked restricted diffusion. An incidental Bartholin gland cyst is noted on the left without enhancement or restricted diffusion (*asterisks*).

HPV.[13,14] Factors that predispose progression of infection to atypia such as diabetes mellitus, obesity, and smoking are also associated with an increased risk of developing malignancy.

Whereas HPV-associated VIN is most common in women under age 50, non-HPV VIN is common in older women and frequently associated with the chronic inflammatory condition of lichen sclerosis.[17]

Less common histologic types include adenocarcinoma, which typically involves the Bartholin glands, and melanoma, which most frequently involves the clitoris or labia minora, and sarcoma.[3,10]

STAGING
Vaginal Cancer

Vaginal cancer is staged according to the 2009 International Federation of Gynecologic Oncology (FIGO) guidelines (**Table 3**).[18] Stage I disease is confined to the vaginal wall, whereas Stage II disease involves the subvaginal tissue. Stage III disease extends to the pelvic wall and/or causes hydronephrosis and also includes spread to regional lymph nodes. Stage IV disease involves adjacent organs or spread beyond the true pelvis.[11,15]

Vulvar Cancer

In 2021, FIGO revised the prior 2009 version of vulvar cancer staging based on the collective data of prognostic factors to determine differentiation of stages and substages (**Table 4**).[19,20] Stage I disease is confined to the vulva with criteria similar to 2009 (except for a change in the depth of invasion measurement).[21] Stage II lesions involve the lower one-third of the urethra, vagina, or anus, similar to the 2009 version. Stage III lesions involve the upper perineal structures and/or

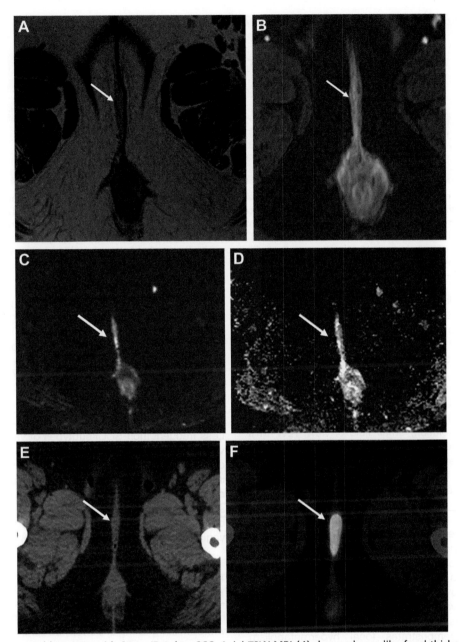

Fig. 8. 32-year-old woman with Stage IB vulvar SCC. Axial T2W MRI (*A*) shows plaque-like focal thickening and nodularity along the right labia minora (*arrow*) measuring approximately 4 cm in length. Axial T1W fat-suppressed postcontrast MRI (*B*) shows diffuse enhancement. Axial DWI (b-800) (*C*) and ADC map (*D*) show improved conspicuity of the lesion with signal significantly different than the adjacent musculature and subcutaneous fat. Axial noncontrast CT (*E*) shows mild soft tissue thickening in the vulva, but the lesion is difficult to detect. Axial fused PET/CT (*F*) shows a hypermetabolic vulvar mass (SUV 13.3).

lymph nodes. A salient change involves reclassification of lesions that extend into the upper two-thirds of the urethra or vagina, bladder, or rectal mucosa to Stage IIIA rather than stage IVA. Stage IV lesions are inseparable from the pelvic bone and/or have fixed, ulcerated regional lymph nodes or distant metastases.

IMAGING FINDINGS
Imaging of Vaginal Cancer

Vaginal cancer may present as a polypoid or lobulated mass or as focal plaque-like thickening and nodularity.[5,6] Thickening may be circumferential and constricting, and the mass may be ulcerated

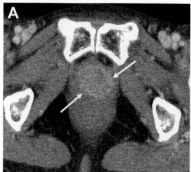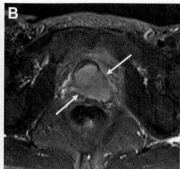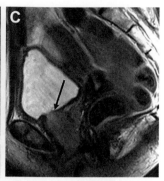

Fig. 9. 68-year-old woman who presented with urinary retention found to have a vaginal adenosquamous carcinoma. Axial contrast-enhanced CT (*A*) shows a 3.5 cm enhancing mass in the vagina (*arrows*). Axial T2W inversion recovery (*B*) and sagittal T2W MRI (*C*) show the intermediate signal mass in the lower one-third of the vagina invading into the bladder mucosa (*arrow*), consistent with FIGO Stage IVA. Bilateral pelvic lymph node sampling at the time of anterior exenteration surgery (including common iliac and obturator lymph nodes) was negative for nodal metastatic disease.

and irregular.[15,21] The signal intensity is typically intermediate on T1-weighted (T1W) MRI and intermediate to high on T2-weighted (T2W) imaging (**Fig. 3**).[6,22] Postcontrast imaging generally demonstrates avid lesion enhancement and dense cellularity, with corresponding high signal on diffusion-weighted imaging (DWI) and low signal on apparent diffusion coefficient (ADC) mapping (see **Fig. 3**).[21,22]

High resolution, small field-of-view T2W MRI aids in assessment of disease beyond the vaginal wall (Stage II or higher) by demonstrating disruption of the low T2 signal muscular layer. Similarly, T2W images may show disruption of the normal target-like appearance of the urethra or low-signal anal sphincter in higher stage disease (**Fig. 4**). Pelvic lymph nodes should be assessed for suspicious features such as heterogeneous signal (including cystic change), enlargement (short axis diameter > 10 mm), and abnormal morphology.

On CT, vaginal malignancy may appear as a soft tissue mass or abnormal soft tissue thickening. PET/CT demonstrates focal hypermetabolism (**Fig. 5**).[21]

Imaging may depict secondary vaginal involvement from cancers arising in adjacent organs (**Fig. 6**). Locoregional recurrence of these tumors can also involve the vagina (**Fig. 7**).[23,24]

Imaging of Vulvar Cancer

Like vaginal cancer, vulvar cancer appears as a mass or focal nodular thickening and is commonly intermediate signal on T1W and intermediate to high signal on T2W MRI.[21,25] Postcontrast T1W fat-suppressed MRI typically shows early arterial enhancement owing to the rich vascularity

supplied by the external and internal pudendal arterial branches.[24,25] DWI provides high sensitivity for detecting disease given the improved signal contrast between tumor and normal tissue.[6,16] PET/CT demonstrates increased metabolic activity within the lesion (**Fig. 8**).[21,25]

Imaging of Other Vaginal and Vulvar Cancers

Less frequent (non-SCC) subtypes of vaginal and vulvar malignancies vary in imaging appearance depending on the cell type but often have similar imaging features as SCC (**Fig. 9**). The paramagnetic effects of melanin that lead to shortened T1 and T2 relaxation times traditionally described in brain melanomas are less frequently observed in vaginal and vulvar melanomas (**Fig. 10**).[15]

TREATMENT AND COMPLICATIONS
Treatment

For vaginal cancer, wide local excision with or without skin grafting is performed for intraepithelial neoplasia and Stage I disease. Adjuvant radiation therapy is often given for close or positive surgical margins. External-beam radiation therapy is considered prior to surgery for bulky Stage I (greater than 4 cm) and higher-grade tumors or those involving the entire vagina. Elective radiation to the pelvic and/or inguinal nodes is often considered for cancers in the lower vagina. Total vaginectomy with vaginal reconstruction may be performed for lesions in the upper vagina.[2] Advanced cases may require pelvic exenteration with or without radiation and chemotherapy. Stage IVB tumors require palliative radiation or chemoradiation.[26]

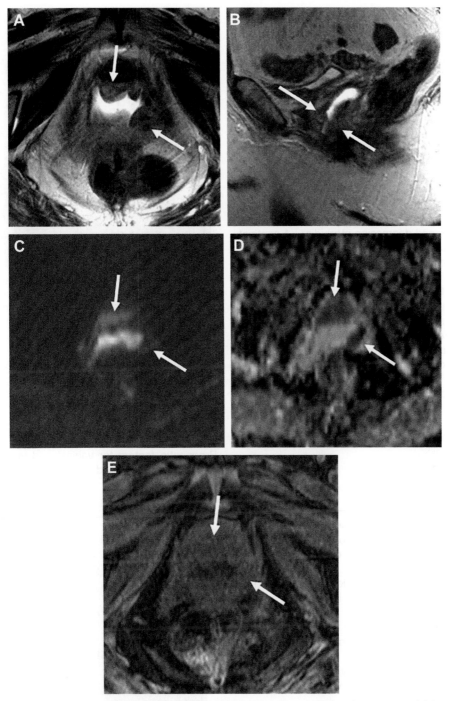

Fig. 10. 84-year-old woman with vaginal bleeding and biopsy-proven vaginal melanoma. Axial (*A*) and sagittal (*B*) T2W MRI and axial DWI (b-1000) (*C*) and ADC map (*D*) demonstrate lobulated intermediate signal soft tissue along the anterior and left lateral vaginal walls with corresponding restricted diffusion (*arrows*). With the vaginal vault distended by aqueous gel, the ADC map is particularly important to scrutinize, as hyperintense fluid may obscure adjacent diffusion abnormalities even on high b-value DWI. Axial T1W fat-suppressed MRI (*E*) shows no intrinsic T1 hyperintensity, a typical feature of vaginal melanomas (*arrows*).

A neovagina is a surgically created conduit for vaginal reconstruction after vaginectomy, commonly performed with a loop of ileum or sigmoid colon (Fig. 11). Early postsurgical complications include hematomas, fluid collections, and abscesses, whereas long-term complications include chronic inflammation, neovaginal strictures, fistulas, and malignancy.[23,27]

Standard primary treatment for vulvar cancer is surgery. Earlier stage disease improves the possibility of curative resection. Laser therapy can be considered for lesions on the intraepithelial neoplastic spectrum. Radical local excision is performed for tumors confined to the vulva with at least a 1 cm margin, generally replacing radical vulvectomy and decreasing morbidity.[1] A sentinel node procedure is increasingly being used for early disease.[19] Inguinofemoral lymph node dissection is performed when the sentinel node is positive for metastasis and/or not detected. Ipsilateral groin node dissection has largely replaced bilateral dissection for small (less than 4 cm), laterally localized (greater than or equal to 2 cm from midline) tumors.[19] Bilateral groin node dissection is indicated with large lateral or medial/midline tumors and positive ipsilateral nodes (see Fig. 4). Adjuvant or neoadjuvant local radiation may be used for Stage II and higher disease.[1] For advanced disease and poor surgical candidates, radiation or chemoradiation therapy is the treatment of choice.[1,11]

COMPLICATIONS

Inflammation from radiation therapy or malignant extension of tumor from the vagina or vulva can lead to fistulous communication with adjacent organs such as the rectum, colon, or bladder. High-resolution T2W MRI is excellent at delineating fistulas as linear fluid-filled tracts (Fig. 12).[27]

Vaginal and vulvar necrosis is a late but morbid complication following pelvic radiation that can lead to infection, hemorrhage, fistula, or perforation. The incidence is approximately 3% to 6% in patients with cervical, vaginal, and vulvar cancers treated with radiation therapy.[28] MRI may show thickened, edematous tissue with an associated focal defect (Fig. 13).

Vaginal stenosis results in scarring and adherence of the vaginal walls. This may occur any time after external beam radiation or brachytherapy for gynecologic or anorectal malignancy, but symptoms typically occur within the first year.[28] On MRI, the vaginal walls may be thickened and coapted with T1 isointense and T2 hypointense signal and delayed enhancement caused by fibrosis. The lower one-third of the vagina is most

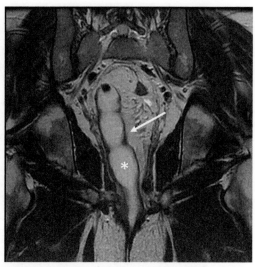

Fig. 11. Normal MRI appearance of a neovagina. Coronal T2W MRI after vaginectomy with intestinal vaginoplasty utilizing sigmoid colon. The neovagina (asterisk) is distended with aqueous gel and appears normal (arrow).

commonly involved, and severe narrowing can lead to distension of the upper vagina and/or or endometrium with fluid or blood products (Fig. 14).

RECURRENCE

Prognostic factors for vaginal and vulvar recurrence primarily depend on disease stage but also

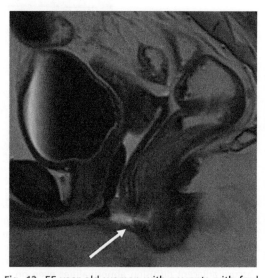

Fig. 12. 55-year-old woman with presents with foul-smelling vaginal discharge 6 months following radiation therapy for vaginal SCC. Sagittal T2W MRI shows a hyperintense fluid-filled tract (arrow) between the posterior vaginal wall and anterior anus, consistent with anovaginal fistula.

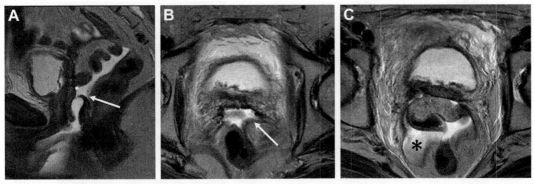

Fig. 13. 77-year-old woman with history of cervical cancer involving the upper vagina status after total abdominal hysterectomy and radiation therapy. Sagittal (*A*) and axial (*B, C*) T2W MRI show a defect at the vaginal cuff (*arrows*) with aqueous gel instilled via the vagina extravasating into the pelvic cavity (*asterisk*), surrounding loops of small bowel, consistent with vaginal necrosis and dehiscence.

include lesion location, patient age, and treatment parameters including radiation dose.[29,30] Although there are no universal established guidelines for routine imaging surveillance after treatment for vaginal or vulvar malignancy, imaging plays an important adjunct role in monitoring patients for complications and recurrence. Recurrent disease commonly demonstrates imaging features similar to that of the original tumor, including intermediate signal on T2W MRI and early tumoral enhancement on T1W postcontrast images (**Fig. 15**). PET/CT and PET/MR can be valuable in helping distinguish recurrent disease from post-treatment and postsurgical changes.

DIFFERENTIAL DIAGNOSIS

Benign lesions can involve the vagina and vulva, occasionally mimicking malignancy. Cysts occur in both the vagina and vulva and generally develop when there is obstruction to outflow of secretions from glands in and around the vagina, including Bartholin and Skene glands and Gartner duct.[31] Cysts are typically hyperintense on T2W MRI and can have variable signal on T1W imaging because of proteinaceous or hemorrhagic contents (**Fig. 16**).[32] These may appear more complex if secondarily infected (see **Fig. 16**). A primary malignancy, such as one arising in a Bartholin gland,

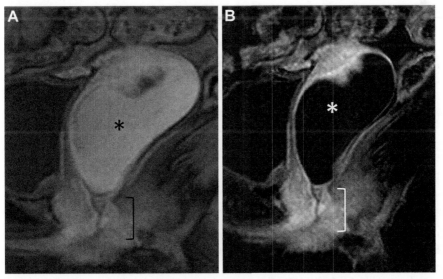

Fig. 14. 50-year-old woman with pelvic pain after radiation therapy for vaginal cancer. Sagittal T1W fat-suppressed (*A*) and postcontrast subtraction MRI (*B*) show coapted anterior and posterior vaginal walls and foreshortened length (*bracket*) with upstream T1 hyperintense hematometrocolpos (*asterisk*). Delayed enhancement of scarring at the vaginal vestibule and vulva with stenotic caliber (*bracket*). Physical examination was consistent with vaginal stenosis.

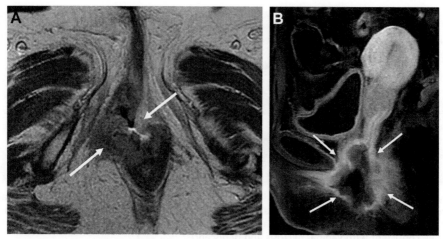

Fig. 15. 42-year-old woman with history of Stage IVB vulvar SCC presents 3 months after completing concurrent chemoradiation with enlarging vulvar ulcer, vaginal discharge, and groin pain. Biopsy showed recurrent SCC. Axial T2W MRI (*A*) shows an ulcerated intermediate signal mass in the vulva and vagina with marked thickening and nodularity (*arrows*). Sagittal T1W fat-suppressed postcontrast MRI (*B*) shows the centrally necrotic mass (*arrows*).

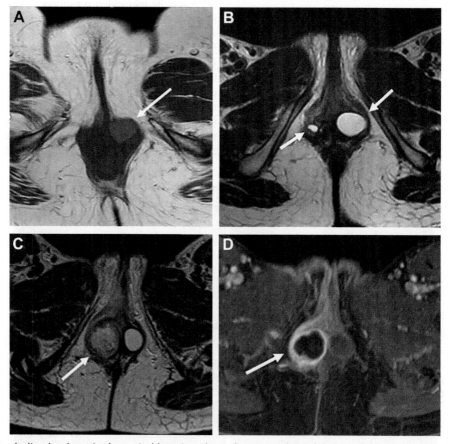

Fig. 16. Bartholin gland cyst in the typical location along the posterolateral aspect of the vagina at or below the level of the symphysis pubis. Axial T2W MRI (*A*) shows an intermediate signal intensity well-circumscribed lesion in the left vagina (*arrow*). T2 signal may be lower than simple fluid because of proteinaceous contents. Axial T2W MRI in a different patient (*B*) with bilateral Bartholin gland cysts (*arrows*). MRI obtained 1 year later (*C*) because of vaginal pain shows significant enlargement of the right cyst and new heterogeneous T2 signal (*arrow*). Axial T1W fat-suppressed postcontrast MRI (*D*) shows a thick, enhancing wall (*arrow*) consistent with clinically proven abscess. An infected Bartholin gland cyst cannot be distinguished from malignancy on imaging alone, and follow-up or tissue sampling is necessary.

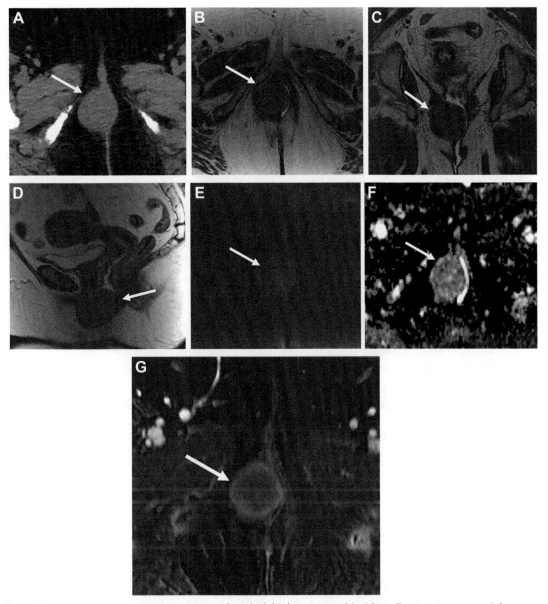

Fig. 17. 76-year-old asymptomatic woman with right labial mass noted incidentally at cystoscopy. Axial noncontrast CT (*A*) shows a rounded right vulvar mass (*arrow*). Axial (*B*), coronal (*C*), and sagittal (*D*) T2W MRI show a low signal intensity, rounded right labial mass. Axial DWI (b-1000) (*E*) and ADC map (*F*) both show low signal (T2 black-out). Axial T1W fat-suppressed postcontrast subtraction MRI (*G*) shows mild peripheral enhancement. A leiomyoma was suggested and confirmed at resection.

typically appears more solid.[31,32] However, if imaging findings are inconclusive, biopsy or excision may be necessary to exclude malignancy.

Benign solid masses in the vagina and vulva can also be mistaken for malignancy. Leiomyomas are benign smooth muscle tumors that rarely occur in the vagina and vulva.[33] These are typically well-circumscribed, pedunculated or intramural masses with vaginal leiomyomas usually involving the midline and anterior vagina. MRI signal intensity can be variable but is most commonly T2 hypointense with postcontrast enhancement. T2 black-out phenomenon has been used to describe low signal on DWI and ADC in uterine leiomyomas, which may also be seen in vaginal and vulvar leiomyomas (**Fig. 17**).[34] Conversely, vaginal leiomyosarcomas may have ill-defined borders and tend to have more heterogeneous signal on T1W and

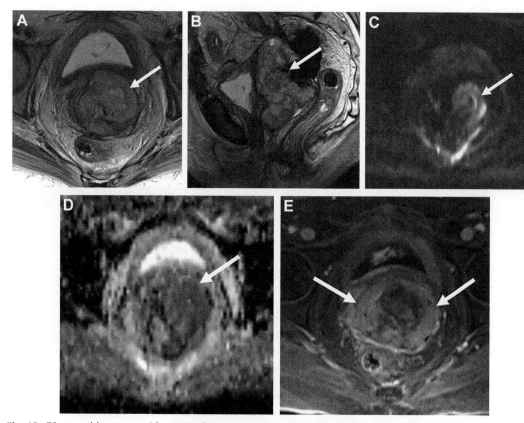

Fig. 18. 70-year-old woman with uterine leiomyosarcoma status after debulking now with vaginal bleeding and biopsy-proven vaginal leiomyosarcoma. Axial (*A*) and sagittal (*B*) T2W MRI show a T2 intermediate lobulated upper vaginal mass (*arrow*). Axial DWI (b-1000) (*C*) and ADC map (*D*) show marked restricted diffusion (*arrows*). Axial T1W fat-suppressed postcontrast MRI (*E*) shows thick, irregular peripheral enhancement and central necrosis (*arrows*).

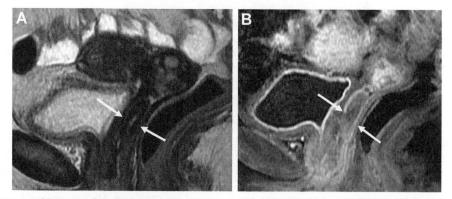

Fig. 19. 51-year-old woman found to have a large vaginal polyp on speculum examination. Sagittal T2W MRI (*A*) shows a predominately low signal 2.4 cm mass in the vagina (*arrows*). Sagittal T1W fat-suppressed postcontrast MRI (*B*) shows no significant internal enhancement (*arrows*). Pathology showed a benign fibroepithelial polyp. Histopathologically, these lesions are covered in squamous epithelium with a central fibrovascular core without atypia.

T2W MRI because of hemorrhage and necrosis (**Fig. 18**).[34] Benign fibroepithelial polyps can occur in the vagina, possibly resulting from local vaginal injury and subsequent granulation tissue response (**Fig. 19**).[35] Other mimics of malignancy include rare lesions such as paragangliomas, hemangiomas, and endometriosis.[19,21]

SUMMARY

Vaginal and vulvar malignancies are rare gynecologic malignancies strongly associated with infection by oncogenic strains of HPV. These malignancies confer significant morbidity, and advanced-stage disease is associated with poor prognosis. Early detection is essential to optimizing patient outcomes, and accurate staging is critical for guiding appropriate management. Excellent soft tissue contrast and anatomic depiction of the complex female pelvic anatomy makes MRI an important tool in the workup of vaginal and vulvar tumors, allowing assessment of local disease extent and evaluation of locoregional lymph nodes. CT and PET/CT are important complementary imaging modalities for the detection of abnormal lymph nodes and distant sites of disease.

CLINICS CARE POINTS

- SCC is the most common type and strongly associated with high risk HPV infection.
- MRI allows depiction of tumor and local extent of disease as well as regional lymph nodes.
- MRI features include focal mass or nodular thickening with intermediate T2 signal, enhancement, and restricted diffusion.
- Lymph node drainage can be variable but most commonly involves the iliac lymph nodes for the upper and middle thirds of the vagina and the inguinofemoral lymph nodes for the lower third of the vagina and vulva.

DISCLOSURE

The authors did not receive support from any organization for the submitted work. The authors have no relevant financial or nonfinancial interests to disclose.

REFERENCES

1. PDQ® Adult Treatment Editorial Board. PDQ vulvar cancer treatment. Bethesda, MD: National Cancer Institute; 2022. Available at: https://www.cancer.gov/types/vulvar/hp/vulvar-treatment-pdq. Accessed May 28, 2022.

2. PDQ® Adult Treatment Editorial Board. PDQ vaginal cancer treatment. Bethesda, MD: National Cancer Institute; 2022. Available at: https://www.cancer.gov/types/vaginal/hp/vaginal-treatment-pdq. Accessed May 28, 2022.

3. Alkatout I, Schubert M, Garbrecht N, et al. Vulvar cancer: epidemiology, clinical presentation, and management options. Int J Womens Health 2015;7: 305–13.

4. Appelbaum AH, Zuber JK, Levi-D'Ancona R, et al. Vaginal anatomy on MRI: New information obtained using distention. South Med J 2018;111(11):691–7.

5. Ferreira DM, Bezerra RO, Ortega CD, et al. Magnetic resonance imaging of the vagina: an overview for radiologists with emphasis on clinical decision making. Radiol Bras 2015;48(4):249–59.

6. Shetty AS, Menias COMR. imaging of vulvar and vaginal cancer. Magn Reson Imaging Clin N Am 2017;25(3):481–502.

7. Viswanathan C, Kirschner K, Truong M, et al. Multimodality imaging of vulvar cancer: staging, therapeutic response, and complications. AJR Am J Roentgenol 2013;200(6):1387–400.

8. Balega J, Van Trappen PO. The sentinel node in gynaecological malignancies. Cancer Imag 2006;6(1): 7–15.

9. Galgano S, Viets Z, Fowler K, et al. Practical considerations for clinical PET/MR imaging. Magn Reson Imaging Clin N Am 2017;25:335–50.

10. Adhikari P, Vietje P, Mount S. Premalignant and malignant lesions of the vagina. Diagn Histopathol 2016;23:28–34.

11. Creasman WT. Vaginal cancers. Curr Opin Obstet Gynecol 2005;17(1):71–6.

12. Sinno AK, Saraiya M, Thompson TD, et al. Human papillomavirus genotype prevalence in invasive vaginal cancer from a registry-based population. Obstet Gynecol 2014;123(4):817–21.

13. Wu X, Matanoski G, Chen VW, et al. Descriptive epidemiology of vaginal cancer incidence and survival by race, ethnicity, and age in the United States. Cancer 2008;113:2873–82.

14. Ugwu AO, Haruna M, Okunade KS, et al. Primary vaginal adenocarcinoma of intestinal-type: case report of a rare gynaecological tumour. Oxf Med Case Reports 2019;(9):omz088.

15. Parikh JH, Barton DP, Ind TE, et al. MR imaging features of vaginal malignancies. Radiographics 2008; 28(1):49–63.

16. Virarkar M, Vulasala S, Daoud T, et al. Vulvar cancer: 2021 revised FIGO staging system and the role of imaging. Cancers 2022;14(9):2264.

17. Ueda Y, Enomoto T, Kimura T, et al. Two distinct pathways to development of squamous cell carcinoma of

the vulva. J Skin Cancer 2011;2011:951250. https://doi.org/10.1155/2011/951250. Epub 2010 Sep 28. PMID: 21188235; PMCID: PMC3003991.

18. Gardner CS, Sunil J, Klopp AH, et al. Primary vaginal cancer: role of MRI in diagnosis, staging and treatment. Br J Radiol 2015;88(1052):20150033.

19. Olawaiye AB, Cuello MA, Rogers LJ. Cancer of the vulva: 2021 update. Int J Gynaecol Obstet 2021; 155(Suppl 1):7–18.

20. Matsuo K, Klar M, Nishio S, et al. Validation of the 2021 FIGO staging schema for advanced vulvar cancer. International Journal of Gynecologic Cancer 2022;32:474–9.

21. Chow L, Tsui BQ, Bahrami S, et al. Gynecologic tumor board: a radiologist's guide to vulvar and vaginal malignancies. Abdom Radiol 2021;46:5669–86.

22. Taylor MB, Dugar N, Davidson SE, et al. Magnetic resonance imaging of primary vaginal carcinoma. Clin Radiol 2007;62(6):549–55.

23. Steiner A, Alban G, Cheng T, et al. Vaginal recurrence of endometrial cancer: MRI characteristics and correlation with patient outcome after salvage radiation therapy. Abdom Radiol (NY) 2020;45(4): 1122–31.

24. Zulfiqar M, Shetty A, Yano M, et al. Imaging of the vagina: Spectrum of disease with emphasis on MRI appearance. Radiographics 2021;41(5):1549–68.

25. Gui B, Persiani S, Miccò M, et al. MRI Staging in locally advanced vulvar cancer: from anatomy to clinico-radiological findings. A multidisciplinary vulvar can team point of view. J Pers Med 2021;11(11): 1219.

26. Rajagopalan MS, Xu KM, Lin JF, et al. Adoption and impact of concurrent chemoradiation therapy for vaginal cancer: a National Cancer Data Base (NCDB) study. Gynecol Oncol 2014;135(3):495–502.

27. Stoker J, Rociu E, Schouten WR, et al. Anovaginal and rectovaginal fistulas. AJR Am J Roentgenol 2002;178(3):737–41.

28. Jia AY, Viswanathan AN. Vaginal necrosis: a rare late toxicity after radiation therapy. Gynecol Oncol 2021 Feb;160(2):602–9.

29. Jhingran A. Updates in the treatment of vaginal cancer. International Journal of Gynecologic Cancer 2022;32:344–51.

30. Zach D, Avall-Lundqvist E, Falconer H, et al. Patterns of recurrence and survival in vulvar cancer: a nationwide population-based study. Gynecol Oncol 2021;161(3):748–54.

31. Tubay M, Hostetler V, Tujo C, et al. Resident and fellow education feature what is that cyst? Common cystic lesions of the female lower genitourinary tract. Radiographics 2014;34(2):427–8.

32. Elsayes KM, Narra VR, Dillman JR, et al. Vaginal masses: magnetic resonance imaging features with pathologic correlation. Acta Radiol 2007;48(8): 921–33.

33. Touimi Benjelloun A, Ziad I, Elkaroini D, et al. Vaginal leiomyoma mimicking a cystocele (report case). Int J Surg Case Rep 2022;93:106955.

34. DeMulder D, Ascher SM. Uterine leiomyosarcoma: can MRI differentiate leiomyosarcoma from benign leiomyoma before treatment? AJR 2018;211: 1405–15.

35. Putran J, Gupta R. Vaginal polyp: an unusual cause of postmenopausal bleeding. Gynecol Surg 2011;8: 49–50.

Adnexal Mass Imaging: Contemporary Guidelines for Clinical Practice

Molly E. Roseland, MD*, Katherine E. Maturen, MD, MS,
Kimberly L. Shampain, MD, Ashish P. Wasnik, MD, Erica B. Stein, MD

KEYWORDS

- Adnexal mass • Ovarian mass • Pelvic ultrasound • O-RADS • Pelvic MRI

KEY POINTS

- First-line imaging for a suspected adnexal mass is pelvic ultrasound with Doppler.
- For sonographically indeterminate adnexal masses, contrast-enhanced pelvic MRI can be used for further characterization.
- American College of Radiology Ovarian-Adnexal Reporting Data System is a comprehensive, pattern-based scoring system for adnexal masses imaged with ultrasound and MRI, classifying lesions into evidence-based risk categories to guide appropriate management.

INTRODUCTION

Adnexal masses are commonly identified on routine imaging of the pelvis, found in 4% to 5% of asymptomatic patients undergoing screening transvaginal ultrasound (US) or computed tomography (CT).[1] Most adnexal masses are benign[2] and consequently at risk for overtreatment, as evidenced by malignancy rates among screening populations which are as low as 0.0005%,[1] with approximately nine gynecologic surgeries performed for each ovarian malignancy diagnosed in the United States.[3] Nonetheless, early recognition of true ovarian malignancies is essential, given the high mortality associated with ovarian cancer[4] and the improved outcomes when patients with ovarian cancer are managed by gynecologic oncologists.[5]

Accurate noninvasive characterization and risk stratification of adnexal masses is thus critical for optimal patient care. Historically, imaging interpretation has been relatively subjective, dependent on specialized clinical expertise,[6] with definitive diagnosis and management often performed by gynecologists via surgery. Today, with increasing imaging utilization, improved access to advanced equipment, and growing acceptance of standardized lexicon and reporting, radiologists play a larger role in guiding appropriate management. Better risk assessment may be able to reduce unnecessary surgeries (as well as associated costs and complications) for benign masses.[7]

To this end, various societies have issued guidelines for imaging, classification, and management of adnexal masses. In this review, the authors summarize these evolving recommendations, with an emphasis on newer publications relevant to practicing radiologists. The authors first discuss preferred imaging modalities and follow-up according to the American College of Radiology (ACR)[8–10] and Society for Radiologists in Ultrasound (SRU).[11,12] They then review the ACR Ovarian-Adnexal Reporting Data System (O-RADS), a set of evidence-based guidelines for risk stratification of adnexal masses by imaging morphology on US[13] and MRI (magnetic resonance imaging).[14]

Michigan Medicine, University of Michigan, University Hospital B1D502D, 1500 East Medical Center Dr., Ann Arbor, MI 48109, USA
* Corresponding author.
E-mail address: mollyroselandmd@gmail.com

Radiol Clin N Am 61 (2023) 671–685
https://doi.org/10.1016/j.rcl.2023.02.002
0033-8389/23/© 2023 Elsevier Inc. All rights reserved.

Imaging Modalities for Evaluation of Adnexal Masses: Guidance from the American College of Radiology and Society for Radiologists in Ultrasound

Pelvic ultrasound

Endorsed by the most recent ACR Appropriateness Criteria[8] and SRU,[11] pelvic US is widely accepted to be the best initial test in an asymptomatic patient with a suspected adnexal mass, regardless of menopausal or pregnancy status.

Transvaginal US is safe, reliable, and low-cost, with sufficient soft tissue resolution to accurately characterize an adnexal mass as cystic or solid. Doppler US (primarily color/power) also plays an important role in differentiating true soft tissue from avascular debris; spectral Doppler may be necessary to differentiate flow from artifact.[11] Transabdominal US is most useful for larger masses or ascites, which may be incompletely imaged transvaginally.

US allows confident diagnosis of many physiologic and benign ovarian lesions with classic US features, such as simple cysts, endometriomas, hemorrhagic cysts, and dermoid cysts.[11] As benign observations comprise most adnexal masses, US may also be routinely used for follow-up, if indicated.[8,11,12] Recommendations for follow-up of low-risk ovarian lesions are found within ACR O-RADS US (described later and detailed in **Tables 1 and 2**),[15] as well as found within SRU consensus documents from 2010 and 2020.[11,12]

US is also highly sensitive for the detection of suspicious features within adnexal masses,[8] with a sensitivity for malignancy reported as high as 100%.[16] Hence, a negative US enables confident exclusion of cancer. However, its specificity is substantially lower, ranging from 46% to 95% and varying based on mass features and interpretation methods. Therefore, US may prompt additional imaging with MRI for better characterization to improve the positive predictive value for malignancy.[8]

Pelvic MRI

In the absence of classic US features, MRI can be used for more definitive characterization of up to 25% of adnexal masses that are considered sonographically indeterminate.[8,17,18]

The ACR (via O-RADS) endorses imaging on a 1.5 or 3-T scanner, using a protocol with the following sequences: T2-weighted (T2W; multiple planes), fat-sensitive (in- and out-of-phase T1, fat-saturated T1 or T2), T1-weighted (T1W) pre-contrast, and T1 post-contrast. Dynamic post-contrast sequences should be obtained with thin slices (3 mm or less) and temporal resolution less than 15 seconds; in the absence of this capability, a single-post contrast sequence at 30 to 40 seconds can be obtained (which may limit risk assessment). Subtraction sequences may also be helpful for intrinsically T1-hyperintense lesions. In addition, diffusion-weighted imaging (DWI) should be obtained with B value greater than 1000. Image quality may be improved with the use of antimotility agents (eg, glucagon).[19–21]

Performed properly, MRI allows for the diagnosis of benign lesions with characteristic appearances, such as dermoid cysts, endometriomas, and fibromas,[17] as well as malignancies, with superior specificity and accuracy compared with US.[21,22] MRI has greater soft-tissue contrast compared with US and CT. It can image the entire adnexa in patients with prior limited US, including those with large body habitus. Larger field-of-view also enables complete characterization of large lesions and a clearer determination of mass origin (eg, extraovarian masses such as pedunculated subserosal uterine fibroids, hydrosalpinges, and or, peritoneal inclusion cysts).[21] Additionally, lack of radiation enables MRI to be safely performed in young or pregnant patients (although gadolinium-based contrast agents should be avoided in pregnancy).[8]

Contrast-enhanced MRI is particularly useful for detection of soft tissue within adnexal masses. For example, Doppler vascularity may be technically difficult to identify within small solid components of large cystic lesions. At MRI, enhancement is readily demonstrable in such tissue, as MRI is sensitive to minimal amounts of gadolinium, and because MRI shows true tissue perfusion rather than flow within discrete blood vessels. Dynamic sequences further allow a determination of enhancement patterns via time-intensity curves (TICs), which are necessary for precise risk assessment.[23,24]

Pelvic CT

CT plays no role in the dedicated workup of adnexal masses due its poor soft tissue resolution in the pelvis.[8] When a previously characterized adnexal mass has clear features of malignancy, contrast-enhanced CT of the abdomen and pelvis and CT of the chest are considered first-line imaging modalities for ovarian cancer staging, given their ability to delineate the extent of distant metastases.[9]

Of course, CT may also be the first modality on which an adnexal mass is initially identified. Updated guidance regarding need for additional imaging is provided by the ACR Incidental Findings Committee in its 2020 white paper,[10] the details of which are beyond the scope of this article.

FDG-PET/CT

Positron emission tomography using F-18-fluorodeoxyglucose (FDG-PET/CT) is not indicated

Table 1
American College of Radiology Ovarian-Adnexal Reporting and Data System (O-RADS) US classifications (version 1, 2020)

O-RADS Score	Risk Category [IOTA Model]	Lexicon Descriptors		Management	
				Pre-menopausal	Post-menopausal
0	Incomplete Evaluation [N/A]	N/A		Repeat study or alternate study	
1	Normal Ovary [N/A]	Follicle defined as a simple cyst ≤ 3 cm		None	N/A
		Corpus Luteum ≤ 3cm			
2	Almost Certainly Benign [< 1%]	Simple cyst	≤ 3 cm	N/A	None
			> 3 cm to 5 cm	None	Follow up in 1 year. *
			> 5 cm but < 10 cm	Follow up in 8 - 12 weeks	
		Classic Benign Lesions	See table on next page for descriptors and management strategies		
		Non-simple unilocular cyst, smooth inner margin	≤ 3 cm	None	Follow up in 1 year * If concerning, US specialist or MRI
			> 3 cm but < 10 cm	Follow-up in 8 - 12 weeks If concerning, US specialist	US specialist or MRI
3	Low Risk Malignancy [1-<10%]	Unilocular cyst (simple or non-simple) ≥ 10 cm		US specialist or MRI Management by gynecologist	
		Typical dermoid cysts, endometriomas, hemorrhagic cysts ≥ 10 cm			
		Unilocular cyst, with irregular inner wall (<3 mm height), any size			
		Multilocular cyst with smooth inner walls/septations, < 10 cm, CS = 1-3			
		Solid lesion with smooth outer contour, any size, CS = 1			
4	Intermediate Risk [10- < 50%]	Multilocular cyst, no solid component	Smooth inner wall, ≥ 10 cm, CS = 1-3	US specialist or MRI Management by gynecologist with gyn-oncologist consultation or solely by gyn-oncologist	
			Smooth inner wall, any size, CS = 4		
			Irregular inner wall ± irregular septation, any size, CS = any		
		Unilocular cyst with solid component	1-3 papillary projections (pp), or solid component that is not a pp, any size, CS= any		
		Multilocular cyst with solid component	Any size, CS = 1-2		
		Solid lesion	Smooth outer contour, any size, CS = 2-3		
5	High Risk [≥ 50%]	Unilocular cyst, ≥ 4 papillary projections, any size, CS = any		Gyn-oncologist	
		Multilocular cyst with solid component, any size, CS = 3-4			
		Solid lesion with smooth outer contour, any size, CS = 4			
		Solid lesion with irregular outer contour, any size, CS = any			
		Ascites and/or peritoneal nodules**			

O-RADS ultrasound risk stratification and management system

Abbreviations: CS, color score; GYN, gynecologic; IOTA, international ovarian tumor analysis; N/A, not applicable.

[a]At a minimum, at least 1-year follow-up showing stability or decrease in size is recommended with consideration of annual follow-up of up to 5 years, if stable. However, there is currently a paucity of evidence for defining the optimal duration or interval of timing for surveillance.

[b]The presence of ascites with category 1 to 2 lesion, must consider other malignant or nonmalignant etiologies of ascites.

Table 2
American College of Radiology Ovarian-Adnexal and Reporting Data System (O-RADS) US classifications (version 1, 2020)

Lexicon Descriptor	Definition	Management	
		Premenopausal	Postmenopausal
Typical hemorrhagic cyst	Reticular pattern: Fine thin intersecting lines representing fibrin strands	≤ 5 cm None	US specialist, gynecologist or MRI
	Retracting clot: An avascular echogenic component with angular, straight, or concave margins	>5 cm but < 10 cm Follow up in 8-12 weeks If persists or enlarges, referral to US specialist, gynecologist, or MRI	US specialist, gynecologist or MRI
Typical dermoid cyst < 10 cm	• Hyperechoic component with acoustic shadowing • Hyperechoic lines and dots • Floating echogenic spherical structures	Optional initial follow up in 8-12 weeks based upon confidence in diagnosis If not removed surgically, annual US follow up should then be considered *	US specialist, gynecologist, or MRI With confident diagnosis, if not removed surgically, annual US follow up should then be considered *
Typical endometriomas < 10 cm	Ground glass/homogeneous low-level echoes	US specialist or MRI if there is enlargement, changing morphology or a developing vascular component	MRI if there is enlargement, changing morphology or a developing vascular component
Simple paraovarian cyst/any size	Simple cyst separate from the ovary that typically moves independent of the ovary when pressure is applied by the transducer	None If not simple, manage per ovarian criteria	Optional single follow up study in 1 year
Typical peritoneal inclusion cyst/any size	Follows the contour of the adjacent pelvic organs or peritoneum, does not exert mass effect and typically contains septations. The ovary is either at the margin or suspended within the lesion.	Gynecologist	Gynecologist
Typical hydrosalpinx/ any size	• Incomplete septation • Tubular • Endosalpingeal folds: Short round projections around the inner wall of a fluid distended tubular structure	Gynecologist	Gynecologist

O-RADS ultrasound risk stratification and management system classic benign lesions (O-RADS 2).
[a]There is currently a paucity of evidence for defining the optimal duration or interval of timing for surveillance. Evidence supports an increasing risk of malignancy in endometriomas following menopause.

for initial adnexal mass imaging. Findings are often nonspecific, given the potential for hypermetabolism in physiologic and common benign adnexal findings, such as uterine fibroids or ovarian follicles and lack of FDG uptake in cystic or necrotic masses.[8,25] It also delivers unnecessary radiation to young and premenopausal women. PET is primarily used for problemsolving for patients with known ovarian cancer.[9] Like traditional CT, PET/CT obtained for other reasons may also reveal incidental adnexal lesions. For example, ovarian hypermetabolism in a postmenopausal woman is considered abnormal and suspicious for malignancy, warranting further evaluation with pelvic US.[17]

ULTRASOUND RISK STRATIFICATION SYSTEMS FOR ADNEXAL MASSES
History of Ultrasound Risk Assessment

Multiple classification systems for adnexal masses have been developed to improve interreader concordance and streamline characterization. Such methods are designed to communicate risk of malignancy for non-simple, non-classic lesions and are typically based on US lesion morphology, with or without additional clinical data.[26]

Several validated algorithms have been proposed by the International Ovarian Tumor Analysis (IOTA) group, a European research consortium among the first to develop and standardize techniques and terminology for adnexal US.[27] The group has also conducted the largest prospective analyses regarding US features and surgical/pathologic outcomes of adnexal masses.

IOTA first proposed the "Simple Rules" (SRs) in 2008, which consist of five benign "B" and five malignant "M" US features.[28] A lesion is considered benign if it has only B features and malignant if only M features; however, if features of both categories exist, it is considered inconclusive. Although SRs have undergone extensive validation, a significant number of lesions are inconclusive (up to 25%), requiring secondary tests for further characterization.[26]

IOTA has also created several statistical models, notably the 2014 Assessment of Different Neoplasias in the Adnexa (ADNEX) risk model,[29] which is uniquely able to estimate the probability of an adnexal mass being benign, borderline, stage I cancer, stage II–IV cancer, or secondary metastatic cancer. ADNEX incorporates three clinical and six US features.[26] Despite its validation and ongoing use in Europe,[29] adoption in North America remains limited.[15]

The SRU has also proposed informal diagnostic criteria and management for "indeterminate,

probably benign" cysts and those "worrisome for malignancy" in its 2010 consensus document.[11] These criteria have been applied in several publications,[30,31] but definitions are incompletely standardized, with limited management recommendations and no formal scoring system.[11,15]

Other investigators have also contributed to this effort. For example, the 2009 Gynecologic-Imaging RADS (GI-RADS)[32] is a 5-point scoring system not affiliated with the ACR.[15] Other algorithms occasionally referenced in the gynecologic literature include the Depriest Morphology Index[33] and the Risk of Malignancy Index (RMI).[34]

American College of Radiology Ovarian-Adnexal Reporting and Data System (O-RADS)

The ACR Ovarian-Adnexal Reporting and Data System (O-RADS) was created to standardize adnexal mass risk assessment, improve interreader agreement in reporting and management, and better define the role of MRI. O-RADS is designed to be a unified, evidence-based system of risk stratification for masses arising in the ovary and fallopian tube, created by a multidisciplinary committee of radiologists, gynecologists, and gynecologic oncologists. The system consists of both US and MRI arms, each with associated lexicons and six numeric risk categories (0–5) indicating risk of malignancy, analogous to other RADS algorithms (eg, BI-RADS for breast imaging). The O-RADS US lexicon was published in 2018,[13] and comprehensive risk categories were released in 2020,[15] with an updated version released in November 2022. The O-RADS MRI lexicon[22] and initial risk stratification[14] were initially released in 2020 to 2021, with a recent guidance article published in 2022.[21]

O-RADS US Lexicon

The O-RADS US lexicon provides a framework of clear, consistent descriptors and definitions,[13] by which adnexal lesions can be classified and assigned a risk category.

Follicles and corpora lutea are "physiologic." Non-physiologic findings are "lesions," including six classic benign lesions: hemorrhagic cysts less than 10 cm, dermoid cysts less than 10 cm, endometriomas less than 10 cm, para-ovarian cysts, peritoneal inclusion cysts, and hydrosalpinges.

For other lesions, the lexicon employs previously validated terminology developed by the IOTA group[27] to designate 5 primary non-classic, non-physiologic lesion types: unilocular cystic ± solid component, multilocular cystic ± solid component, and solid (>80% solid component).

Lesion size is defined as maximum lesion diameter. Solid lesions are further described by their external contour (smooth vs irregular) and internal tissue (presence or absence of shadowing). Cystic lesions are described by their inner margin (smooth, irregular, or with papillary projections [solid nodules >3 mm]) and fluid contents (anechoic or hyperechoic). Lesion vascularity is assessed in cyst walls or solid tissue via color score (CS), a scale of 1 to 4 indicating no flow, minimal low, moderate flow, or very strong flow, respectively, on color Doppler, based on radiologist subjective assessment. Additional terms describe extraovarian findings, free fluid, and peritoneal nodules.

O-RADS US Risk Categories, Management Recommendations, and Resources

O-RADS US proposes six risk categories[15]: 0 (incomplete), 1 (normal ovary/physiologic findings), 2 (almost certainly benign; less than 1% malignancy risk), 3 (low risk of malignancy, 1% to <10%), 4 (intermediate risk, 10% to <50%), and 5 (high risk, 50% or greater).

Specific morphologic criteria for each category were determined following analysis of data from the prospective IOTA phase 1 to 3 trials, which included a large cohort of European patients who underwent US followed by surgery/histologic diagnosis for an adnexal mass. This analysis established associations of individual lexicon descriptors with malignancy.[15]

Detailed risk category criteria for O-RADS US Version 1 (2020) are shown in **Tables 1** and **2**, also presented in Andreotti and colleagues.[15] Updated, color-coded, printable tables are

available online at the ACR O-RADS Web site (https://www.acr.org/Clinical-Resources/Reporting-and-Data-Systems/O-Rads). The "ACR Guidance App," available for iPhone and Android, also allows for streamlined calculation of risk scores in practice. A recent review in *AJR*, authored by members of the O-RADS US committee, provides a thorough summary and educational guide for new users.[35]

In general, increased soft tissue and greater vascularity are associated with a higher risk of malignancy within the O-RADS US algorithm. A few key points further summarize the original 2020 system.[15] Classic benign lesions less than 10 cm (simple cysts, endometriomas, dermoid cysts, hemorrhagic cysts) are considered O-RADS US 2, upgraded to O-RADS US 3 if greater than 10 cm. Classic non-ovarian lesions (hydrosalpinges peritoneal inclusion cysts, para-ovarian cysts) are always considered benign, O-RADS US 2. Unilocular cystic lesions are scored progressively higher with increasing soft tissue, ranging from O-RADS US 2 (entirely simple) to 3 (irregular wall), 4 (<4 papillary projections), and 5 (>4 papillary projections). **Figs 1** and **2** illustrate examples of O-RADS US 5 and O-RADS US 3 unilocular cystic lesions, respectively. Multilocular cystic lesions are scored at least O-RADS US 3 (smooth walls), upgraded to 4 or 5 based on progressively increasing vascularity, wall irregularity, and/or soft tissue. **Fig. 3** shows an O-RADS US 3 multilocular cystic lesion with MRI correlation. Solid lesions are also scored a minimum of O-RADS US 3 (smooth, no flow), upgraded to 4 with increasing vascularity or 5 with irregular margins. Lesions that are uncharacterizable by US (due to large

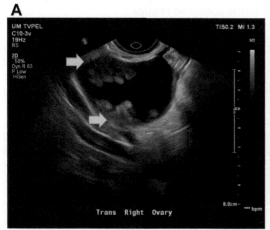 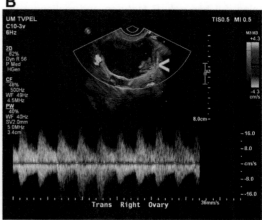

Fig. 1. A 40-year-old premenopausal woman with a unilocular cystic adnexal lesion with greater than 4 papillary projections (*yellow arrows*) on grayscale US (*A*) and moderately increased vascularity (*green arrowhead*) on color Doppler (color score [CS] 3) (*B*), O-RADS US 5. Surgically resected, pathologically proven seromucinous borderline tumor.

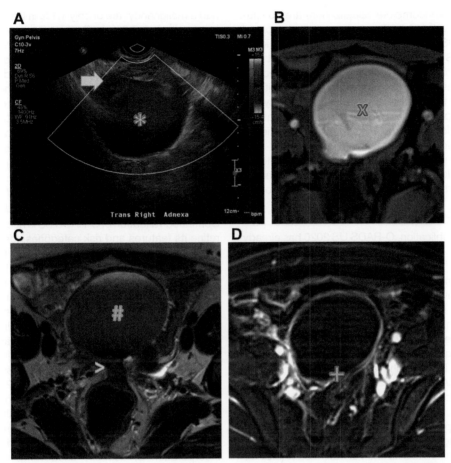

Fig. 2. A 35-year-old premenopausal woman with a unilocular cystic adnexal lesion with low-level internal echoes (*asterisk*) and irregular inner wall (*yellow arrow*) on US (*A*), suggestive of endometrioma, but technically O-RADS US 3 (low risk). Subsequent MRI (*B*, axial T1W; *C*, axial T2W; *D*, axial T1-fat-saturated subtraction) shows classic endometrioma: hyperintense on T1WI (red X in *B*), hypointense with shading on T2WI (# in *C*), smooth, thin enhancing walls (+ in *D*), O-RADS MRI 2, almost certainly benign. Dependent debris and fibrotic endometriotic plaque tethering ovary to rectum (*green arrowhead* in *C*) account for atypical US appearance. Subsequent surgery (for endometriosis) confirmed benign endometrioma.

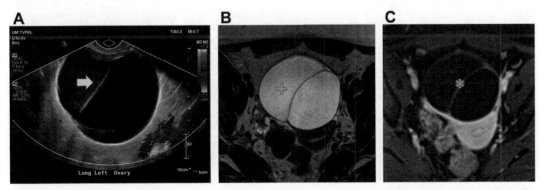

Fig. 3. A 23-year-old premenopausal woman with a multilocular cystic adnexal lesion with smooth walls (*yellow arrow*) and no vascularity by US (color score [CS] 1) (*A*), O-RADS US 3, low risk. Subsequent MRI (*B*, axial T2W; *C*, axial T1-fat-saturated post-contrast) shows a multilocular cystic lesion containing simple fluid (+ in *B*), with smooth, thin wall enhancement (* in *C*) and no soft tissue component, O-RADS MRI 3, low risk. Patient underwent left oophorectomy for ovarian torsion, with pathology showing benign serous cystadenoma.

size or poor/incomplete visualization) are considered O-RADS US 0. **Fig. 4** shows an example of an O-RADS 0 lesion further characterized by MRI.

O-RADS US has several unique features. It provides specific management and/or referral recommendations for each risk category. Although it can be applied to any adnexal mass, regardless of symptoms and patient risk factors, recommendations are designed for asymptomatic, average-risk patients, and therefore may be modified as clinically indicated. If multiple or bilateral lesions are identified, they should be scored individually, with management dictated by the lesion with the highest score.[35]

O-RADS US Validation

Since its publication, O-RADS US 2020 has already been the subject of multiple recent validation studies,[16,36–42] assessing its diagnostic performance among variable international populations, often relative to other risk stratification systems.[43]

A large meta-analysis[36] shows O-RADS US to have a high-pooled sensitivity and moderate-pooled specificity (97% and 77%, respectively), as well as high accuracy, with AUC (area under the curve) of 0.97. Basha and colleagues[37] notably found O-RADS US to have a higher sensitivity than GI-RADS or IOTA SRs (97% compared with 93% and 92%, respectively), as well as higher AUC (0.98 compared with 0.97 and 0.94), whereas Hack and colleagues[38] determined O-RADS US to have a comparable AUC to the ADNEX model (0.91 vs 0.95). O-RADS US interreader agreement has also been found to be high,[38,42] regardless of experience level,[41] similar to GI-RADS, ADNEX, and SRs.[37,41]

Malignancy rates by risk category largely fall within expected ranges,[37–40] although some tend toward their lower limits. For example, O-RADS US 3 had a malignancy rate of only 1.1% in Cao and colleagues[40] and 2.8% in Basha and colleagues,[37] compared with the expected 1% to 10% range. Likewise, O-RADS US 4 had a malignancy rate of 11.6% in Jha and colleagues,[39] compared with the expected 10% to 50% range. However, these findings may be expected given the emphasis on sensitivity for O-RADS US and the express intent of its authors to detect more malignancies and avert complications of missed ovarian cancer.[15]

O-RADS US Ongoing Research and Future Modifications

Continued validation of O-RADS US is necessary to refine its features and risk categories, ideally with larger, prospective, multicenter studies. Inclusion of patients imaged outside of cancer centers, who may have a lower risk of malignancy, is essential to refine scoring for routine use in the community. Data from the newest IOTA 5 trial (assessing conservative management for lower risk adnexal lesions) are also expected to provide valuable data to assess O-RADS US performance.[15]

The ACR O-RADS US committee issued an updated risk table in November 2022, before formal publication of this review. According to Phillips and colleagues,[43] lexicon definitions for benign and physiologic lesions are expanded and clarified. Changes to risk stratification allow incorporation of acoustic shadowing, a benign finding associated with fibrous tumors that may enable "downgrading" of solid lesions.[38] Additional changes add subcategories for O-RADS US 4, given new data indicating a relatively lower risk of malignancy in multilocular cysts without solid components and smooth solid lesions.[40]

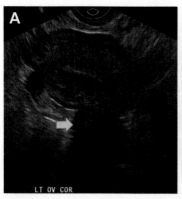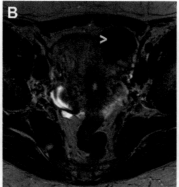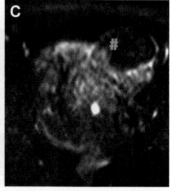

Fig. 4. A 41-year-old premenopausal woman with a poorly visualized, shadowing left adnexal mass (*yellow arrow*) by US (*A*), O-RADS US 0. Subsequent MRI (*B*, axial T2W; *C*, axial diffusion-weighted sequence with B-value 1800; *D*, axial T1-fat-saturated post-contrast) shows a homogeneous, T2-hypointense mass (*green arrowhead* in *B*) without impeded diffusion (# in *C*), considered "T2/DWI dark," diagnostic of a benign fibroma, O-RADS MRI 2. The patient was managed conservatively.

MRI RISK STRATIFICATION FOR ADNEXAL MASSES: AMERICAN COLLEGE OF RADIOLOGY OVARIAN-ADNEXAL REPORTING AND DATA SYSTEM MRI
O-RADS MRI History and Evidence Basis

ADNEX MR, proposed by Thomassin-Naggara and colleagues in 2013, was the first validated, formal MRI risk stratification system for adnexal masses,[23] and is the evidence basis and conceptual foundation for O-RADS MRI.

The development of ADNEX MR followed a similar trajectory to other ACR RADS systems. An initial lexicon of MRI features was proposed, and criteria for five evidence-based risk categories were established, based on the results of a retrospective analysis of European patients with MRI-confirmed adnexal masses and subsequent diagnosis confirmation (via surgery or long-term imaging follow-up). A multivariate model identified lexicon features with the highest positive and negative likelihood ratios for malignancy, which was used as the basis for scoring.[23] Its initial publication reported high accuracy, sensitivity, and specificity.

The prospective, multicenter EURAD study in 2020[24] further validated the predictive value of the ADNEX MR score among a larger cohort of women across Europe (1130 patients), providing sufficient evidence to establish the O-RADS MRI score. Accuracy was high (AUC 0.93–0.96), with good agreement among radiologists with different experience levels. Sensitivity and specificity also remained relatively high (93% and 91%, respectively). Of note, the system was highly effective for excluding malignancy, with a negative predictive value of 98%, indicating that a lesion with a score of 2 to 3 is very unlikely to represent malignancy.[21]

O-RADS MRI Lexicon

Following a review of the relevant literature, the ACR O-RADS committee created a consensus O-RADS MRI lexicon, available online (https://www.acr.org/-/media/ACR/Files/RADS/O-RADS/O-RADS-MR-Lexicon-Terms-Table.pdf) and detailed in Reinhold and colleagues' recent 2021 review.[22] Terms are organized into seven key components.

First, analogous to O-RADS US, an adnexal observation should be assigned a type/category: physiologic or non-physiologic (lesion). Again, lesions may be unilocular cystic ± solid component, multilocular cystic ± solid component, or solid (>80%).

Other basic features should be then assessed, including size (maximum diameter), contour (smooth or irregular), and signal intensity. Signal intensity may be homogeneous or heterogeneous and can be described on T2W, T1W, and DWI sequences. For T2W-imaging (T2WI), hyperintense signal refers to signal that is similar to cerebrospinal fluid (CSF), hypointense signal refers to signal that is similar or less intense than iliopsoas muscle, and intermediate signal refers to signal that is higher than muscle but less than CSF. For T1W-imaging (T1WI), hyperintense signal refers to signal that is similar to fat, hypointense signal refers to signal that is similar to CSF, and intermediate signal refers to signal that is similar to or higher than muscle. High DWI signal refers to signal intensity greater than fluid.

If cystic, fluid descriptors should be used. Simple fluid is similar to CSF. Non-simple fluid may be hemorrhagic (variable signal intensity/debris), endometriotic (hyperintense on T1WI, hypointense-intermediate with shading on T2WI), proteinaceous (variably hypointense on T2WI), or fat/lipid-containing (hyperintense on T1WI with dropout on fat-saturated sequences).

If enhancing solid tissue is present, it can be a papillary projection (protrusion with stalk, acute angle with wall), mural nodule (focal protrusion >3 mm, obtuse angle to wall), irregular septation (variable thickness), or larger solid portion. Vascularized soft tissue should be differentiated from "other solid components," including smooth septations, blood clots, or Rokitansky nodules in dermoids, which are not considered true "solid tissue."

Lesion walls, septations, or solid enhancing tissue should be assessed with dynamic contrast-enhanced sequences (DCE) and a TIC. Low-risk TICs demonstrate slow, progressive enhancement, less than the outer myometrium; intermediate-risk curves demonstrate a moderate initial rise, slower or equal to myometrium, followed by a plateau, and high-risk curves demonstrate a steep initial rise, faster than myometrium, followed by a plateau. If DCE is not available, a visual assessment of enhancement relative to myometrium can be performed at 30 to 40 seconds post-injection. If the uterus is absent, only low versus intermediate/high-risk curves can be identified based on absence or presence of a plateau on a TIC.

Finally, other adnexal findings can be described, including presence of free fluid, hydrosalpinges, peritoneal inclusion cysts, or peritoneal thickening/nodularity.

O-RADS MRI Concepts, Risk Categories, and Resources

Authors are careful to note that O-RADS MRI should only be applied to average risk patients without acute symptoms. It provides a score with estimated malignancy risk to inform referring clinicians, but does not suggest management, unlike O-RADS US.[21]

The complete details of the O-RADS MRI scores and risk categories are provided in **Table 3**,

Table 3
American College of Radiology Ovarian-Adnexal Reporting and Data System (O-RADS) MRI classifications (version 1, September 2020)

O-RADS MRI Score	Risk Category	Positive Predictive Value for Malignancy[a]	Lexicon Description
0	Incomplete Evaluation	N/A	N/A
1	Normal Ovaries	N/A	No ovarian lesion Follicle defined as simple cyst ≤ 3 cm in a premenopausal woman Hemorrhagic cyst ≤ 3 cm in a premenopausal woman Corpus luteum +/- hemorrhage ≤ 3 cm in a premenopausal woman
2	Almost Certainly Benign	<0.5%^	Cyst: Unilocular- any type of fluid content • No wall enhancement • No enhancing solid tissue* Cyst: Unilocular – simple or endometriotic fluid content • Smooth enhancing wall • No enhancing solid tissue Lesion with lipid content** • No enhancing solid tissue Lesion with "dark T2/dark DWI" solid tissue • Homogeneously hypointense on T2 and DWI Dilated fallopian tube - simple fluid content • Thin, smooth wall/endosalpingeal folds with enhancement • No enhancing solid tissue Para-ovarian cyst – any type of fluid • Thin, smooth wall +/- enhancement • No enhancing solid tissue
3	Low Risk	~5%^	Cyst: Unilocular – proteinaceous, hemorrhagic or mucinous fluid content*** • Smooth enhancing wall • No enhancing solid tissue Cyst: Multilocular - Any type of fluid, no lipid content • Smooth septae and wall with enhancement • No enhancing solid tissue Lesion with solid tissue (excluding T2 dark/DWI dark) • Low risk time intensity curve on DCE MRI Dilated fallopian tube – • Non-simple fluid: Thin wall /folds • Simple fluid: Thick, smooth wall/ folds • No enhancing solid tissue
4	Intermediate Risk	~50%^	Lesion with solid tissue (excluding T2 dark/DWI dark) • Intermediate risk time intensity curve on DCE MRI • If DCE MRI is not feasible, score 4 is any lesion with solid tissue (excluding T2 dark/DWI dark) that is enhancing ≤ myometrium at 30-40s on non-DCE MRI Lesion with lipid content • Large volume enhancing solid tissue
5	High Risk	~90%^	Lesion with solid tissue (excluding T2 dark/DWI dark) • High risk time intensity curve on DCE MRI • If DCE MRI is not feasible, score 5 is any lesion with solid tissue (excluding T2 dark/DWI dark) that is enhancing > myometrium at 30-40s on non-DCE MRI Peritoneal, mesenteric or omental nodularity or irregular thickening with or without ascites

Abbreviations: DCE, dynamic contrast enhancement with a time resolution of 15 s or less; DWI, diffusion-weighted images.

[a]Approximate PPV based on data from Thomassin-Naggara, et al O-RADS MRI Score for Risk Stratification of Sonographically Indeterminate Adnexal Masses. JAMA Network Open. 2020;3(1):e1919896. Please note that the PPV provided applies to the score category overall and not to individual characteristics. Definitive PPV are not currently available for individual characteristics. The PPV values for malignancy include both borderline tumors and invasive cancers.

[b]Solid tissue is defined as a lesion component that enhances and conforms to one of these morphologies: papillary projection, mural nodule, irregular septation/wall, or other larger solid portions.

[c]Minimal enhancement of Rokitansky nodules in lesion containing lipid does not change to O-RADS MRI 4.

[d]Hemorrhagic cyst ≤3 cm in premenopausal woman is O-RADS MRI 1.

From American College of Radiology Committee on O-RADS (Ovarian and Adnexal). O-RADS MRI Assessment Categories version 1 (2020). Available at: https://www.acr.org/-/media/ACR/Files/RADS/O-RADS/O-RADS-MR-Risk-Stratification-System-Table-September-2020.pdf. Accessed Aug 10 2022.

identical to a printable version of the risk table available on the ACR O-RADS website.[44] An online calculator is also available at https://www.oradsmricalc.com/, and several thorough recent reviews have been published by members of the O-RADS MRI committee.[19-21].

A few general concepts help to clarify the risk table. O-RADS MRI score 2 encompasses almost certainly benign lesions, including most unilocular cysts, endometriomas (unilocular or multilocular), fibromas (homogeneous T2/DWI dark), and dermoid cysts (intralesional fat). O-RADS MRI 2 examples are provided in **Figs. 2** (endometrioma) and **4** (fibroma). O-RADS MRI 3 (low risk) includes smooth multilocular cysts without solid tissue, smooth enhancing *non-simple* unilocular cysts (proteinaceous or hemorrhagic), and solid lesions with low-risk enhancement. **Fig. 3** shows an example of an O-RADS MRI 3 multilocular cystic lesion. O-RADS MRI 4 and 5 both contain solid tissue, differentiated based on TIC (intermediate and high-risk, respectively). **Fig. 5** illustrates an O-RADS MRI 4 lesion with associated intermediate-risk TIC. Fat-containing masses with large enhancing tissue components are also considered O-RADS MRI 4, as these may represent malignant degeneration of a dermoid cyst (or a rare immature teratoma). In the absence of DCE, masses with solid tissue enhancing equal to or less than myometrium at 30 to 50 seconds are considered O-RADS MRI 4, whereas those enhancing greater than myometrium are O-RADS MRI 5.[21] Concurrent findings of peritoneal carcinomatosis are also scored as O-RADS MRI 5, regardless of imaging features

of the primary ovarian lesion(s), as illustrated in **Fig. 6**.

Risk scores also do not preclude assignment of a precise imaging diagnosis, when possible, such as dysgerminoma, lymphoma, or borderline tumors. An example of a serous borderline tumor with classic features (hyperintense papillary architecture with hypointense internal branching on T2WI)[45] is included in **Fig. 5**.

O-RADS MRI Current Research, Validation, and Future Directions

Several additional studies of the EURAD cohort have been released since the initial O-RADS MRI publication. To identify potential scoring pitfalls, a follow-up study by Thomassin-Naggara and colleagues assessed the frequency and causes of misclassified lesions.[24] Incorrect diagnoses occurred in only 9% of cases, commonly resulting in upgrading benign lesions to potentially malignant O-RADS MRI 4 or 5. This was often related to confusion using the lexicon, such as interpreting enhancement in a dermoid cyst as suspicious "solid tissue," or misinterpretation of TICs. These are errors that may be averted in practice using the new, refined O-RADS MRI lexicon. Wengert and colleagues also confirmed that O-RADS MRI score was significantly more accurate using TICs compared to visual assessment among the EURAD cohort.[46]

Two recent publications have validated the use of O-RADS MRI outside Europe,[47,48] demonstrating a high sensitivity (91%–96%), specificity (94%–96%), and accuracy (94%–95%). There is a need for further research assessing the

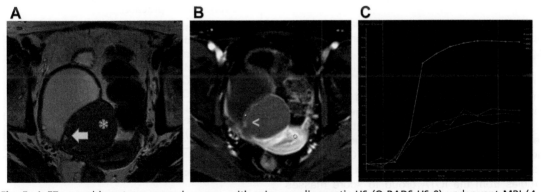

Fig. 5. A 57-year-old postmenopausal woman with prior nondiagnostic US (O-RADS US 0) underwent MRI (*A*, axial T2W; *B*, axial T1-fat-saturated post-contrast), showing a unilocular cystic adnexal lesion containing non-simple fluid (* in *A*) and multiple enhancing papillary projections (*green arrowhead in B*). Mass has classic features of serous borderline tumor, with hyperintense papillary projections with hypointense stalks on T2WI (*yellow arrow in A*). Time-intensity curves (TICs) of both normal myometrium and papillary projections (*C*, white TIC = myometrium; colored TICs = papillary projections) show papillary projections have an intermediate risk curve, O-RADS MRI 4, intermediate risk. The adnexal mass was resected with pathology confirming serous borderline tumor.

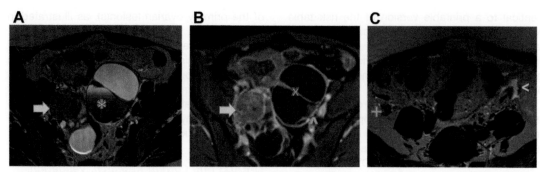

Fig. 6. A 48-year-old premenopausal woman with prior nondiagnostic US underwent pelvic MRI (*A and C*, axial T2W; *B*, axial T1-fat-saturated post-contrast), showing a solid, enhancing right adnexal mass (*yellow arrow* in *A*, *B*) and a multilocular cystic left adnexal lesion containing non-simple fluid (* in *A*) with thickened, enhancing walls (red X in *B*) and papillary projections (*blue arrowhead* in *B*). There are associated findings of peritoneal carcinomatosis, with peritoneal nodules (+ in *C*) and ascites (*green arrowhead* in *C*), O-RADS MRI 5, high risk. Surgically debulked, with pathology confirming high-grade serous carcinoma.

interreader reliability and diagnostic performance of O-RADS MRI within North America.

Other studies have suggested potential modifications to O-RADS MRI criteria, particularly for the intermediate risk category, proposing additional features of cystic masses that may be more suggestive of malignancy (larger size, more locules, impeded diffusion),[49] or suggesting defined ADC (apparent diffusion coefficient) thresholds.[50] Two upcoming trials using O-RADS MRI are also currently in process, including ASCORDIA in France, evaluating whether the system can help avert unnecessary surgeries for benign lesions, and another in the United Kingdom, assessing the value of adding MRI to the intial treatment for ovarian cancer.[21] The results of these ongoing studies are likely to inform future iterations of O-RADS MRI.

SUMMARY AND CONCLUSIONS

Evidence-based guidelines are available to guide appropriate imaging, risk assessment, and management for adnexal masses.

The ACR and SRU endorse pelvic US as the preferred initial imaging modality to characterize most adnexal masses. For lesions that remain indeterminate, pelvic MRI is performed.

Various classification and risk stratification systems have been developed to help interpret adnexal imaging findings. ACR O-RADS US uses terminology and data from prior large studies from the IOTA group to score masses from 0 to 5 based on the risk of malignancy, with associated management recommendations. ACR O-RADS MRI expands on an existing risk model (ADNEX-MR), scoring adnexal masses on a scale of 0 to 5 based on the risk of malignancy. The governing concept of O-RADS is consistent across modalities: solid tissue with

abundant vascularity confers the highest risk of malignancy.

CLINICS CARE POINTS

- Guidance from the American College of Radiology (ACR) Appropriateness Criteria suggests pelvic ultrasound (US) for initial evaluation of an adnexal mass. Pelvic MRI can be performed if US is indeterminate.

- The ACR O-RADS provides a unified algorithm for classifying adnexal masses by both US and MRI, using consistent terminology and risk categories to standardize reporting and guide appropriate management. An increasing body of evidence supports Ovarian-Adnexal Reporting and Data System (O-RADS) use in routine clinical practice.

- Adnexal lesions with larger soft tissue components and high vascularity/enhancement receive the highest scores in both O-RADS US and MRI systems. Specific criteria for each risk category are readily available on the ACR O-RADS website, with numerous other resources available for new users (review articles, phone applications, and online calculators).

DISCLOSURES

M.E. Roseland, E.B. Stein, K.L. Shampain: Nothing to disclose.

DISCLOSURE

K.E. Maturen: Royalties, Elsevier Inc and Wolters Kluwer NV (unrelated to article). A.P. Wasnik:

None related to this article. Unrelated disclosures include royalties, Elsevier Inc; royalties, intellectual property, licensed by the University of Michigan to Applied Morphomics, Inc; and research support, payable to the University of Michigan from Sequana Medical, NV.

REFERENCES

1. Buys SS, Partridge E, Greene MH, et al. Ovarian cancer screening in the Prostate, Lung, Colorectal and Ovarian (PLCO) cancer screening trial: findings from the initial screen of a randomized trial. Am J Obstet Gynecol 2005;193(5):1630–9.

2. Hack K, Glanc P. The Abnormal Ovary: Evolving Concepts in Diagnosis and Management. Obstet Gynecol Clin N Am 2019;46(4):607–24.

3. Siegel RL, Miller KD, Jemal A. Cancer statistics. CA Cancer J Clin 2019;69(1):7–34.

4. Webb PM, Jordan SJ. Epidemiology of epithelial ovarian cancer. Best Pract Res Clin Obstet Gynaecol 2017;41:3–14.

5. Woo YL, Kyrgiou M, Bryant A, et al. Centralisation of services for gynaecological cancers - a Cochrane systematic review. Gynecol Oncol 2012;126(2):286–90.

6. Sokalska A, Timmerman D, Testa AC, et al. Diagnostic accuracy of transvaginal ultrasound examination for assigning a specific diagnosis to adnexal masses. Ultrasound Obstet Gynecol 2009;34(4):462–70.

7. Froyman W, Wynants L, Landolfo C, et al. Validation of the Performance of International Ovarian Tumor Analysis (IOTA) Methods in the Diagnosis of Early Stage Ovarian Cancer in a Non-Screening Population. Diagnostics 2017;7(2). https://doi.org/10.3390/diagnostics7020032.

8. Expert Panel on Women's I, Atri M, Alabousi A, et al. ACR Appropriateness Criteria((R)) Clinically Suspected Adnexal Mass, No Acute Symptoms. J Am Coll Radiol 2019;16(5S):S77–93.

9. Expert Panel on Women's I, Kang SK, Reinhold C, et al. ACR Appropriateness Criteria((R)) Staging and Follow-Up of Ovarian Cancer. J Am Coll Radiol 2018;15(5S):S198–207.

10. Patel MD, Ascher SM, Horrow MM, et al. Management of Incidental Adnexal Findings on CT and MRI: A White Paper of the ACR Incidental Findings Committee. J Am Coll Radiol 2020;17(2):248–54.

11. Levine D, Brown DL, Andreotti RF, et al. Management of asymptomatic ovarian and other adnexal cysts imaged at US: Society of Radiologists in Ultrasound Consensus Conference Statement. Radiology 2010;256(3):943–54.

12. Levine D, Patel MD, Suh-Burgmann EJ, et al. Simple Adnexal Cysts: SRU Consensus Conference Update on Follow-up and Reporting. Radiology 2019;293(2):359–71.

13. Andreotti RF, Timmerman D, Benacerraf BR, et al. Ovarian-Adnexal Reporting Lexicon for Ultrasound: A White Paper of the ACR Ovarian-Adnexal Reporting and Data System Committee. J Am Coll Radiol 2018;15(10):1415–29.

14. Thomassin-Naggara I, Poncelet E, Jalaguier-Coudray A, et al. Ovarian-Adnexal Reporting Data System Magnetic Resonance Imaging (O-RADS MRI) Score for Risk Stratification of Sonographically Indeterminate Adnexal Masses. JAMA Netw Open 2020;3(1):e1919896.

15. Andreotti RF, Timmerman D, Strachowski LM, et al. O-RADS US Risk Stratification and Management System: A Consensus Guideline from the ACR Ovarian-Adnexal Reporting and Data System Committee. Radiology 2020;294(1):168–85.

16. Hiett AK, Sonek JD, Guy M, et al. Performance of IOTA Simple Rules, Simple Rules risk assessment, ADNEX model and O-RADS in differentiating between benign and malignant adnexal lesions in North American women. Ultrasound Obstet Gynecol 2022;59(5):668–76.

17. Anthoulakis C, Nikoloudis N. Pelvic MRI as the "gold standard" in the subsequent evaluation of ultrasound-indeterminate adnexal lesions: a systematic review. Gynecol Oncol 2014;132(3):661–8.

18. Van Calster B, Timmerman D, Bourne T, et al. Discrimination between benign and malignant adnexal masses by specialist ultrasound examination versus serum CA-125. J Natl Cancer Inst 2007;99(22):1706–14.

19. Sadowski EA, Maturen KE, Rockall A, et al. Ovary: MRI characterisation and O-RADS MRI. Br J Radiol 2021;94(1125). 20210157.

20. Sadowski EA, Stein EB, Thomassin-Naggara I, et al. O-RADS MRI After Initial Ultrasound for Adnexal Lesions: AJR Expert Panel Narrative Review. AJR Am J Roentgenol 2022. https://doi.org/10.2214/AJR.22.28084.

21. Sadowski EA, Thomassin-Naggara I, Rockall A, et al. O-RADS MRI Risk Stratification System: Guide for Assessing Adnexal Lesions from the ACR O-RADS Committee. Radiology 2022;303(1):35–47.

22. Reinhold C, Rockall A, Sadowski EA, et al. Ovarian-Adnexal Reporting Lexicon for MRI: A White Paper of the ACR Ovarian-Adnexal Reporting and Data Systems MRI Committee. J Am Coll Radiol 2021;18(5):713–29.

23. Thomassin-Naggara I, Aubert E, Rockall A, et al. Adnexal masses: development and preliminary validation of an MR imaging scoring system. Radiology 2013;267(2):432–43.

24. Thomassin-Naggara I, Belghitti M, Milon A, et al. O-RADS MRI score: analysis of misclassified cases in

a prospective multicentric European cohort. Eur Radiol 2021;31(12):9588–99.

25. Forstner R, Thomassin-Naggara I, Cunha TM, et al. ESUR recommendations for MR imaging of the sonographically indeterminate adnexal mass: an update. Eur Radiol 2017;27(6):2248–57.

26. Moro F, Esposito R, Landolfo C, et al. Ultrasound evaluation of ovarian masses and assessment of the extension of ovarian malignancy. Br J Radiol 2021;94(1125):20201375.

27. Timmerman D, Valentin L, Bourne TH, et al. Terms, definitions and measurements to describe the sonographic features of adnexal tumors: a consensus opinion from the International Ovarian Tumor Analysis (IOTA) Group. Ultrasound Obstet Gynecol 2000;16(5):500–5.

28. Timmerman D, Testa AC, Bourne T, et al. Simple ultrasound-based rules for the diagnosis of ovarian cancer. Ultrasound Obstet Gynecol 2008;31(6):681–90.

29. Van Calster B, Van Hoorde K, Valentin L, et al. Evaluating the risk of ovarian cancer before surgery using the ADNEX model to differentiate between benign, borderline, early and advanced stage invasive, and secondary metastatic tumours: prospective multicentre diagnostic study. BMJ 2014;349:g5920.

30. Maturen KE, Blaty AD, Wasnik AP, et al. Risk Stratification of Adnexal Cysts and Cystic Masses: Clinical Performance of Society of Radiologists in Ultrasound Guidelines. Radiology 2017;285(2):650–9.

31. Patel-Lippmann KK, Sadowski EA, Robbins JB, et al. Comparison of International Ovarian Tumor Analysis Simple Rules to Society of Radiologists in Ultrasound Guidelines for Detection of Malignancy in Adnexal Cysts. AJR Am J Roentgenol 2020;214(3):694–700.

32. Amor F, Alcazar JL, Vaccaro H, et al. GI-RADS reporting system for ultrasound evaluation of adnexal masses in clinical practice: a prospective multicenter study. Ultrasound Obstet Gynecol 2011;38(4):450–5.

33. DePriest PD, Shenson D, Fried A, et al. A morphology index based on sonographic findings in ovarian cancer. Gynecol Oncol 1993;51(1):7–11.

34. Jacobs I, Oram D, Fairbanks J, et al. A risk of malignancy index incorporating CA 125, ultrasound and menopausal status for the accurate preoperative diagnosis of ovarian cancer. Br J Obstet Gynaecol 1990;97(10):922–9.

35. Strachowski LM, Jha P, Chawla TP, et al. O-RADS for Ultrasound: A User's Guide, From the AJR Special Series on Radiology Reporting and Data Systems. AJR Am J Roentgenol 2021;216(5):1150–65.

36. Vara J, Manzour N, Chacon E, et al. Ovarian Adnexal Reporting Data System (O-RADS) for Classifying Adnexal Masses: A Systematic Review and Meta-Analysis. Cancers 2022;14(13). https://doi.org/10.3390/cancers14133151.

37. Basha MAA, Metwally MI, Gamil SA, et al. Comparison of O-RADS, GI-RADS, and IOTA simple rules regarding malignancy rate, validity, and reliability for diagnosis of adnexal masses. Eur Radiol 2021;31(2):674–84.

38. Hack K, Gandhi N, Bouchard-Fortier G, et al. External Validation of O-RADS US Risk Stratification and Management System. Radiology 2022;304(1):114–20.

39. Jha P, Gupta A, Baran TM, et al. Diagnostic Performance of the Ovarian-Adnexal Reporting and Data System (O-RADS) Ultrasound Risk Score in Women in the United States. JAMA Netw Open 2022;5(6):e2216370.

40. Cao L, Wei M, Liu Y, et al. Validation of American College of Radiology Ovarian-Adnexal Reporting and Data System Ultrasound (O-RADS US): Analysis on 1054 adnexal masses. Gynecol Oncol 2021;162(1):107–12.

41. Lai HW, Lyu GR, Kang Z, et al. Comparison of O-RADS, GI-RADS, and ADNEX for Diagnosis of Adnexal Masses: An External Validation Study Conducted by Junior Sonologists. J Ultrasound Med 2022;41(6):1497–507.

42. Pi Y, Wilson MP, Katlariwala P, et al. Diagnostic accuracy and inter-observer reliability of the O-RADS scoring system among staff radiologists in a North American academic clinical setting. Abdom Radiol (NY) 2021;46(10):4967–73.

43. Phillips CH, Guo Y, Strachowski LM, et al. The Ovarian/Adnexal Reporting and Data System for Ultrasound: From Standardized Terminology to Optimal Risk Assessment and Management. Can Assoc Radiol J 2022;13. https://doi.org/10.1177/08465371221108057. 8465371221108057.

44. American College of Radiology Committee on O-RADS™ (Ovarian and Adnexal). O-RADS MRI Assessment Categories version 1. 2020. Available at: https://www.acr.org/-/media/ACR/Files/RADS/O-RADS/O-RADS-MR-Risk-Stratification-System-Table-September-2020.pdf. Accessed August 10, 2022.

45. Tsuboyama T, Sato K, Ota T, et al. MRI of Borderline Epithelial Ovarian Tumors: Pathologic Correlation and Diagnostic Challenges. Radiographics 2022;220068.

46. Wengert GJ, Dabi Y, Kermarrec E, et al. O-RADS MRI Classification of Indeterminate Adnexal Lesions: Time-Intensity Curve Analysis Is Better Than Visual Assessment. Radiology 2022;303(2):E28.

47. Aslan S, Tosun SA. Diagnostic accuracy and validity of the O-RADS MRI score based on a simplified MRI protocol: a single tertiary center retrospective study. Acta Radiol 2021. https://doi.org/10.1177/02841851211060413. 2841851211060413.

48. Pereira PN, Yoshida A, Sarian LO, et al. Assessment of the performance of the O-RADS MRI score for the evaluation of adnexal masses, with technical notes. Radiol Bras 2022;55(3):137–44.

49. Assouline V, Dabi Y, Jalaguier-Coudray A, et al. How to improve O-RADS MRI score for rating adnexal masses with cystic component? Eur Radiol 2022; 32(9):5943–53.

50. Hottat NA, Badr DA, Van Pachterbeke C, et al. Added Value of Quantitative Analysis of Diffusion-Weighted Imaging in Ovarian-Adnexal Reporting and Data System Magnetic Resonance Imaging. J Magn Reson Imaging 2022;56(1):158–70.

MR Imaging of Gynecologic Tumors
Pearls, Pitfalls, and Tumor Mimics

Michela Lupinelli, MD[a],*, Martina Sbarra, MD[b],
Aoife Kilcoyne, MBCCh, BAO[c,d], Aradhana M. Venkatesan, MD[e],
Stephanie Nougaret, MD, PhD[f,g]

KEYWORDS

- Gynecologic malignancies • Endometrial cancer • Cervical cancer • Ovarian cancer • MR imaging
- Pitfalls • Tumor mimics

KEY POINTS

- In patients with endometrial cancer, MR imaging allows accurate detection of crucial prognostic factors. Common pitfalls are in the detection of myometrial invasion, cervical stroma, and vaginal invasion and in the distinction between direct adnexal spread and ovarian metastasis.
- In patients with cervical cancer, MR imaging is fundamental to treatment planning providing important information about tumor size, parametrial invasion, and vaginal infiltration. Difficulties can arise in the evaluation of small tumors, parametrial and vaginal invasion.
- When an adnexal mass is classified as sonographically indeterminate, MR imaging adds valuable evidence on the various components, particularly the presence of solid tissue. In this case, particular attention should be paid in the distinction between solid and non-solid tissue and in the identification of peritoneal carcinomatosis.
- A wide variety of pathologies in the pelvis can mimic a gynecologic tumor, but the presence of specific MR imaging features can maximize diagnostic accuracy.

INTRODUCTION

Gynecologic malignancies lead to nearly half a million deaths around the world annually.[1] Accurately quantifying disease burden and expediting the appropriate first line treatment is important for optimal clinical outcomes. Management pathways are highly dependent on tumor staging and therefore high-quality pre-treatment imaging assessment is essential. MR imaging has an increasing role at diagnosis and in guiding the management of patients with gynecologic malignancies due to its exquisite anatomical detail and ability to quantify tumor burden and response to treatment.[2–4] As such, MR imaging has been incorporated into many gynecologic cancer guidelines to assess tumor burden.[5–7]

The aim of this article is to demonstrate how MR imaging can be useful in the risk stratification and management of patients with endometrial, cervical, and ovarian cancer. There is a specific focus on the most common pitfalls and tumor

[a] Department of Radiology, Morgagni-Pierantoni Hospital, Via Carlo Forlanini 34, 47121, Forlì, Italy; [b] Unit of Diagnostic Imaging, Fondazione Policlinico Universitario Campus Bio-medico, Via Alvaro Del Portillo, 200, Roma 00128, Italy; [c] Department of Radiology, Massachusetts General Hospital, 55 Fruit Street, Boston, MA 02114, USA; [d] Harvard Medical School, Boston, MA, USA; [e] Department of Abdominal Imaging, Division of Diagnostic Imaging, The University of Texas MD Anderson Cancer Center, 1400 Pressler Street, Houston, TX 77030, USA; [f] Department of Radiology, IRCM, Montpellier Cancer Research Institute, Montpellier 34090, France; [g] INSERM, U1194, University of Montpellier, Montpellier 34295, France
* Corresponding author.
E-mail address: michela.lupinelli@auslromagna.it

Radiol Clin N Am 61 (2023) 687–711
https://doi.org/10.1016/j.rcl.2023.02.011
0033-8389/23/© 2023 Elsevier Inc. All rights reserved.

mimics that radiologists should be aware of when evaluating patients with gynecologic malignancy.

ENDOMETRIAL CANCER

Endometrial cancer (EC) is the sixth most common cancer in women worldwide[1]

Pelvic MR imaging is recommended by the American College of Radiology (ACR) and European Society of Urogenital Radiology (ESUR) Guidelines[3,8] for pre-operative evaluation of EC as it allows risk stratification through the assessment of myometrial invasion (MI), in conjunction with tumor grade, histology, and molecular subtype. Moreover, it plays a key role in the assessment of cervical stroma invasion (CSI), the identification of suspicious lymph nodes, adjuvant treatment planning in locally advanced disease,

---

(4 cm in some centers if exophytic), tumor distance $\geq$1 cm from the internal os (0.5 cm in some centers) and with <50% CSI. Treatment options include cone biopsy for stage IA1 disease and radical trachelectomy (cervical excision with uterovaginal anastomosis) for stages IA2 and IB1.[26]

MR imaging has demonstrated great accuracy in the assessment of crucial factors to determine eligibility for FST (tumor size, distance to the internal cervical os, PMI, and lymph node metastases).[4,50,54,55] The internal os, an important landmark for FST consideration, is defined as the waist of the uterus at which the low-SI cervical stroma becomes intermediate-SI myometrium on sagittal T2WI.[4,50]

The addition of DWI enables visualization of small tumors and assessment of the depth of CSI, increasing tumor margin conspicuity as compared to evaluation based upon T2WI alone. The addition of DWI in the sagittal plane, specifically, facilitates the assessment of tumor size especially cranio-caudal length, and tumor extent including tumor-to-internal cervical os distance.[4,7,50]

The use of multi-phase contrast-enhanced MR imaging is optional but useful to identify small tumors with early enhancement within the otherwise hypoenhancing stroma.[4,7,50]

FST in OC

In pre-menopausal women, most common ovarian neoplasms are primary germ cell tumors (mature or immature teratomas) and epithelial borderline tumors. Invasive epithelial OCs and sex-cord stromal tumors are less common.[40]

For a patient who wishes to preserve her fertility, surgical staging with unilateral salpingo-oophorectomy and preservation of the contralateral ovary and uterus can be proposed.[56] This is only feasible when low-grade stage IA epithelial carcinomas, any stage malignant germ cell tumors, sex-cord stromal tumors, and borderline tumors are present.[56]

Surgery remains the basis of the initial management of all ovarian neoplasms, allowing systematic staging and tumor resection to obtain an accurate histologic diagnosis, but MR imaging plays an important role in the selection of those patients who may benefit from FST, namely in identifying specific T1 and T2 features to guide the histologic diagnosis (eg, the presence of fat, blood, or solid components) and identifying the presence of extra-ovarian disease which contraindicates FST.[4]

Box 1
Fertility-sparing treatment in patients with gynecologic malignancies

FST in EC

10% of EC occurs in pre-menopausal women.[1] Treatment options for patients who wish to preserve their fertility can be considered in endometrium-confined disease.[49] The presence of genetic risk factors, MI, CSI, ovarian or lymph node metastases contraindicates the possibility of FST.[49] MR imaging is mandatory in the staging of these patients as it can confirm endometrium-confined disease, by evaluating the presence of an uninterrupted low-SI subendometrial layer on T2WI and a continuous layer of early enhancement on multi-phase contrast-enhanced MR imaging (35–50 s) that represents the intact junctional zone which excludes MI.[4,50] Occasionally, in pre-menopausal patients, subendometrial enhancement may be absent. In this case, the inner surface of the enhanced myometrium should be smooth and sharply demarcated to confirm endometrium-confined disease.[4]

FST in CC

CC represents the third most common neoplasm among women of childbearing age.[1]

FST is appropriate in selected candidates with CCs and endorsed by both the European Society Guidelines (ESMO, ESGO/ESTRO/ESP) and National Cancer Care Network.[4,26,51–53] Candidates eligible for FST are those with squamous cell carcinoma or usual-type (HPV-related) adenocarcinoma, tumor size $\leq$2 cm

Abbreviations: CC, cervical cancer; CSI, cervical stroma invasion; DWI, diffusion-weighted imaging; EC, endometrial cancer; ESGO, European society of gynecological oncology; ESMO, European society of medical oncology; ESP, European society of pathology; ESTRO, European society of radiation oncology; FST, fertility-sparing treatment; HPV, human papilloma virus; MI, myometrial invasion; MR imaging, magnetic resonance imaging; OC, ovarian cancer; PMI, parametrial invasion; SI, signal intensity; WI, weighted imaging.

and fertility sparing treatment (FST) planning.[3,8] The role of MR imaging in FST planning is depicted in **Box 1.** A representative MR imaging protocol for EC[3] is summarized in **Table 1.**

On T2-weighted imaging (T2WI), EC is of intermediate-to-high signal intensity (SI), appearing hyperintense compared to the myometrium and associated with restricted diffusion on diffusion-weighted imaging (DWI). Generally, EC enhances earlier than normal endometrium but later than adjacent myometrium, thus appearing hypointense on post-contrast images compared to the adjacent myometrium.[9]

Common pitfalls and their mitigations are illustrated in **Table 2.**

Pearls

Myometrial invasion

The degree of MI correlates with lymphovascular space invasion (LVSI), nodal metastasis, tumor recurrence, and prognosis.[10] MR imaging accuracy in the evaluation of the depth of MI ranges from 83% to 92%, especially when T2-weighted imaging (T2-WI), DWI, and post-contrast sequences are examined together.[11,12] It is essential to understand that disruption of the inner myometrial layer, the junctional zone, is indicative of MI.[13] Additional important concepts pertinent to the evaluation of MI in EC are summarized in **Box 2.**

Cervical stroma invasion

The presence of CSI is associated with a higher risk of LVSI and lymph nodes metastases, with the presence of CSI consistent with a Federation of Gynecology and Obstetrics (FIGO) stage II tumor.[14] To accurately diagnose CSI, the low-SI of the cervical stroma must be disrupted by the intermediate-SI of the endometrial tumor on T2WI.[3] On DWI, CSI is suggested by the presence of high-SI tissue on T2WI that disrupts the cervical stroma, associated with corresponding low-SI on apparent diffusion coefficient (ADC) map. On

---

Table 1
Representative MR imaging protocol for endometrial cancer

	EC
T1 sequences of the pelvis	Axial plane T1WI of the pelvis is optional.
T2 sequences of the pelvis	Sagittal T2WI of the pelvis is recommended. • Small-FOV[a] axial oblique (perpendicular to the endometrial cavity) T2WI is recommended. • Small-FOV[a] coronal oblique (parallel to the endometrial cavity) T2WI is optional. Slice thickness ≤ 4 mm is recommended. Fat saturation is not recommended.
DWI sequences	DWI-MR imaging is recommended. A minimum of 2 b values is recommended (low b = 0–50 s/mm, high b = 800–1000 s/mm)
Contrast-enhanced imaging	Fat-saturated contrast-enhanced T1W sequences are recommended. Images can be acquired via multi-phase contrast-enhanced imaging or as a single sequence 2 min and 30 s after contrast administration.
Lymph node and kidney evaluation	Axial T2WI from the renal hila to the pubic symphysis is recommended. Axial DWI from the renal hila to the pubic symphysis is recommended in patients with grade 3 endometrioid and non-endometrioid tumors.

Abbreviations: DWI, diffusion-weighted imaging; FOV, field-of-view; WI, weighted imaging.
[a] Recommended FOV: 24 to 26 cm; Matrix: 256 to 320 × 256 to 320.

Table 2
MR imaging pitfalls in the evaluation of endometrial cancer

	Pitfall	HOW to Resolve It
Myometrial invasion	Myometrium compressed by the tumor	On *T2WI, DWI and multi-phase contrast-enhanced MR imaging*: To exclude MI, the junctional zone must be seen as an uninterrupted low SI line on T2WI and DWI and as an uninterrupted hyperintense line on early phase contrast-enhanced MR imaging.
	Tumor isointense on T2WI	*DWI* will show restricted tumor diffusion, allowing the differentiation of pathologic from normal tissue.
	Leiomyomas or adenomyosis	*DWI and contrast-enhanced MR imaging* can improve tumor delineation
	Cornual tumor extension	*DWI and contrast-enhanced MR imaging* can help better delineate the tumor in the uterine corna where the myometrium is thinner
Cervical stroma invasion	The tumor protrudes into the cervical canal or distends it without CSI	On *DWI*, CSI is suggested by the presence of a high SI mass (with low-SI on ADC maps) disrupting the cervical stroma. On *multi-phase contrast-enhanced MR imaging*, CSI is suggested when the normal enhancement is disrupted by a hypoenhancing tumor, best assessed on delayed phase images (4–5 min).
EC with ovarian metastases vs. synchronous primary cancers of the ovary	The distinction between direct adnexal spread or ovarian metastasis	On *T2WI, DWI and contrast-enhanced MR imaging*: *Ovarian Metastasis:* When a large endometrial tumor is associated with a small ovarian lesion; when bilateral ovarian involvement is present or when the ovarian and uterine masses are morphologically similar *Synchronous primary ovarian malignancy:* When a small, low-grade endometrial tumor and a large unilateral complex ovarian mass (with or without endometriosis) are present
Vaginal involvement	The presence of small vaginal implants	Vaginal wall implants will be associated with wall thickening, and are

(continued on next page)

Table 2 (continued)		
	Pitfall	**HOW to Resolve It**
		intermediate-to-high SI on *T2WI*, associated with restricted diffusion on *DWI*. *DWI* is also helpful to detect small vaginal implants that are subtle on T2WI.
Fertility sparing treatment	Assessment of endometrium-confined disease when subendometrial enhancement is not present	Endometrium-confined disease will demonstrate an uninterrupted low-SI subendometrial layer on *T2WI* and a continuous layer of enhancement on early phase *contrast-enhanced MR imaging* (35–50 s) exclude MI. When subendometrial enhancement is not present, the inner surface of the enhanced myometrium should be smooth and sharply demarcated.

Abbreviations: ADC, apparent diffusion coefficient; DWI, diffusion-weighted imaging; SI, signal intensity; WI, weighted imaging.

contrast-enhanced MR imaging, CSI is demonstrated when the normal enhancement is disrupted by a hypoenhancing tumor, best assessed on delayed phase images (4–5 min after contrast injection)[3] (**Fig. 3**).

Pitfalls

Myometrial invasion

- *Myometrium compressed by the tumor:* To exclude MI in situations where the tumor compresses the myometrium, the junctional zone must be seen as an uninterrupted low-SI line on T2WI and DWI and as an uninterrupted hyperintense line on early phase contrast-enhanced MR imaging.[9]
- *Tumor isointense on T2WI:* When EC appears isointense on T2WI, thus less distinguishable, DWI will demonstrate restricted tumor diffusion, allowing the differentiation of pathologic from normal tissue.[15]
- *Leiomyomas or adenomyosis:* Adenomyosis leads to increased thickness of the junctional zone. In this setting, DWI and multi-phase contrast-enhanced MR can improve tumor delineation.[16]
- *Cornual tumor extension:* When tumor extends into the uterine cornu where the myometrium is thinner, the addition of multi-phase contrast-enhanced MR imaging and

DWI can significantly improve pre-operative staging accuracy.[17]

Cervical stroma invasion
The presence of tumor extension into the endocervical canal alone is not diagnostic of CSI and the diagnosis can only be made if disruption of the cervical stroma is present.[3] Occasionally, the tumor can invade cervical stroma through the adjacent myometrium without endocervical mucosal invasion.[9]

Direct adnexal spread or ovarian metastasis
Distinguishing EC with ovarian metastases from synchronous primary cancers of the ovary is clinically significant as it affects prognosis.[18] Although an important distinction, this diagnosis can be a challenge to make on imaging. When a large EC is associated with a small ovarian lesion, when bilateral ovarian involvement is present or when there is morphologic similarity between ovarian and uterine masses, the possibility of an ovarian metastasis should be raised. However, a small, low-grade EC detected in the presence of a large unilateral complex ovarian mass (with or without endometriosis) raises a greater likelihood of a synchronous primary ovarian malignancy.[19]

Vaginal involvement
Vaginal involvement can occur by direct spread or secondary to the presence of vaginal metastasis

("drop metastases"). When implants are small, DWI and contrast-enhanced MR imaging are particularly helpful in their detection.[3]

Mimics

Endometrial hyperplasia or polyps

Benign conditions, such as endometrial hyperplasia or polyps, can mimic an EC. Pedunculated lesions or intra-tumoral cystic changes are seen more frequently in endometrial polyps than in EC, but such morphologic features on T2WI alone may not be enough to differentiate these lesions.[20] The use of DWI and the analysis of ADC values can help in this scenario.[21]

On occasion, a submucosal leiomyoma may be mistaken for EC on transvaginal ultrasound. In this case, the low-SI of leiomyomas on T2WI allows for differentiation between these lesions.[20]

CERVICAL CANCER

Globally, cervical cancer (CC) is the fourth most common cancer in women, and the most common gynecologic malignancy worldwide.[1]

According to the ACR and the ESUR guidelines,[7,22] pelvic MR imaging is recommended in the pre-operative staging of CC as it is particularly accurate for the detection of tumor size and parametrial infiltration (PMI) and provides useful information on local spread to adjacent structures and lymph-node status.[23] A representative MR imaging protocol[7] for CC is summarized in **Table 3.**

Box 2
Myometrial invasion in endometrial cancer

MI is a fundamental prognostic factor in EC. According to the International FIGO staging system,[14] EC is staged IA when MI is absent or less than 50% and IB when more than 50% invasion into myometrium is present.

The depth of MI is defined as the ratio between the distance from the inner edge of the myometrium to maximum tumor extension into the myometrium and total myometrial thickness (Figs. 1 and 2).

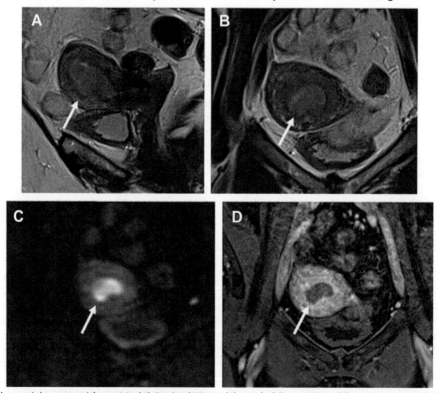

Fig 1 Endometrial tumor without MI. (*A*) Sagittal T2WI, (*B*) axial oblique T2WI, (*C*) axial DWI and (*D*) gadolinium-enhanced axial T1W fat-saturated images. (*A, B*) The T2 low-SI of the inner myometrial layer, the junctional zone, remains visible and well-demarcated, indicative of disease confined to the endometrium (*arrows*). (*C*) On DWI the junctional zone appears smooth and sharply demarcated (*arrows*). (*D*) On post-contrast imaging, the junctional zone demonstrates early enhancement and appears uninterrupted (*arrow*).

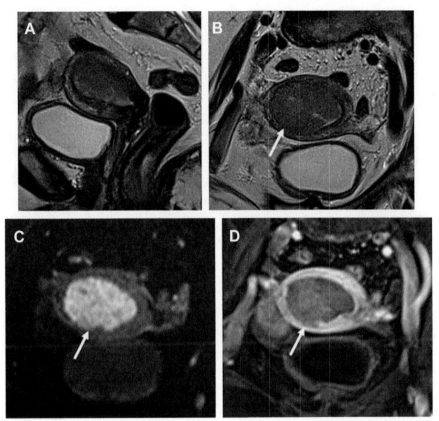

Fig 2 Endometrial tumor with MI. (*A*) Sagittal T2WI, (*B*) axial oblique T2WI, (*C*) axial DWI, and (*D*) gadolinium-enhanced axial T1W fat-saturated images. (*A, B*) The T2 low-SI of the junctional zone is disrupted in the right posterior aspect of the uterine body (*arrows*). (*C, D*) Tumor margins are ill-defined and spiculated on DWI and contrast-enhanced MR imaging (*arrows*). (*D*) The early enhanced junctional zone is interrupted on post-contrast image (*arrow*).

Abbreviations: DWI, diffusion-weighted image; FIGO, International Federation of Gynecology and Obstetrics; MI, myometrial invasion; SI, signal intensity; WI, weighted image.

On MR imaging, CC appears as an intermediate-to-high-SI lesion on T2WI with disruption of the low-SI cervical stroma and restricted diffusion on DWI (high-SI on high b-value DWI and low-SI on the ADC map). Possible MR imaging pitfalls and their mitigations are depicted in **Table 4**.

Pearls

Tumor size

The excellent soft tissue contrast and multi-planar capability of MR imaging facilitate great accuracy in the assessment of tumor size, with precision superior to computed tomography (CT) and clinical examination.[24] Tumor size represents a major prognostic factor in CC, with important consequences for treatment.[25] Tumors <4 cm can be treated surgically with radical hysterectomy whereas larger tumors are treated with concurrent chemo-radiation therapy.[26]

Vaginal infiltration

CC frequently involves the upper-third vagina by direct contiguous spread, which corresponds to FIGO stage IIA disease.[27] Skip lesions in the distal vagina are more commonly seen in recurrent CC. To correctly diagnose vaginal infiltration, segmental disruption of the three-layered vaginal wall by an intermediate-to-high SI soft tissue must be demonstrated on T2WI[28] (**Fig. 4**).

Parametrial invasion

The identification of tumor spread beyond the cervix is of outmost importance for treatment planning and prognosis and denotes FIGO stage IIB: tumors staged ≥ IIB are excluded from definitive surgical management or FST.[26]

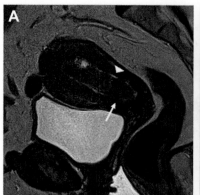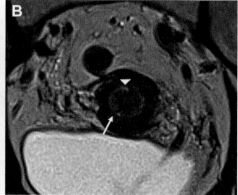

Fig. 3. Cervical stromal invasion of EC. (A) Sagittal T2WI and (B) axial oblique T2WI show a T2 intermediate-SI endometrial tumor distending the endometrial cavity with widening of the internal uterine os (arrows). The tumor distends the cervical canal, but the T2 hypointense cervical stroma ring is uninterrupted and a rim of high-SI on T2WI is seen around the mass (arrowheads). This is consistent with EC without cervical stroma invasion. SI, signal intensity; WI, weighted image.

MR imaging is the optimal imaging modality for the detection of PMI, with an overall accuracy of 94%[29](**Box 3**).

Pitfalls

Early/microinvasive or small tumors
Stage IA is microinvasive and cannot be delineated on MR imaging.[27] Tumors <2 cm (stages IB1 and IB2) can sometimes be difficult to delineate on MR imaging, particularly in young patients, in whom hormonal changes may result in a higher SI of the cervix on T2WI, similar to that of the tumor. In these situations, the addition of DWI and contrast-enhanced imaging increases MR imaging accuracy, with reported sensitivity and specificity of, respectively, 90% and 98% for the staging of early IB1 tumors.[20]

Table 3
Representative MR imaging protocol for cervical cancer

	CC
T1 sequences of the pelvis	Axial plane T1WI of the pelvis without and with fat saturation is recommended.
T2 sequences of the pelvis	Sagittal T2WI of the pelvis is recommended. • Small-FOV[a] axial oblique (perpendicular to the cervix or short axis) T2WI is recommended. • Small-FOV[a] coronal oblique (parallel to the cervix or long axis) T2WI is optional. Slice thickness ≤ 4 mm is recommended. Fat saturation is not recommended.
DWI sequences	DWI-MR imaging is recommended A minimum of 2 b values is recommended (low b = 0–50 s/mm, high b = 800–1000 s/mm)
Contrast-enhanced imaging	Contrast administration is optional.
Lymph node and kidney evaluation	Axial T2WI from the renal hila to the pubic symphysis is recommended. Axial DWI from the renal hila to the pubic symphysis is recommended.

Abbreviations: DWI, diffusion-weighted imaging; FOV, field-of-view; WI, weighted imaging.
[a] Recommended FOV: 20 to 24 cm; Matrix: 256 × 256.

Table 4
MR imaging pitfalls in the evaluation of cervical cancer

	Pitfall	HOW to Resolve It
Early/microinvasive or small tumors	Small tumors can be difficult to delineate in young patients (higher SI of the cervix on T2WI)	*DWI and multi-phase contrast-enhanced MR imaging* sequences help delineate small tumors, which show restricted diffusion on DWI and early enhancement on multi-phase contrast-enhanced MR imaging.
Parametrial invasion	Overestimation of PMI on T2WI due to edema or inflammation	Adequately planned images obtained perpendicular to the long axis of the cervix are fundamental to accurately depict PMI. The addition of *DWI* can help differentiate between pathological tissue (high SI on high b-value DWI and low-SI on ADC map) and edema/inflammation (high SI both on high b-value DWI and on ADC map).
Vaginal involvement	Overestimation of vaginal involvement in the vaginal fornices	To correctly assess vaginal involvement, the integrity of vaginal walls must be disrupted by a soft-tissue mass on *T2WI* and *DWI*.
Fertility sparing treatment	Difficult identification of small tumors, PMI, and measurement of tumor-to-internal cervical os distance	*DWI* helps in the assessment of small tumors and cervical stromal invasion. Also, the addition of *DWI in the sagittal plane* facilitates the measurement of tumor size in the craniocaudal length and tumor-to-internal cervical os distance. The use of *multi-phase contrast-enhanced MR imaging* is optional but useful to identify small tumors with earlier enhancement within the otherwise hypoenhancing stroma.

Abbreviations: DWI, diffusion-weighted imaging; PMI, parametrial invasion; SI, signal intensity; WI, weighted imaging.

Parametrial invasion

A common pitfall is the overestimation of PMI on T2WI, due to edema/inflammation at the level of the cervical stroma.[23]

Accurate depiction of PMI relies on adequately planned images obtained perpendicular to the long axis of the cervix and the addition of DWI to T2WI, with higher sensitivity (81% vs 75%) and specificity (97% vs 85%) compared with the use of T2WI alone.[29,30]

Vaginal involvement

Assessment of involvement of vaginal fornices is often overestimated at MR imaging.[7]

When vaginal invasion is suspected, instillation of ultrasound gel to distend the vaginal canal can be helpful, due to its high SI on T2WI.[7]

To correctly assess vaginal involvement, the integrity of the vaginal wall must be disrupted. When a tumor compresses the fornices without invasion, a rim of high SI on T2WI can be seen

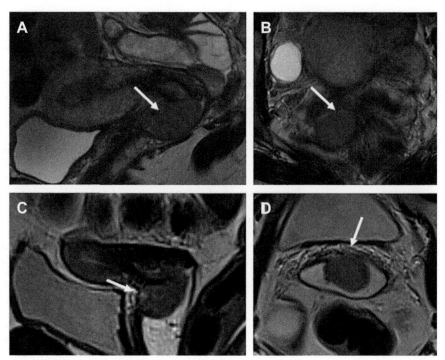

Fig. 4. Vaginal involvement of CC. (*A*) Sagittal T2WI and (*B*) axial oblique T2WI show a CC without vaginal involvement. Images show tumor extension into the vagina, compressing the fornices without invasion. A rim of high SI on T2WI can be seen around the mass and confirms the cervical-confined disease (*arrows*). (*C*) Sagittal T2WI and (*D*) axial oblique T2WI show a cervical tumor with vaginal involvement. The three-layered anterior vaginal fornix is no longer visible and replaced by tumor (*arrows*).SI, signal intensity; WI, weighted image.

around the periphery of the mass, improving the radiologist's confidence to exclude vaginal involvement[7,31] (see **Fig. 4**).

Mimics

Cervical polyp

Cervical polyps represent one of the most common causes of intermenstrual vaginal bleeding in perimenopausal women. They are polypoid growths into the cervical canal with a predominantly glandular structure with a fibrous core[20] (**Fig. 7**)

Adenoma malignum

Adenoma malignum (or minimal deviation adenocarcinoma, MDA) is a subtype of mucinous adenocarcinoma of the cervix with a poor prognosis, accounting for 3% of all cervical adenocarcinomas.[1] It appears as a multicystic lesion in the endocervical glands, with a very high SI on T2WI and slight hyperintensity on T1WI. Distinguishing MDA from Nabothian cysts relies on the identification of a solid component with restricted diffusion on DWI and enhancement on contrast-enhanced imaging[32] (**Fig. 8**).

OVARIAN CANCER

Ovarian cancer (OC) is the most lethal of all gynecological malignancies with high-grade serous ovarian carcinoma being responsible for the majority of cases.[1]

When evaluating an ovarian mass, the initial imaging modality of choice is transvaginal ultrasound. In most cases, this allows characterization of the mass through the "International Ovarian Tumor Analysis Simple Rules,"[33] but up to 20% to 25% of adnexal masses remain indeterminate after initial sonographic evaluation.[34,35]

MR imaging can help assess the risk of malignancy, determine the site of origin of a large pelvic mass, or when FST is being considered.[36] A representative MR imaging protocol[37] is summarized in **Table 5**.

The ACR Ovarian-Adnexal Reporting and Data Systems (O-RADS) MR imaging Committee has developed a lexicon and risk stratification system for MR imaging-based evaluation of adnexal lesions, to score them from almost certainly benign (O-RADS-MR 2) to high risk (O-RADS-MR 5). An O-RADS-MR 1 score represents a completely normal ovary without lesions (**Table 6**).[38]

Box 3
Parametrial invasion in cervical cancer

The parametrium is the fat tissue surrounding the uterus located between the two layers of the broad ligament that contains lymph nodes, lymphatics, and blood vessels.[57]

Tumor spread beyond the cervix with invasion of the parametrium denotes FIGO stage IIB disease.[27]

On MR imaging, the normal cervical stroma demonstrates low SI and must appear uninterrupted on axial oblique T2WI. Preservation of a stromal rim thickness of >3 mm excludes PMI.[23]

The presence of focal or diffuse full-thickness disruption of the cervical stromal ring associated with at least one ancillary feature (a spiculated tumor-to-parametrium interface, a soft tissue nodule in the parametrium or tumor encasement of the uterine vessels) confirms the diagnosis of PMI.[7,29,57] DWI should be obtained in the axial oblique plan with the same orientation, FOV, and slice thickness as the axial oblique T2WI, to enable side-by-side interpretation and/or image fusion[7] (Figs. 5 and 6).

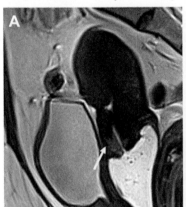
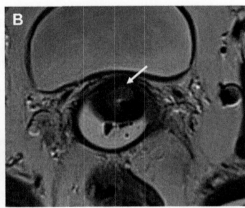

Fig 5 Cervical tumor without PMI. (*A*) Sagittal T2WI and (*B*) axial oblique T2WI show a cervical tumor without parametrial invasion. (*B*) Focal disruption of the T2 hypointense cervical stromal stroma ring in the anterior aspect of the cervix (*arrow*). However, the ring is only partially interrupted and its edges are sharp.

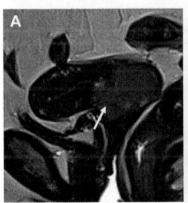
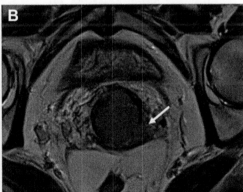

Fig 6 Cervical tumor with PMI. (*A*) Sagittal T2WI and (*B*) axial oblique T2WI illustrate a CC with parametrial invasion. (*B*) Full-thickness disruption of the T2 hypointense cervical stromal ring is demonstrated (*arrow*). Here, the interface between tumor and parametrium appears ill-defined and spiculated.

Abbreviations: DWI, diffusion-weighted image; FIGO, International Federation of Gynecology and Obstetrics; FOV, field-of-view; MR imaging, magnetic resonance imaging; PMI, parametrial invasion; SI, signal intensity; WI, weighted image.

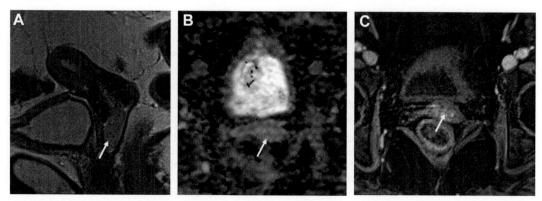

Fig. 7. Pelvic MR imaging performed for the evaluation of suspected CC. (*A*) Sagittal T2WI shows a soft tissue mass originating from the cervical canal with polypoid extension into the vaginal canal (*arrow*). (*B*) Axial DWI show no diffusion restriction within the lesion (*arrow*) and (*C*) axial post-contrast image shows no pathologic contrast enhancement (*arrow*). These features are compatible with a cervical polyp. CC, cervical cancer; DWI, diffusion-weighted image; MR imaging, magnetic resonance imaging; WI, weighted image.

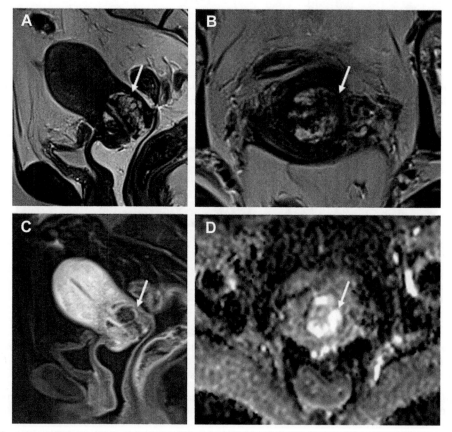

Fig. 8. Adenoma malignum. (*A*) Sagittal T2WI, (*B*) axial oblique T2WI, (*C*) gadolinium-enhanced sagittal T1W fat-saturated image, and (*D*) axial DWI show a multicystic endocervical lesion, with high-SI on T2WI (*A, B, arrows*). (*C, D*) Sagittal T1 fat-suppressed MR imaging (*C*) and axial DWI (*D*) demonstrate the heterogenous contrast enhancement due to the presence of solid and cystic components (*arrow* in *C*) associated with restricted diffusion on DWI (*arrow* in *D*). These features are typical of adenoma malignum. DWI, diffusion-weighted image; SI, signal intensity; WI, weighted image.

Table 5
Representative MR imaging protocol for sonographically indeterminate adnexal masses

	Adnexal Mass
Basic MR sequences	• T1 sequences: axial T1WI of the pelvis is recommended • T2 sequences: sagittal and axial T2WI of the pelvis are recommended
Problem-solving sequences	• FS T1W is recommended when evaluating a high SI T1 mass (T1 "bright" mass) • Axial oblique or coronal oblique T2W of the corpus of the uterus is recommended to better understand the site of origin of a low-SI T2 mass (T2 "dark" solid mass) • DWI and contrast-enhanced MR imaging are recommended to delineate the imaging features of a T2 "dark" solid, cystic-solid, or solid mass

Abbreviations: DWI, diffusion-weighted imaging; WI, weighted imaging.

Common difficulties a radiologist can face with a sonographically indeterminate adnexal mass are summarized in **Table 7**.

Pearls

Characterization of a lesion (benign or malignant)
To better characterize sonographically indeterminate adnexal masses, an algorithmic approach can be used, based on the depiction of fluid and solid components.[37] An algorithm is illustrated in **Box 4**.

Uncertain origin
MR imaging is also helpful in the evaluation of a large pelvic lesion of uncertain origin to assess for ovarian versus nonovarian origin.[38] To accurately identify the ovary, it is recommended to identify the right and left gonadal veins. If a gonadal vein joins a pelvic mass, the origin is ovarian.[39] Other useful signs to search for are the absence of a normal-appearing ipsilateral ovary and the beak sign, defined as sharp angles between the ovary and a mass, with the mass deforming the edges of the ovary into a beak shape.[39]

Peritoneal dissemination and whole-body MR imaging
About 60% of all OCs and 80% of serous carcinomas are discovered at an advanced stage (FIGO stage III or IV),[40] with implications regarding the likelihood of successful primary cytoreductive surgery and, consequently, on prognosis.[36] CT is the recommended modality for staging of OC. However, there is a role for MR imaging in the depiction of peritoneal carcinomatosis, in particular, when DWI and contrast-enhanced MR imaging are studied together.[36]

Whole-body MR imaging (WB-MR imaging) is not routinely used in clinical practice, but several studies have demonstrated its high accuracy in the detection of peritoneal, mesenteric, and serosal metastases.[41–43]

Pitfalls

Be aware that diffusion-weighted imaging is not specific to ovarian tumor
Lesions containing fat, blood, and pus may demonstrate restriction diffusion, thus, the presence of restricted diffusion in an ovarian lesion is not specific (**Figs. 10** and **11**).

How to identify a solid portion
A common pitfall is to misdiagnose non-solid tissue (O-RADS-MR imaging 2–3) as solid tissue and overstage a lesion as O-RADS-MR imaging 4 to 5.[44,45] Solid component refers to any non-fluid component of a lesion and is not synonymous with solid tissue.

• Solid tissue is defined as exhibiting post-contrast enhancement and conforms to one of the following morphologies: papillary projections, mural nodules, irregular septations/walls, and solid component.
• Other solid components (not solid tissue) include the presence of a smooth wall/septation, clot, debris, and fat within a lesion.

DWI may be useful in this setting as a solid tissue exhibits restricted diffusion on high b-value DWI and low-SI on the ADC map (see **Fig. 10**).

Conversely, not all masses associated with solid tissue may warrant contrast administration. A "dark-dark appearance", that is, hypointensity on T2WI (collagen) and DWI, on both low and high b-value images, is indicative of benign pathology

Table 6
Ovarian-Adnexal Reporting and Data System (O-RADS) MR imaging risk stratification system

O-RADS MR Imaging Score	Risk Category	Positive Predictive Value for Malignancy	Lexicon Description
0	Evaluation	N/A	N/A
1	Normal Ovaries	N/A	No ovarian lesion Follicle defined as simple cyst ≤ 3 cm in a pre-menopausal woman Hemorrhagic cyst ≤ 3 cm in pre-menopausal woman Corpus luteum ± hemorrhage ≤ 3 cm in pre-menopausal woman
2	Almost Certainly Benign	< 0.5%[a]	Cyst: Unilocular—any type of fluid content • No wall enhancement • No enhancing solid tissue[b] Cyst: Unilocular—simple or endometriotic fluid content • Smooth enhancing wall • No enhancing solid tissue Lesion with lipid content[c] • No enhancing solid tissue Lesion with "dark T2/dark DWI" solid tissue • Homogeneously hypointense on T2 and DWI Dilated fallopian tube-simple fluid content • Thin, smooth wall/endosalpingeal folds with enhancement • No enhancing solid tissue Para-ovarian cyst—any type of fluid • Thin, smooth wall ± enhancement • No enhancing solid tissue
3	Low Risk	~ 5%[a]	Cyst Unilocular—proteinaceous, hemorrhagic, or mucinous fluid content[d] • Smooth enhancing wall • No enhancing solid tissue Cyst: Multilocular—any type of fluid, no lipid content • Smooth septae and wall with enhancement • No enhancing solid tissue Lesion with solid tissue (excluding T2 dark/DWI dark) • Low risk time-intensity curve on DCE-MR imaging Dilated fallopian tube- • Non-simple fluid: Thin wall/folds • Simple fluid: Thick, smooth wall/folds • No enhancing solid tissue
4	Intermediate Risk	~ 50%[a]	Lesion with solid tissue (excluding T2 dark/DWI dark)

| 5 | High Risk | $\sim 90\%$[a] | • Intermediate risk time-intensity curve on DCE-MR imaging
• If DCE-MR imaging is not feasible, score 4 is any lesion with solid tissue (excluding T2 dark/DWI dark) that is enhancing $\leq$ myometrium at 30–40s on non-DCE-MR imaging
Lesion with lipid content
• Large volume enhancing solid tissue

Lesion with solid tissue (excluding T2 dark/DWI dark)
• High risk time-intensity curve on DCE-MR imaging
• If DCE-MR imaging is not feasible score 5 is any lesion with solid tissue (excluding T2 dark/DWI dark) that is enhancing > myometrium at 30–40s on non-DCE-MR imaging
Peritoneal, mesenteric, or omental nodularity or irregular thickening with or without ascites |

Abbreviations: DCE, dynamic contrast enhancement with a time resolution of 15 s or less; DWI, diffusion-weighted images; MR imaging, magnetic resonance imaging.

[a] Approximate PPV based on data from Thomassin-Naggara, et al. O-RADS MR imaging Score for Risk Stratification of Sonographically Indeterminate Adnexal Masses. JAMA Network Open. 2020;3(1):e1919896. Please note that the PPV provided applies to the score category overall and not to individual characteristics. Definitive PPV are not currently available for individual characteristics. The PPV values for malignancy include both borderline tumors and invasive cancers.

[b] Solid tissue is defined as a lesion component that enhances and conforms to one of these morphologies: papillary projection, mural nodule, irregular septation/wall or other larger solid portions.

[c] Minimal enhancement of Rokitansky nodules in lesion containing lipid does not change to O-RADS MR imaging 4.

[d] Hemorrhagic cyst $\leq$3 cm in pre-menopausal woman is O-RADS MR imaging 1.

From American College of Radiology Committee on O-RADS™ (Ovarian and Adnexal). O-RADS MRI Assessment Categories version 1 (2020). Available at: https://www.acr.org/-/media/ACR/Files/RADS/O-RADS/O-RADS-MR-Risk-Stratification-System-Table-September-2020.pdf. Accessed Nov 15 2022.

Table 7
MR imaging pitfalls in the evaluation of sonographically indeterminate adnexal mass

Pitfall		Mitigations
Be aware that DWI is not specific to ovarian tumor	Fat, blood, and pus may demonstrate restricted diffusion	*T1WI* can help identify fat and blood. Pus appears hyperintense on *T2WI* thus distinguishable from solid tissue
How to identify a solid portion	Distinguishing solid from non-solid tissue	On *contrast-enhanced MR imaging*, solid tissue is a solid component that enhances after contrast medium administration and has one of the following morphologic characteristics: papillary projections, mural nodules, irregular septations/walls, or a solid portion. On *DWI*, a solid lesion has restricted diffusion, with increased SI high b-value DWI and low-SI on ADC map.
Analysis of perfusion curves	Curve analysis misinterpretation	• If solid tissue is small: Avoid analysis of movement artifact by carefully repositioning the ROI over the mass on each phase. • If enhancement is weak: Analyze the presence of a potential plateau and avoid including in the ROI the analysis of external myometrium. • If the solid tissue is mixed and the cystic content is bright on T1WI: look at the subtraction sequence.
	Absence of myometrium	In case of an absent myometrium: • If there is no plateau associated with the TIC, the TIC is low-risk (O-RADS MR 3) • If the TIC demonstrates a plateau, it is unclear if this is an intermediate- or high-risk TIC. Thus, the score is O-RADS-MR 4
	Non-availability of TIC or DCE sequences	If DCE sequences are not available and/or the TIC is not feasible, look at post-contrast images: • If SI of solid tissue greater than that of the myometrium, the lesion is classified as O-RADS MR 5 • If SI of solid tissue is less than that of the myometrium, the lesion is classified as O-RADS MR 4

| Peritoneal carcinomatosis | Hepatic peritoneal implants can be mistaken for hepatic metastasis | *Morphologic evaluation* is essential for the correct diagnosis: a well-defined, biconvex shape and peripheral location are typical for hepatic surface implants, whereas an ill-defined, circular shape, partially, or completely surrounded by liver tissue is characteristic of intraparenchymal metastases. |

Abbreviations: DCE, dynamic contrast-enhanced; DWI, diffusion-weighted imaging; SI, signal intensity.

Box 4
Characterization of an adnexal lesion (benign or malignant)

The ACR O-RADS MR Imaging Committee has developed a lexicon and risk stratification system for MR imaging-based evaluation of adnexal lesions, with the aim to improve communication between radiologists and clinicians. It relies on the evaluation of lesion origin, morphology, SI on conventional sequences, on high b-value DWI, and enhancement kinetics on post-contrast imaging. According to O-RADS descriptors, fluid components may be simple or non-simple (hemorrhagic, proteinaceous, endometriotic, fat- or lipid-containing) depending on their T1 and T2 SI[38]. Solid components include solid tissue (papillary projections, mural nodules, irregular septations or walls or a large solid portion) or nonsolid tissue (smooth septations or walls, blood clot, non-enhancing debris, fibrin strands, and fat).[44,45]

To better characterize a sonographically indeterminate adnexal masses, an algorithmic approach can be used[37] (Fig. 9).

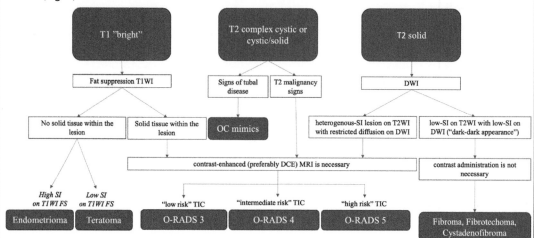

Fig. 9. Diagnostic algorithm. (Adapted from Forstner R, Thomassin-Naggara I, Cunha TM, et al. ESUR recommendations for MR imaging of the sonographically indeterminate adnexal mass: an update [published correction appears in Eur Radiol. 2017 Jun;27(6):2258]. Eur Radiol. 2017;27(6):2248-2257.).

First, identifying the intrinsic T1WI and T2WI signal characteristics of the mass helps to partition adnexal masses into three groups: T1 "bright" masses, T2 solid masses, and complex cystic or cystic-solid masses.

- A T1 "bright" lesion may contain blood (endometriotic or hemorrhagic cyst) or fat (teratoma) and fat-saturated T1WI will help distinguish these etiologies. If there is no solid component within the lesion, it represents an O-RADS-MR 2 lesion, whereas when solid tissue is detected, further evaluation must be performed for a complex cystic/mixed cystic-solid mass.

- When a T2 solid mass is present, demonstrating a homogenous low SI on T2WI with low SI on high b-value DWI ("dark-dark appearance"), it is most likely benign (fibroma, fibrotechoma, cystadenofibroma). In this case, contrast administration can be avoided.[37,44,45]

- When a T2 solid mass presents as a heterogenous-SI lesion on T2WI or when a complex cystic or cystic-solid mass is present, further assessment of the solid component through contrast-enhanced (preferably DCE) MR imaging is necessary.[37,38,45]

A purely cystic lesion with no solid component can be confidently considered benign.

Post-contrast sequences can be obtained as a DCE acquisition or as a nondynamic contrast acquisition, acquired pre-contrast and at 30 to 40 s following contrast injection.[38,45]

Abbreviations: DWI, diffusion-weighted image; MR imaging, magnetic resonance imaging; O-RADS, Ovarian-Adnexal Reporting and Data Systems; SI, signal intensity; TIC, time-intensity curves.

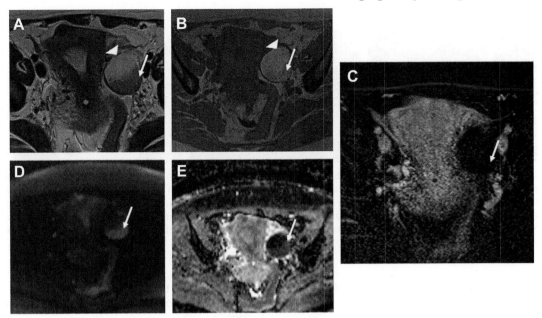

Fig. 10. Endometrioma. (*A*) Axial T2WI, (*B*) axial T1WI, (*C*) axial gadolinium-enhanced subtracted T1W fat-saturated image, (*D*) axial DWI, and (*E*) axial ADC map show a unilocular T1 hyperintense lesion in the left ovary (high SI on T2WI and high SI on T1WI) (*A, B, arrowheads*). In the posterior portion of the lesion, a solid component is seen (*arrows*). (*C–E*) The component shows no contrast enhancement on the subtraction sequence (*C, arrow*) and does not demonstrate restricted diffusion, since the high SI on DWI corresponds to high SI on ADC map (*D, E, arrows*), therefore, compatible with non-solid tissue (clot). The collective findings are consistent with a left endometrioma. ADC, apparent diffusion coefficient; DWI, diffusion-weighted image; SI, signal intensity; WI, weighted image.

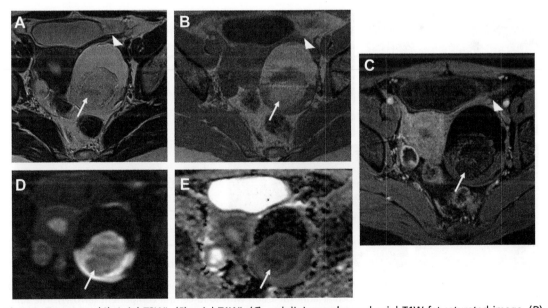

Fig. 11. Teratoma. (*A*) Axial T2WI, (*B*) axial T1WI, (*C*) gadolinium-enhanced axial T1W fat-saturated image, (*D*) axial DWI, and (*E*) axial ADC map demonstrate a unilocular fat-containing lesion in the left ovary (high-SI on T2WI, high-SI on T1WI and low-SI on T1W fat-saturated image) (*A–C, arrowheads*). A solid component with eccentric growth is seen within the lesion (*arrows*). (*C–E*) The mass exhibits mild contrast enhancement (*C, arrow*), restricted diffusion (high-SI on DWI and low-SI on ADC map) (*D, E, arrows*), compatible with a Rokitansky nodule. The collective imaging findings are consistent with a mature left ovarian teratoma. ADC, apparent diffusion coefficient; DWI, diffusion-weighted image; SI, signal intensity; WI, weighted image.

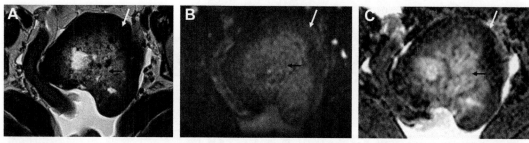

Fig. 12. Torsed ovarian fibroma. (*A*) Axial oblique T2WI, (*B*) axial DWI, and (*C*) ADC map show a lesion with low-SI on T2WI, on DWI and on ADC map ("dark/dark appearance"), typical of benign lesions (*white arrows*). The low-SI on ADC map of a T2 low-SI lesion is known as "T2 blackout effect". The central part of the lesion (*black arrows*) demonstrates higher SI on T2WI, on DWI and on ADC map due to the presence of edema. These findings are consistent with a torsed fibroma. ADC, apparent diffusion coefficient; DWI, diffusion-weighted image; SI, signal intensity; WI, weighted image.

and contrast administration can be avoided[44,45] (**Figs. 12** and **13**).

Analysis of perfusion curves
Specific tips to avoid curve misinterpretation are described in **Table 7** and **Box 5**.

Peritoneal carcinomatosis
Cardiac and respiratory movements and suscepti-bility artifacts from air can markedly degrade image quality, particularly for hepatic surface im-plants and peritoneal implants on the bowel surface.[42]

Also, it is essential not to mistake hepatic perito-neal implants for hepatic metastasis as this will change disease staging (stage IIIC vs stage IVB, respectively).[46] Diagnostic accuracy necessitates careful morphologic evaluation: a well-defined, biconvex shape and peripheral location are typical for hepatic surface implants, versus an ill-defined,

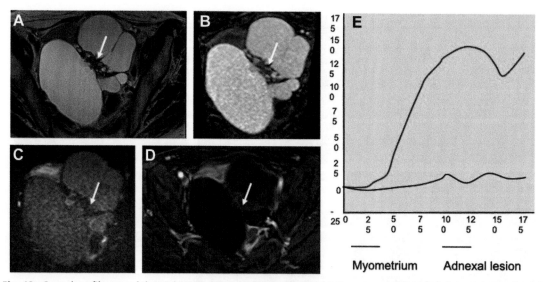

Fig. 13. Cystadenofibroma. (*A*) Axial T2WI, (*B*) axial DWI, (*C*) axial ADC map, and (*D*) gadolinium-enhanced axial T1W fat-saturated images show a multilocular adnexal lesion with solid central component (*arrows*). The solid component has slightly inhomogeneous low-SI on T2WI, on DWI, and on ADC map ("dark/dark appearance") and mild contrast enhancement. (*E*) The time-intensity curve of the solid tissue (*blue line*) compared to that of the myometrium (*red line*) demonstrates a slow and progressive uptake, lower than that of the myometrium ("low-risk TIC"). The presence of slightly inhomogeneous SI on T2WI and contrast enhancement represents an O-RADS MR 3 lesion. Histopathologic analysis after resection confirmed cystoadenofibroma. ADC, apparent diffu-sion coefficient; DWI, diffusion-weighted image; MR, magnetic resonance; O-RADS, Ovarian-Adnexal Reporting and Data Systems; SI, signal intensity; TIC, time-intensity curve; WI, weighted image.

Box 5
Analysis of perfusion curves in sonographically indeterminate adnexal masses

In the characterization of sonographically indeterminate adnexal masses, the identification of solid tissue within the lesion is of fundamental importance. The degree of enhancement of the solid tissue compared with that of the outer myometrium can help identify three types of time-intensity curves (TIC): a slow and progressive uptake ("low-risk TIC"), typical of benign lesions, an early uptake later than that of the myometrium followed by a plateau ("intermediate-risk TIC"), typical of borderline/malignant lesions, or an avid and early contrast uptake more than that of the myometrium followed by a plateau ("high-risk TIC"), typical of malignant tumors.[38,45]

TIC analysis is misinterpreted in 6.1% of misclassified O-RADS cases in the study from Thomassin-Naggara and colleagues[58] Most errors included failure to recognize a shoulder and plateau between low and intermediate-risk TIC (no confusion was found between high-risk TIC vs intermediate and low-risk) (Fig 14 and 15).

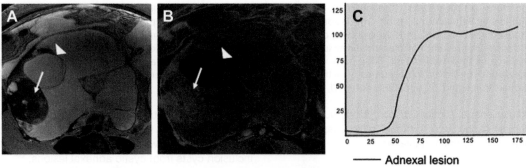

Adnexal lesion

In case of an absent myometrium, adnexal TIC must be interpreted alone.

Fig. 14. In case of an absent myometrium, adnexal TIC must be interpreted alone: (A) Axial T2WI and (B) gadolinium-enhanced axial T1W fat-saturated image. There is a large multilocular adnexal lesion with thick septa and a nodule with eccentric growth (arrows). The lesion demonstrates high SI on T2WI and low SI on T1W fat-saturated image, with a drop of SI within the lesion (arrowheads). Septa and nodule present contrast enhancement after gadolinium administration. (C) The time-intensity curve of the solid nodule (blue line) demonstrates early uptake followed by a plateau. The uterus is absent due to previous hysterectomy, therefore, no comparison can be made between this curve and that of the myometrium. In this case, an intermediate-risk TIC and high-risk TIC are both possible and cannot be differentiated. Thus, the lesion is rated O-RADS MR 4. Histopathologic analysis after surgical removal confirmed mucinous borderline tumor.

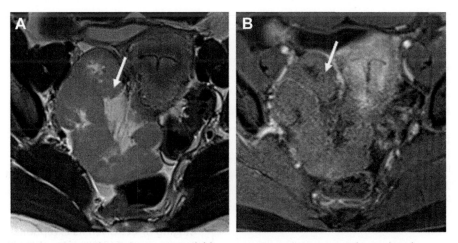

In case DCE-MR imaging and/or TIC are not available, post-contrast images must be analyzed.

Fig 15. In case DCE-MR imaging and/or TIC are not available, post-contrast images must be analyzed: (A) Axial T2WI and (B) gadolinium-enhanced axial T1W fat-saturated image. There is a large lesion in the right ovary. It demonstrates contrast enhancement after gadolinium administration and is therefore solid (arrows). (B) DCE-MR sequences and TIC were not available: the SI of the solid tissue is inferior to that of the myometrium. This is an O-RADS MR 4 lesion. The lesion was surgically resected and consistent with a dysgerminoma.

Abbreviations: DCE, dynamic contrast-enhanced; MR, magnetic resonance; O-RADS, Ovarian-Adnexal Reporting and Data Systems; SI, signal intensity; TIC, time-intensity curve; WI, weighted image.

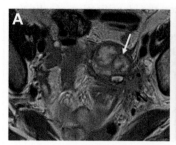 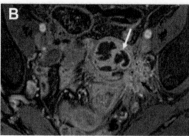 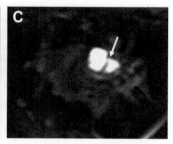

Fig. 16. Actinomycosis. Pelvic MR imaging performed to evaluate suspected ovarian tumor with peritoneal carcinomatosis. (*A*) Axial T2WI, (*B*) gadolinium-enhanced axial T1W fat-saturated image, and (*C*) axial DWI show a multilocular left adnexal lesion. The lesion demonstrates thick walls and septa and is filled with fluid with intermediate-to-high SI on T2WI and DWI, due to the presence of pus (*A–C, white arrows*). The left lateral pelvic fascia is thickened and spiculated solid tissue is seen invading the left obturator space (*A–C, black arrows*). The presence of thick-walled fluid-filled mass with tubular morphology suggest a tubo-ovarian abscess; cytologic assessment confirmed the presence of actinomycosis. DWI, diffusion-weighted image; MR imaging, magnetic resonance imaging; SI, signal intensity; WI, weighted image.

circular shape, partially or completely surrounded by liver tissue, which should raise suspicion for intraparenchymal metastases.[23]

Mimics

Tubo-ovarian abscess

A tubo-ovarian abscess is a complex infectious mass, involving the tubo-ovarian complex, that can present as a cystic or complex cystic mass and hence be mistaken for a neoplasm. At MR imaging, its classic appearance is a thick-walled fluid-filled mass, with heterogenous or high SI on T2WI and internal gas bubbles. The tubular morphology helps in distinguishing hydrosalpinx or pyosalpinx from a primary adnexal neoplasm[39] (**Fig. 16**).

Mucocele of the appendix/pseudomyxoma peritonei

Mucocele of the appendix is a mucinous dilatation of the appendix, due to epithelial proliferation, inflammation, or obstruction.[47] It appears as a tubular fluid-filled structure connected to the base of the cecum.[47] A mucinous adenocarcinoma of the appendix presents enhancing nodules or irregular mural thickening and may be associated with peritoneal seeding (pseudomyxoma peritonei). The presence of scalloped hepatic and splenic borders and bowel displacement by implants can help distinguish mucinous implants from cystic ovarian metastases.[39]

Peritoneal inclusion cyst

Peritoneal inclusion cysts are cystic lesions without true cyst walls, with their margins formed by peritoneal adhesions and the margins of adjacent organs.[48] The ovary is typically closely associated with a peritoneal inclusion cyst, located centrally or eccentrically within the cyst,

suspended and entrapped by the peritoneal adhesions, ("spider in a web" appearance). The lack of a perceptible cyst wall helps distinguish peritoneal inclusion cysts from cystic adnexal lesions.[39]

SUMMARY

Pelvic MR imaging plays a crucial role in the pretreatment evaluation of patients with common gynecologic malignancies, allowing accurate staging for endometrial and cervical cancers and serving as a problem-solving tool for patients with complex adnexal masses. However, MR imaging is not free from potential pitfalls and challenges, and the radiologist should be aware of these when evaluating pelvic MR imaging studies, to maximize diagnostic accuracy and the appropriate management of patients.

CLINICS CARE POINTS

- MR imaging is the modality of choice for the pre-treatment evaluation of patients with gynecologic neoplasms, informing patient management and tailored treatment.

- MR imaging delineates fundamental prognostic factors for EC with a high degree of accuracy. It also plays a crucial role in the staging of CC. Given its exceptional soft tissue contrast, MR imaging also allows for the characterization of sonographically indeterminate adnexal masses.

- MR imaging for the assessment of gynecologic malignancies is not free from interpretive challenges, notably in the evaluation of myometrial, vaginal, cervical stromal, and parametrial invasion and in the identification of solid tissue in sonographically indeterminate adnexal mass.

DISCLOSURE

A.M. Venkatesan receives grant funding from the University of Texas MD Anderson Cancer Center Institutional Research Grant Program, the University of Texas MD Anderson Cancer Center Radiation Oncology Strategic Initiatives Pilot Grant Program, the Oden Institute for Computational Engineering and Sciences, UTMDACC & Texas Advanced Computing Center (TACC) Oncological Data & Computational Sciences Grant Program, and the Department of Defense.

REFERENCES

1. Sung H, Ferlay J, Siegel RL, et al. Global Cancer Statistics 2020: GLOBOCAN Estimates of Incidence and Mortality Worldwide for 36 Cancers in 185 Countries. CA Cancer J Clin 2021;71(3):209–49.

2. Lakhman Y, D'Anastasi M, Miccò M, et al. Second-Opinion Interpretations of Gynecologic Oncologic MRI Examinations by Sub-Specialized Radiologists Influence Patient Care. Eur Radiol 2016;26(7): 2089–98.

3. Nougaret S, Horta M, Sala E, et al. Endometrial Cancer MRI staging: Updated Guidelines of the European Society of Urogenital Radiology. Eur Radiol 2019;29(2):792–805.

4. McEvoy SH, Nougaret S, Abu-Rustum NR, et al. Fertility-sparing for young patients with gynecologic cancer: How MRI can guide patient selection prior to conservative management. Abdom Radiol 2017; 42(10):2488–512.

5. Colombo N, Creutzberg C, Amant F, et al. ESMO-ESGO-ESTRO consensus conference on endometrial cancer: Diagnosis, treatment and follow-up. Ann Oncol 2016;27(1):16–41.

6. Kubik-Huch RA, Weston M, Nougaret S, et al. European Society of Urogenital Radiology (ESUR) Guidelines: MR Imaging of Leiomyomas. Eur Radiol 2018; 28(8):3125–37.

7. Manganaro L, Lakhman Y, Bharwani N, et al. Staging, recurrence and follow-up of uterine cervical cancer using MRI: Updated Guidelines of the European Society of Urogenital Radiology after revised FIGO staging 2018. Eur Radiol 2021;31(10): 7802–16.

8. Reinhold C, Ueno Y, Akin EA, et al. ACR Appropriateness Criteria® Pretreatment Evaluation and Follow-Up of Endometrial Cancer. J Am Coll Radiol 2020;17(11):S472–86.

9. Nougaret S, Lakhman Y, Vargas HA, et al. From Staging to Prognostication: Achievements and Challenges of MR Imaging in the Assessment of Endometrial Cancer. Magn Reson Imaging Clin N Am 2017;25(3):611–33.

10. Wang J, Xu P, Yang X, et al. Association of Myometrial Invasion With Lymphovascular Space Invasion, Lymph Node Metastasis, Recurrence, and Overall Survival in Endometrial Cancer: A Meta-Analysis of 79 Studies With 68,870 Patients. Front Oncol 2021; 11(October):1–11.

11. Luna C, Balcacer P, Castillo P, et al. Endometrial cancer from early to advanced-stage disease: an update for radiologists. Abdom Radiol 2021; 46(11):5325–36.

12. Manfredi R, Mirk P, Maresca G, et al. Local-Regional Staging of Endometrial Carcinoma: Role of MR Imaging in Surgical Planning. Radiology 2004;231(2): 372–8.

13. Fujii S, Kido A, Baba T, et al. Subendometrial enhancement and peritumoral enhancement for assessing endometrial cancer on dynamic contrast enhanced MR imaging. Eur J Radiol 2015;84(4):581–9.

14. Lewin SN. Revised FIGO Staging System for Endometrial Cancer. Clin Obstet Gynecol 2011;54(2): 215–8.

15. Beddy P, Moyle P, Kataoka M, et al. Evaluation of depth of myometrial invasion and overall staging in endometrial cancer: Comparison of diffusion-weighted and dynamic contrast-enhanced MR imaging. Radiology 2012;262(2):530–7.

16. Utsunomiya D, Notsute S, Hayashida Y, et al. Endometrial Carcinoma in Adenomyosis: Assessment of Myometrial Invasion on T2-Weighted Spin-Echo and Gadolinium-Enhanced T1-Weighted Images. Am J Roentgenol 2004;182(2):399–404.

17. Sala E, Crawford R, Senior E, et al. Added value of dynamic contrast-enhanced magnetic resonance imaging in predicting advanced stage disease in patients with endometrial carcinoma. Int J Gynecol Cancer 2009;19(1):141–6.

18. Wang T, Zhang X, Lu Z, et al. Comparison and analysis of the clinicopathological features of SCEO and ECOM. J Ovarian Res 2019;12(1):10.

19. Willmott F, Allouni KA, Rockall A. Radiological manifestations of metastasis to the ovary. J Clin Pathol 2012;65(7):585–90.

20. Otero-García MM, Mesa-Álvarez A, Nikolic O, et al. Role of MRI in staging and follow-up of endometrial and cervical cancer: pitfalls and mimickers. Insights Imaging 2019;10(1). https://doi.org/10.1186/s13244-019-0696-8.

21. Moharamzad Y, Davarpanah AH, Yaghobi Joybari A, et al. Diagnostic performance of apparent diffusion coefficient (ADC) for differentiating endometrial carcinoma from benign lesions: a systematic review and meta-analysis. Abdom Radiol 2021;46(3): 1115–28.

22. Siegel CL, Andreotti RF, Cardenes HR, et al. ACR appropriateness criteria ® pretreatment planning of invasive cancer of the cervix. J Am Coll Radiol 2012;9(6):395–402.

23. Sala E, Rockall AG, Freeman SJ, et al. The added role of MR imaging in treatment stratification of patients with gynecologic malignancies: What the radiologist needs to know. Radiology 2013;266(3):717–40.

24. Mitchell DG, Snyder B, Coakley F, et al. Early invasive cervical cancer: Tumor delineation by magnetic resonance imaging, computed tomography, and clinical examination, verified by pathologic results, in the ACRIN 6651/GOG 183 intergroup study. J Clin Oncol 2006;24(36):5687–94.

25. Wagner AE, Pappas L, Ghia AJ, et al. Impact of tumor size on survival in cancer of the cervix and validation of stage IIA1 and IIA2 subdivisions. Gynecol Oncol 2013;129(3):517–21.

26. Cibula D, Pötter R, Planchamp F, et al. The European Society of Gynaecological Oncology/European Society for Radiotherapy and Oncology/European Society of Pathology Guidelines for the Management of Patients With Cervical Cancer. Int J Gynecol Cancer 2018;28(4):641–55.

27. Bhatla N, Berek JS, Cuello Fredes M, et al. Revised FIGO staging for carcinoma of the cervix uteri. Int J Gynecol Obstet 2019;145(1):129–35.

28. Parikh JH, Barton DPJ. Ind TEJ., et al. MR Imaging Features of Vaginal Malignancies. Radiographics 2008;28(1):49–63.

29. Woo S, Suh CH, Kim SY, et al. Magnetic resonance imaging for detection of parametrial invasion in cervical cancer: An updated systematic review and meta-analysis of the literature between 2012 and 2016. Eur Radiol 2018;28(2):530–41.

30. Park JJ, Kim CK, Park SY, et al. Parametrial invasion in cervical cancer: Fused T2-weighted imaging and high-b-value diffusion-weighted imaging with background body signal suppression at 3 T. Radiology 2015;274(3):734–41.

31. Salib MY, Russell JHB, Stewart VR, et al. 2018 figo staging classification for cervical cancer: Added benefits of imaging. Radiographics 2020;40(6):1807–22.

32. Sugiyama K, Takehara Y. MR findings of pseudoneoplastic lesions in the uterine cervix mimicking adenoma malignum. Br J Radiol 2007;80(959):878–83.

33. Timmerman D, Testa AC, Bourne T, et al. Simple ultrasound-based rules for the diagnosis of ovarian cancer. Ultrasound Obstet Gynecol 2008;31(6):681–90.

34. Timmerman D, Van Calster B, Testa A, et al. Predicting the risk of malignancy in adnexal masses based on the Simple Rules from the International Ovarian Tumor Analysis group. Am J Obstet Gynecol 2016;214(4):424–37.

35. Sadowski EA, Paroder V, Patel-Lippmann K, et al. Indeterminate Adnexal Cysts at US: Prevalence and Characteristics of Ovarian Cancer. Radiology 2018;287(3):1041–9.

36. Kang SK, Reinhold C, Atri M, et al. ACR Appropriateness Criteria ® Staging and Follow-Up of Ovarian Cancer. J Am Coll Radiol 2018;15(5):S198–207.

37. Forstner R, Thomassin-Naggara I, Cunha TM, et al. ESUR recommendations for MR imaging of the sonographically indeterminate adnexal mass: an update. Eur Radiol 2017;27(6):2248–57.

38. Sadowski EA, Thomassin-Naggara I, Rockall A, et al. O-RADS MRI Risk Stratification System: Guide for Assessing Adnexal Lesions from the ACR O-RADS Committee. Radiology 2022;303(1):35–47.

39. Nougaret S, Nikolovski I, Paroder V, et al. MRI of Tumors and Tumor Mimics in the Female Pelvis: Anatomic Pelvic Space–based Approach. Radiographics 2019;39(4):1205–29.

40. Torre LA, Trabert B, DeSantis CE, et al. Ovarian cancer statistics, 2018. CA Cancer J Clin 2018;68(4):284–96.

41. Tunariu N, Blackledge M, Messiou C, et al. What's New for Clinical Whole-body MRI (WB-MRI) in the 21st Century. Br J Radiol 2020;93(1115):20200562.

42. Rizzo S, De Piano F, Buscarino V, et al. Pre-operative evaluation of epithelial ovarian cancer patients: Role of whole body diffusion weighted imaging MR and CT scans in the selection of patients suitable for primary debulking surgery. A single-centre study. Eur J Radiol 2020;123(December 2019):108786.

43. Michielsen K, Vergote I, Op De Beeck K, et al. Whole-body MRI with diffusion-weighted sequence for staging of patients with suspected ovarian cancer: A clinical feasibility study in comparison to CT and FDG-PET/CT. Eur Radiol 2014;24(4):889–901.

44. Thomassin-Naggara I, Poncelet E, Jalaguier-Coudray A, et al. Ovarian-Adnexal Reporting Data System Magnetic Resonance Imaging (O-RADS MRI) Score for Risk Stratification of Sonographically Indeterminate Adnexal Masses. JAMA Netw Open 2020;3(1):1–14.

45. Reinhold C, Rockall A, Sadowski EA, et al. Ovarian-Adnexal Reporting Lexicon for MRI: A White Paper of the ACR Ovarian-Adnexal Reporting and Data Systems MRI Committee. J Am Coll Radiol 2021;18(5):713–29.

46. Javadi S, Ganeshan DM, Qayyum A, et al. Ovarian Cancer, the Revised FIGO Staging System, and the Role of Imaging. Am J Roentgenol 2016;206(6):1351–60.

47. Koga H, Aoyagi K, Honda H, et al. Appendiceal mucocele: sonographic and MR imaging findings. Am J Roentgenol 1995;165(6):1552.

48. Vallerie AM, Lerner JP, Wright JD, et al. Peritoneal Inclusion Cysts: A Review. Obstet Gynecol Surv 2009; 64(5):321–34.

49. Concin N, Creutzberg CL, Vergote I, et al. ESGO / ESTRO / ESP Guidelines for the management of patients with endometrial carcinoma. Virchows Arch 2021;478(2):153–90.

50. Moro F, Bonanno GM, Gui B, et al. Imaging modalities in fertility preservation in patients with gynecologic cancers. Int J Gynecol Cancer 2021;31(3): 323–31.

51. Colombo N, Carinelli S, Colombo A, et al. Cervical cancer: ESMO clinical practice guidelines for diagnosis, treatment and follow-up. Ann Oncol 2012; 23(SUPPL. 7). https://doi.org/10.1093/annonc/mds268.

52. Bradley K., Frederick P., Reynolds R.K., et al., Cervical Cancer, Version 1.2022, NCCN Clinical Practice Guidelines in Oncology, *J Natl Compr Cancer Netw*, 17(1),2022, 64-84.

53. Bentivegna E, Gouy S, Maulard A, et al. Oncological outcomes after fertility-sparing surgery for cervical cancer: a systematic review. Lancet Oncol 2016; 17(6):e240–53.

54. Stein EB, Hansen JM, Maturen KE. Fertility-Sparing Approaches in Gynecologic Oncology: Role of Imaging in Treatment Planning. Radiol Clin North Am 2020;58(2):401–12.

55. Butterfield N, Smith JR. Role of Imaging in Fertility-spar- ing Treatment of. Gynecologic 2016;1: 2214–33.

56. Colombo N, Sessa C, Bois A Du, et al. ESMO-ESGO consensus conference recommendations on ovarian cancer: Pathology and molecular biology, early and advanced stages, borderline tumours and recurrent disease. Int J Gynecol Cancer 2019;29(4):728–60.

57. Valentini AL, Gui B, Miccò M, et al. MRI anatomy of parametrial extension to better identify local pathways of disease spread in cervical cancer. Diagnostic Interv Radiol 2016;22(4):319–25.

58. Thomassin-Naggara I, Belghitti M, Milon A, et al. O-RADS MRI score: analysis of misclassified cases in a prospective multicentric European cohort. Eur Radiol 2021;31(12):9588–99.

PET/MRI in Gynecologic Malignancy

Matthew Larson, MD, PhD[a], Petra Lovrec, MD[b], Elizabeth A. Sadowski, MD[c], Ali Pirasteh, MD[d],*

KEYWORDS

- PET • MRI • Ovarian cancer • Cervical cancer • Endometrial cancer

KEY POINTS

- PET/MRI can be used for initial staging, treatment response assessment, and surveillance of gynecologic malignancies, with PET and MRI having synergic roles in the assessment of disease extent.
- Simultaneous PET/MRI allows for both whole-body and dedicated pelvis imaging in a single imaging session.
- Effective utilization of PET/MRI with the goal of time-efficient image acquisitions and streamlined workflow requires institutional expertise in both PET and MRI.

INTRODUCTION

The majority of patients with gynecologic malignancies undergo imaging during the course of their care, whether at the time of initial diagnosis/staging, for assessment of treatment response, and/or for surveillance. The most commonly utilized imaging tools in management of gynecologic malignancies are computed tomography (CT), positron emission tomography (PET) most commonly performed with ^{18}F-fluorodeoxyglucose (FDG), and magnetic resonanceimaging (MRI). By providing excellent soft tissue contrast and detailed delineation of the anatomy, MRI is the preferred modality in evaluation of local tumor extent for gynecologic malignancies. However, PET is preferred in evaluation of nodal disease as it increases diagnostic accuracy compared to anatomic imaging alone.[1–6] Hence, simultaneous PET/MRI can evaluate gynecologic malignancies in one imaging session and can be used instead of separate pelvis MRI and PET/CT exams. Although a growing body of literature supports the utility of this approach,[7,8] PET/MRI utilization is associated with several challenges, including scanner availability, technical aspects of imaging protocols, regional/institutional expertise, and reimbursement. In this article, we will provide a review of the technical aspects of PET/MRI, a summary of the utility of PET/MRI in the management of gynecologic malignancies, and our approach to using this platform.

TECHNICAL OVERVIEW OF PET/MRI
Advantages

Many of the technical advantages of PET/MRI (compared to PET/CT) are relevant to gynecologic malignancies. In contrast to PET/CT, where PET is acquired after a whole-body CT, simultaneous PET/MRI scanners provide concurrent acquisition of MRI and PET. The presence of PET detectors at

a Department of Radiology, University of Wisconsin-Madison School of Medicine and Public Health, 600 Highland Avenue, E3/352, Madison, WI 53792, USA; b Department of Radiology, Loyola University Medical Center, 2160 First Avenue, Maywood, IL 60153, USA; c Departments of Radiology, Obstetrics and Gynecology, University of Wisconsin-Madison School of Medicine and Public Health, 600 Highland Avenue, E3/372, Madison, WI 53792-3252, USA; d Departments of Radiology and Medical Physics, University of Wisconsin-Madison School of Medicine and Public Health, 1111 Highland Avenue, WIMR II 2423, Madison, WI 53705, USA
* Corresponding author.
E-mail address: pirasteh@wisc.edu

Radiol Clin N Am 61 (2023) 713–723
https://doi.org/10.1016/j.rcl.2023.02.013

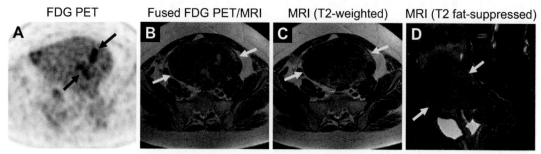

Fig. 1. MRI characterizes benign findings that are FDG-avid on PET. A patient with stage IA2 cervical cancer diagnosed by loop electrosurgical excision procedure (positive margins) underwent FDG PET for initial staging. Axial PET (*A*) and axial fused PET/T2-weighted MRI (*B*) did not identify residual cervical or metastatic disease, but did demonstrate foci of FDG uptake (*A, arrows*) within in a uterine mass (*B, arrows*). Axial T2 (*C*) and sagittal T2 fat-suppressed (*D*) MRI images delineate features of the mass, including heterogeneous T2-hypointensity similar to that of skeletal muscles without an invasive, infiltrative tumor margin and confinement to the uterine serosa (*C, D, arrows*). These findings are consistent with a benign intramural leiomyoma. As a result, the patient was able to undergo curative hysterectomy.

the isocenter of the PET/MRI scanner minimizes the probability of misregistration between PET and MRI images. PET/MR imaging provides an up to 80% reduction in radiation exposure as compared to PET/CT, which is particularly relevant to young patients of child-bearing age.[9] A non-contrast PET/MRI is preferred over PET/CT for patients who are unable to receive intravenous contrast or among those in whom radiation exposure should be avoided as much as possible (eg, pregnant patients and those with compromised renal function).[10] This approach leverages the advantages of MRI in providing a detailed depiction of anatomy and the pathology, even without intravenous contrast, along with the advantages of PET, which permits differentiation between benign and potentially malignant entities.[11,12] Moreover,

as a result of its excellent soft tissue contrast, MRI can differentiate between malignant and benign entities that are FDG-avid.[7] For example, uterine leiomyomata, the endometrium during the ovulatory and menstrual phases, and the ovaries (in premenopausal patients) may demonstrate avid FDG uptake, which can be confidently characterized as benign normal findings by MRI (**Figs. 1** and **2**).

Limitations

One limitation of current PET/MRI platforms is the diameter of the scanner bore; while the scanner size is equal to other regular-sized current MRI platforms, it does not accommodate patients who need a wide-bore scanner and/or suffer from claustrophobia, especially after the

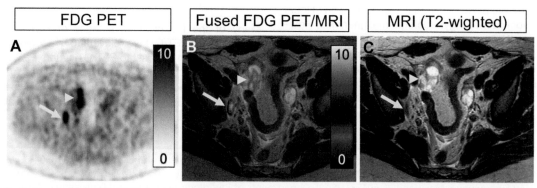

Fig. 2. In a patient with cervical cancer, a right pelvic sidewall nodal metastasis demonstrates abnormal uptake on PET/MRI, as seen on standalone axial PET (*A*) and fused FDG PET/MRI (*B*) (*arrows*). Of note, this lymph node would not be considered suspicious on MRI as the lymph node measures only 0.5 cm in short-axis diameter, as seen on the corresponding axial T2-weighted MRI (*C, arrow*). Conversely, while the uptake in the right adnexal region (*A, arrowhead*) might be considered suspicious on PET due to its FDG avidity, it was confidently characterized as benign/physiologic ovarian uptake on axial T2-weighted MRI, as it corresponded to a normal ovary containing physiologic follicles (*B, C, arrowheads*).

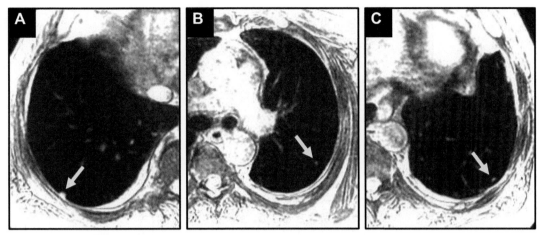

Fig. 3. MRI-based detection of lung nodules. High-resolution axial 3D T1-weighted gradient-echo MRI with a short echo time can be obtained in a single breath-hold during PET/MRI, enabling detection of even sub-centimeter lung nodules (*A–C, arrows*).

placement of receiver surface coils. Hence, some patients would need to undergo separate PET/CT and MRI exams on a wide-bore MRI platform. In addition, current PET/MRI systems operate at a 3.0 T field strength. Although 3.0 T platforms are favorable over 1.5 T in many aspects, offering higher signal-to-noise ratio and shorter scan times through accelerated image acquisition techniques, patients harboring certain medical devices/implants may only be able to undergo MRI at 1.5 T. Another disadvantage of PET/MRI is in the evaluation of lung nodules. This is relevant in the setting of gynecologic malignancies, as PET with MRI of the lungs can miss sub-centimeter lung nodules. High-resolution CT of the chest remains the most sensitive modality for detection of lung nodules. Hence, if evaluation of the lungs is desired, a separate CT of the chest should be considered in addition to PET. Advances in MRI

acquisition techniques have narrowed the gap between MRI and CT for detection of actionable lung nodules, and these techniques can be used in the setting of PET/MRI for evaluation of gynecologic malignancies (**Fig. 3**).[13,14]

PET/MRI PROTOCOL

In our group's approach, whole-body PET/MRI follows dedicated pelvis MRI in the same imaging session (**Fig. 4**). Patients are asked to fast for 4–6 hours before the exam except for small amounts of water with medications. The serum blood glucose level is checked before FDG administration and should be ≤ 200 mg/mL. Diabetic patients are asked to withhold insulin or oral hypoglycemic medications for 6 hours before their appointment. The FDG dose is 0.14 mCi/kg for adults, with minimum and maximum dose limits of 10 and 25 mCi,

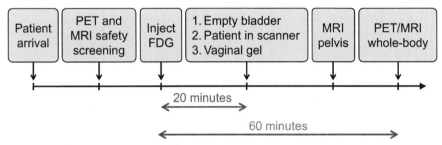

Fig. 4. Schematic workflow for PET/MRI. After arrival, patients undergo standard pre-PET evaluation and MRI safety screening; 20 minutes after intravenous administration of FDG, the patient empties their bladder and is placed on the PET/MRI scanner table. Vaginal gel is inserted for cervical and endometrial cancer cases. Dedicated MRI of the pelvis is performed first. Whole-body PET/MRI follows immediately after, performed 60 minutes post-FDG injection.

Table 1
Example of imaging protocol for MRI pelvis + PET/MRI whole-body

Pulse Sequence	TR (ms)	TE (ms)	NSA	FA	Slice Thickness/Gap (mm)	Matrix	FOV (mm)
Dedicated pelvis MRI							
Coronal 2D T2 SSFSE	min	80	1	90	5.0/0	320 × 224	500 × 500
Sagittal 2D T2 FSE	6000	102	2	111°	2.9/0.3	384 × 256	280 × 238
Axial 2D T2 FSE	4800	102	2	111°	2.9/0.3	384 × 224	320 × 320
Axial DWI (b = 0, 500 s/mm²)	6800	min	4	90°	4.5/0.5	192 × 192	320 × 320
Sagittal DWI* (b = 0, 500 s/mm²)	6800	min	6	90°	4.0/0.5	128 × 128	280 × 280
Axial 3D T1 Dixon pre-contrast and post-contrast	5.7	1.2, 2.4	1	15°	3.6/0	240 × 224	360 × 288
Sagittal 3D T1 Dixon post-contrast	6.4	1.2, 2.3	1	15°	3.6/0	216 × 224	320 × 256
Lungs							
Axial 3D T1 (breath-held)	2.1	0.9	1	4°	2.6/0	320 × 288	460 × 414
PET/MRI: skull-base to thigh							
• 5–6 PET beds (depending on patient height)							
MRAC	40	1.67,2.3	1	5°	5.2/0	256 × 128	500 × 380
Axial 3D T1 Dixon (head/neck station)	5.2	1.2, 2.3	1	10°	3.0/0	300 × 300	340 × 340
• 3 min per PET bed							
Axial 3D T1 Dixon (chest/abdomen/pelvis)	5.2	1.2, 2.3	1	10°	3.8/0	300 × 300	500 × 400
• In each PET bed, the following MRI images are acquired							
Axial T2 FRFSE Dixon	3000	110	2	111°	4/0.4	320 × 256	500 × 400

Abbreviations: DWI, diffusion-weighted imaging; FR-FSE, fast-recovery fast spin-echo; FSE, fast spin-echo; min, minimum; MRAC, MR-based attenuation correction; NSA, number of signal averages; SSFSE, single-shot fast spin-echo; TE, echo time; TR, repetition time.
*Sagittal DWI is performed only for endometrial cancer patients without prior hysterectomy.

respectively. Patients empty their bladder before entering the PET/MRI suite both for comfort and to help optimize PET image quality by minimizing the amount of FDG accumulated in the bladder. **Table 1** summarizes our image acquisition protocol. For whole-body PET/MRI, MRI images are acquired simultaneously with PET, with the goal of MR acquisition time not exceeding the PET time. MRI images must serve at least two purposes: attenuation correction and anatomic localization of abnormalities seen on PET. We achieve this aim through three MRI pulse sequences in each PET bed: Dixon-based MR attenuation correction (MRAC) as well as 3D T1-weighted and 2D T2-weighted images, both with Dixon fat suppression. We also acquire a single breath-hold axial 3D T1-weighted image through the chest for detection of pulmonary nodules (see **Fig. 3**).[8]

Efficient utilization of PET/MRI requires a different approach than the one typically taken toward individual PET and MRI exams. With concomitant PET imaging, a modified, shortened-pelvis MR acquisition can still obtain adequate diagnostic information. For example, fat-suppressed T2-weighted images of the pelvis as well as the post-contrast images of the lower abdomen (often acquired as part of dedicated pelvis MR imaging) can be eliminated as they are acquired as part of the whole-body PET/MR exam. This reduction in scan time leads to decreased patient discomfort and motion, and directly translates to higher image quality. The described approach to combined whole-body PET/MRI and pelvis MRI requires only 1 hour of scanner table time, minimizes the likelihood of PET and MRI misregistration through using a simultaneous PET/MRI acquisition, and achieves consistent radiotracer uptake times of approximately 60 minutes for the whole-body PET/MRI

exam. It is important that PET and MRI technologists work hand-in-hand. PET technologists inject the radiotracer and are trained to perform the MRI safety screening. Although scanning is carried out by the MRI technologists, post-processing and transferring of images is a joint effort. Two separate exams are generated: (1) a whole-body PET/MRI, which is interpreted by nuclear medicine physicians or radiologists certified to interpret PET, and (2) a dedicated pelvis MRI, which is interpreted by abdominal radiologists. Although the two exams are interpreted separately, the readers communicate to ensure concordance between the two reports.

UTILITY OF PET/MRI IN GYNECOLOGIC MALIGNANCIES
Cervical Cancer

MRI plays a key role in local staging of the primary cervical cancer, and it is integrated into the 2018 International Federation of Gynecology and Obstetrics (FIGO) staging system.[15–17] Although early disease may be diagnosed on histopathology from biopsy or excision, imaging guides treatment by identifying locally invasive or metastatic disease.[16,18] MRI is preferred over CT in evaluation of pelvic organs due to its superior tissue contrast resolution; this is especially relevant to cervical cancer (**Figs. 5** and **6**).[19,20] Furthermore, the primary tumor stage directly correlates with the probability of nodal metastases, with higher stages associated with worse prognoses.[21,22] FDG PET outperforms MRI and CT for detection of lymph node and distant cervical cancer metastases (see **Fig. 2**; **Fig. 7**).[1–4] Prior single-center studies have demonstrated a successful single-session approach using PET/MR, when pelvic MRI and whole-body PET are needed to respectively stage

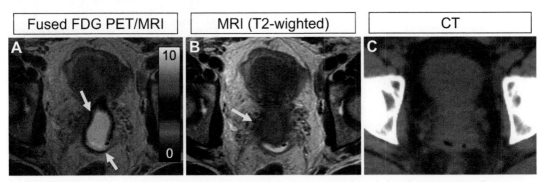

| Fused FDG PET/MRI | MRI (T2-wighted) | CT |

Fig. 5. PET/MRI assessment of parametrial invasion in cervical cancer. Although fused FDG PET/MRI demonstrates avid FDG uptake in the region of a cervical mass (*A, arrows*), parametrial invasion can only be seen on T2-weighted MRI (*B, arrow*) due to high tissue contrast and spatial resolution. Axial CT of the pelvis (*C*) is unable to confidently depict the tumor or its anatomic extent.

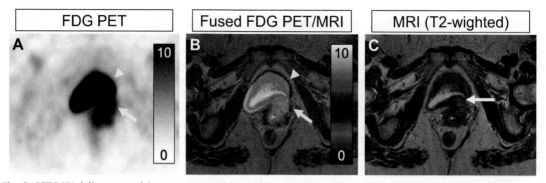

| FDG PET | Fused FDG PET/MRI | MRI (T2-wighted) |

Fig. 6. PET/MRI delineates pelvic tumor extent in cervical cancer. A patient with a new diagnosis of cervical cancer underwent PET/MRI for initial staging. Axial PET (*A*) and fused FDG PET/MRI (*B*) demonstrate abnormal uptake at the level of the cervical mass (*A, B, arrows*) that is inseparable from the activity of the excreted radiotracer in the urinary bladder (*A, B, arrowheads*), limiting the ability to discern bladder wall invasion by tumor. Axial T2-weighted MRI image (*C*) demonstrates a clear invasion of the posterior bladder wall by the cervical mass (*C, arrow*).

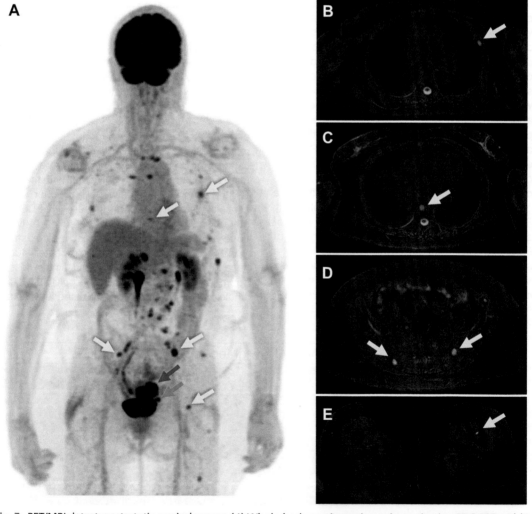

Fig. 7. PET/MRI detects metastatic cervical cancer. (*A*) Whole-body maximum intensity projection FDG PET and (*B–E*) fused PET/axial fat-suppressed T2-weighted MRI images in a patient with a new diagnosis of cervical cancer demonstrate an avid cervical mass (*A, red arrow*) and an adjacent pelvic nodal metastasis (*A, blue arrow*). In addition, widespread osseous metastases are demonstrated, including metastases to the left femur, bony pelvis, spine, and ribs (*A–E, yellow arrows*).

MRI	FDG PET	Fused PET/MRI

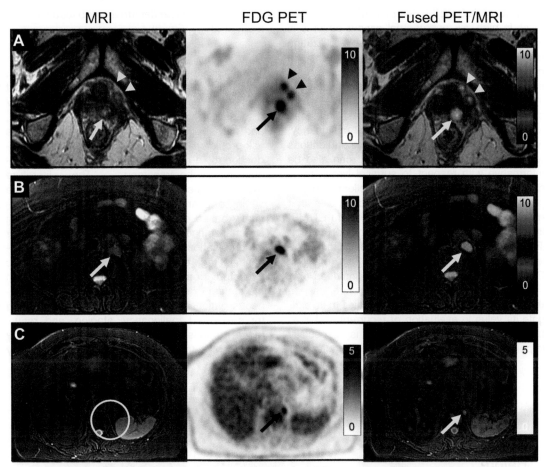

Fig. 8. PET/MRI guides management for recurrent disease. A patient with FIGO stage IB, grade 1 endometrioid carcinoma underwent curative-intent hysterectomy and adjuvant brachytherapy. Six months later, a pelvic exam revealed a mass. Oligorecurrent disease was suspected and surgery vs definitive radiotherapy was considered. (*A*) Restaging FDG PET/MRI, as illustrated by axial T2WI of the lower pelvis (*left panel*), corresponding axial PET (*middle panel*), and fused PET/MR imaging (*right panel*) demonstrated additional sites of disease recurrence in the vagina (*A, arrows*) and two retropubic nodules (*A, arrowheads*). (*B, C*) PET/MRI images of the abdomen, as illustrated by axial T2 fat-suppressed MRI images of the lower abdomen (*left panels*), corresponding axial PET (*middle panels*), and fused PET/MRI (*right panels*), also revealed left para-aortic and upper abdominal nodal metastatic disease (*B and C, arrows*), for which systemic treatment was recommended. Of note, one of the upper abdominal lymph nodes was only visible on PET (*C, circle*).

the primary tumor and evaluate the extent of metastatic disease.[23–25] PET/MRI has demonstrated a higher diagnostic accuracy than CT or MRI alone for the pre-treatment staging of cervical cancer.[26,27] When evaluating for tumor recurrence, PET/CT has been reported to impact patient management through successful detection of local recurrence and distant metastases.[28] Data on efficacy of PET/MRI in the same setting are limited; one study demonstrated that PET and MRI provide complementary information in assessment of treatment response or recurrent tumor, but in a small population that included 15 cervical cancer, 9 ovarian cancer, and 6 endometrial cancer

patients, where disease-specific data were not reported.[29]

Endometrial cancer

Initial diagnosis of endometrial cancer is established by endometrial sampling, with surgery performed to stage most patients. For those patients with high-risk histologic subtypes and grades, further staging may be needed to determine local tumor extent and presence of metastases. MRI is the widely accepted modality used for assessment of myometrial invasion and extra-uterine tumor spread and can guide the extent of surgery and nonsurgical treatment planning.[30]

The utility of FDG PET in detection of nodal metastases in high-risk endometrial cancer patients is established.[31] Literature supports the utilization of FDG PET/MRI for detection/staging of the primary tumor,[32] with favorable accuracy as compared to PET/CT for detection of myometrial invasion.[33–37] A non-contrast PET/MRI has a similar diagnostic accuracy to contrast-enhanced MRI for evaluation of endometrial malignancy, which is beneficial to those with contraindications to intravenous contrast.[38] PET/MRI can also be informative with respect to surgical lymph node dissection planning given its excellent negative predictive value.[32,39] There are no studies that have specifically investigated the role of PET/MRI in assessment of recurrent endometrial cancer. The aforementioned study by Kitajima and colleagues reporting the complementary roles of PET and MRI for recurrent disease included only six endometrial cancer patients.[29] Hence, despite the potential of PET/MRI, future studies to investigate its value in evaluation of recurrent endometrial cancer are needed. This is especially important because the extent of metastatic and/or recurrent disease determines subsequent treatment strategy (**Fig. 8**).

Ovarian cancer

The initial staging of ovarian cancer is surgical, which dictates the remainder of the treatment course.[40] Women with suspected stage IIIC or IV disease undergo a CT of the chest, abdomen, and pelvis, and those with a high peri-operative risk profile or a low likelihood of achieving cytoreduction to <1 cm of residual disease receive neoadjuvant chemotherapy.[41] The literature evaluating the role of PET/MR imaging in the setting of ovarian cancer is scarce and predominantly based on single-center studies that often summarize findings for PET/MRI in ovarian cancer in combination with results for other pelvic malignancies (eg, cervical and endometrial cancer). One study comparing PET/MRI to MRI and CT in the setting of ovarian cancer among a heterogeneous patient population (ie, patients presenting for suspected malignancy, staging, and recurrence) demonstrated superior diagnostic accuracy of PET/MRI for characterization of the primary

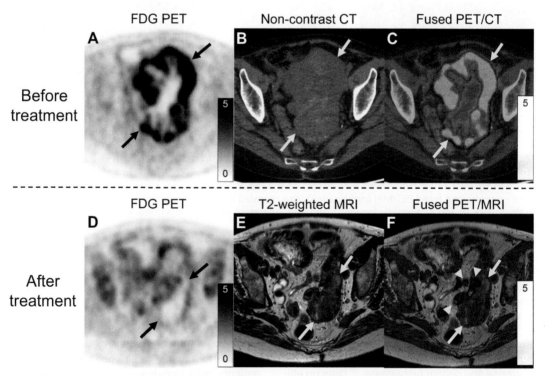

Fig. 9. PET/MRI for response assessment in ovarian cancer. (*A*) axial FDG PET, (*B*) axial non-contrast CT, and (*C*) fused PET/CT images from a pre-treatment PET/CT in a patient with high-grade serous carcinoma of the left ovary demonstrated an avid pelvic mass (*A and C, arrows*) that is difficult to distinguish from the surrounding structures on CT (*B, arrows*). (*D*) axial FDG PET, (*E*) axial T2-weighted MRI, and (*F*) fused images from the PET/MRI performed after systemic therapy demonstrate markedly decreased size and resolved FDG uptake of the mass (*D-F, arrows*). PET/MRI also confirmed that the low-level uptake around the mass was benign and corresponded to the adjacent bowel loops (*F, arrowheads*).

lesion and for M staging.[42] In one report of 31 ovarian cancer patients, the peritoneal carcinomatosis index assessed using PET/MRI was superior to that measured by diffusion-weighted imaging (DWI) alone, which suggests that PET/MRI may be a useful tool when evaluating patients for upfront surgical cytoreduction.[43] In the evaluation of patients with recurrent disease, PET/MRI has demonstrated favorable sensitivity over PET/CT or MRI alone among studies that evaluated ovarian cancer patients alongside other gynecologic malignancies.[29,44–46] Lastly, PET/MRI can also aid in the assessment of ovarian cancer response to treatment (**Fig. 9**).

Oligometastatic and oligorecurrent disease

Distinguishing patients with oligometastatic or oligorecurrent disease from those who present with widespread metastatic/recurrent often impacts treatment decisions.[47] For example, in the appropriate population with oligometastatic cervical cancer, targeted radiotherapy can achieve favorable outcomes,[48,49] while avoiding the potential toxicities of system chemotherapy. Several nonimaging clinical variables (eg, serum tumor markers in the setting of ovarian cancer or aggressive histology of the primary tumor) factor into whether a patient will benefit from an extensive imaging workup to assess for oligometastatic or oligorecurrent disease. That said, imaging is typically of vital importance for the assessment of recurrent disease, as the distribution of tumor recurrence can be unpredictable, given the heterogeneous behavior of cervical, endometrial, and ovarian tumors. The current literature discussed above supports the diagnostic performance and the complementary roles of PET and MRI in evaluation of gynecologic malignancies. Hence, the potential of simultaneous PET/MRI to accurately establish the oligometastatic or oligorecurrent state of disease (in one imaging session) is promising, but in need of further prospective, multi-site validation.

SUMMARY

The current body of literature supports the individual value of PET and MRI as well as their complementary nature in evaluation of gynecologic malignancies. Although several reports support the utilization of simultaneous PET/MRI in this setting, the majority of the current literature consists of single-center studies with no prospective trials on large and homogeneous patient cohorts to validate the apparent potential of PET/MRI. As clinical PET/MRI scanners become more available, the potential to execute such multi-center studies becomes more feasible. Successful implementation of a PET/MRI program, which overcomes the technical and logistical challenges of this combined modality, necessitates a multidisciplinary approach by radiologists, nuclear medicine physicians, and surgical/medical/radiation oncologists. Comprehensive imaging prior, during, and after treatment can help tailor treatment strategy, thereby, maximizing therapeutic benefit in patients with gynecologic malignancies.

DISCLOSURES

A. Pirasteh: Departmental research support (GE Healthcare) and KL2 Award Number TR002374. No other disclosures relevant to this work. M. Larson, E. Ssdowski, and P. Lovrec: No relevant disclosures.

REFERENCES

1. Grigsby PW, Siegel BA, Dehdashti F. Lymph node staging by positron emission tomography in patients with carcinoma of the cervix. J Clin Oncol 2001; 19(17):3745–9.
2. Choi HJ, Ju W, Myung SK, et al. Diagnostic performance of computer tomography, magnetic resonance imaging, and positron emission tomography or positron emission tomography/computer tomography for detection of metastatic lymph nodes in patients with cervical cancer: Meta-analysis. Cancer Sci 2010;101(6):1471–9.
3. Pandharipande PV, Choy G, del Carmen MG, et al. MRI and PET/CT for triaging stage IB clinically operable cervical cancer to appropriate therapy: decision analysis to assess patient outcomes. AJR Am J Roentgenol 2009;192(3):802–14.
4. Liu B, Gao S, Li S. A Comprehensive Comparison of CT, MRI, Positron Emission Tomography or Positron Emission Tomography/CT, and Diffusion Weighted Imaging-MRI for Detecting the Lymph Nodes Metastases in Patients with Cervical Cancer: A Meta-Analysis Based on 67 Studies. Gynecol Obstet Invest 2017;82(3):209–22.
5. Yoshida Y, Kurokawa T, Kawahara K, et al. Incremental benefits of FDG positron emission tomography over CT alone for the preoperative staging of ovarian cancer. AJR Am J Roentgenol 2004;182(1):227–33.
6. Reinhardt MJ, Ehritt-Braun C, Vogelgesang D, et al. Metastatic lymph nodes in patients with cervical cancer: detection with MR imaging and FDG PET. Radiology 2001;218(3):776–82.
7. Sadowski EA, Pirasteh A, McMillan AB, et al. PET/MR imaging in gynecologic cancer: tips for differentiating normal gynecologic anatomy and benign pathology versus cancer. Abdom Radiol (NY) 2022; 47(9):3189–204.

8. Ohliger MA, Hope TA, Chapman JS, et al. PET/MR Imaging in Gynecologic Oncology. Magn Reson Imaging Clin N Am 2017;25(3):667–84.

9. Melsaether AN, Raad RA, Pujara AC, et al. Comparison of Whole-Body F-18 FDG PET/MR Imaging and Whole-Body F-18 FDG PET/CT in Terms of Lesion Detection and Radiation Dose in Patients with Breast Cancer. Radiology 2016;281(1):193–202.

10. Ishiguro T, Nishikawa N, Ishii S, et al. PET/MR imaging for the evaluation of cervical cancer during pregnancy. BMC Pregnancy Childbirth 2021;21(1):7.

11. Lee SI, Catalano OA, Dehdashti F. Evaluation of Gynecologic Cancer with MR Imaging, F-18-FDG PET/CT, and PET/MR Imaging. J Nucl Med 2015;56(3):436–43.

12. Beiderwellen K, Grueneisen J, Ruhlmann V, et al. F-18 FDG PET/MRI vs. PET/CT for whole-body staging in patients with recurrent malignancies of the female pelvis: initial results. Eur J Nucl Med Mol Imaging 2015;42(1):56–65.

13. Burris NS, Johnson KM, Larson PEZ, et al. Detection of Small Pulmonary Nodules with Ultrashort Echo Time Sequences in Oncology Patients by Using a PET/MR System. Radiology 2016;278(1):239–46.

14. Cieszanowski A, Lisowska A, Dabrowska M, et al. MR Imaging of Pulmonary Nodules: Detection Rate and Accuracy of Size Estimation in Comparison to Computed Tomography. PLoS One 2016;11(6):e0156272.

15. Merz J, Bossart M, Bamberg F, et al. Revised FIGO Staging for Cervical Cancer - A New Role for MRI. Rofo-Fortschr Gebiet Rontgenstrahlen Bildgeb Verfahr 2020;192(10):937–44.

16. Bhatla N, Aoki D, Sharma DN, et al. Cancer of the cervix uteri. Int J Gynecol Obstet 2018;143:22–36.

17. Corrigendum to "Revised FIGO staging for carcinoma of the cervix uteri" Int J Gynecol Obstet 145(2019) 129-135. Int J Gynaecol Obstet 2019;147(2):279–80.

18. Network NCC. Cervical Cancer (Version 1.2021). Available at: https://www.nccn.org/professionals/physician_gls/pdf/cervical.pdf. Accessed October 15, 2020.

19. Hricak H, Gatsonis C, Chi DS, et al. Role of imaging in pretreatment evaluation of early invasive cervical cancer: Results of the Intergroup Study American College of Radiology Imaging Network 6651-Gynecologic Oncology Group 183. J Clin Oncol 2005;23(36):9329–37.

20. Bipat S, Glas AS, van der Velden J, et al. Computed tomography and magnetic resonance imaging in staging of uterine cervical carcinoma: a systematic review. Gynecol Oncol 2003;91(1):59–66.

21. Benedetti-Panici P, Maneschi F, D'Andrea G, et al. Early cervical carcinoma. Cancer 2000;88(10):2267–74.

22. Ditto A, Martinelli F, Lo Vullo S, et al. The Role of Lymphadenectomy in Cervical Cancer Patients: The Significance of the Number and the Status of Lymph Nodes Removed in 526 Cases Treated in a Single Institution. Ann Surg Oncol 2013;20(12):3948–54.

23. Grueneisen J, Schaarschmidt BM, Heubner M, et al. Integrated PET/MRI for whole-body staging of patients with primary cervical cancer: preliminary results. Eur J Nucl Med Mol Imaging 2015;42(12):1814–24.

24. Sarabhai T, Schaarschmidt BM, Wetter A, et al. Comparison of F-18-FDG PET/MRI and MRI for pre-therapeutic tumor staging of patients with primary cancer of the uterine cervix. Eur J Nucl Med Mol Imaging 2018;45(1):67–76.

25. Nazir A, Matthews R, Chimpiri AR, et al. Fluorodeoxyglucose positron-emission tomography-magnetic resonance hybrid imaging: An emerging tool for staging of cancer of the uterine cervix. World J Nucl Med 2021;20(2):150–5.

26. Tsuyoshi H, Tsujikawa T, Yamada S, et al. Diagnostic Value of (18)F-FDG PET/MRI for Revised 2018 FIGO Staging in Patients with Cervical Cancer. Diagnostics 2021;11(2):202.

27. Steiner A, Narva S, Rinta-Kiikka I, et al. Diagnostic efficiency of whole-body (18)F-FDG PET/MRI, MRI alone, and SUV and ADC values in staging of primary uterine cervical cancer. Cancer Imag 2021;21(1):16.

28. Mittra E, El-Maghraby T, Rodriguez CA, et al. Efficacy of 18F-FDG PET/CT in the evaluation of patients with recurrent cervical carcinoma. Eur J Nucl Med Mol Imaging 2009;36(12):1952–9.

29. Kitajima K, Suenaga Y, Ueno Y, et al. Value of fusion of PET and MRI in the detection of intra-pelvic recurrence of gynecological tumor: comparison with F-18-FDG contrast-enhanced PET/CT and pelvic MRI. Ann Nucl Med 2014;28(1):25–32.

30. Maheshwari E, Nougaret S, Stein EB, et al. Update on MRI in Evaluation and Treatment of Endometrial Cancer. Radiographics 2022;42(7):2112–30.

31. Atri M, Zhang Z, Dehdashti F, et al. Utility of PET/CT to Evaluate Retroperitoneal Lymph Node Metastasis in High-Risk Endometrial Cancer: Results of ACRIN 6671/GOG 0233 Trial. Radiology 2017;283(2):450–9.

32. Ironi G, Mapelli P, Bergamini A, et al. Hybrid PET/MRI in Staging Endometrial Cancer: Diagnostic and Predictive Value in a Prospective Cohort. Clin Nucl Med 2022;47(3):e221–9.

33. Queiroz MA, Kubik-Huch RA, Hauser N, et al. PET/MRI and PET/CT in advanced gynaecological tumours: initial experience and comparison. Eur Radiol 2015;25(8):2222–30.

34. Schwartz M, Gavane SC, Bou-Ayache J, et al. Feasibility and diagnostic performance of hybrid PET/MRI compared with PET/CT for gynecological malignancies: a prospective pilot study. Abdominal Radiology 2018;43(12):3462–7.

35. Kitajima K, Suenaga Y, Ueno Y, et al. Value of fusion of PET and MRI for staging of endometrial cancer:

Comparison with F-18-FDG contrast-enhanced PET/CT and dynamic contrast-enhanced pelvic MRI. Eur J Radiol 2013;82(10):1672–6.

36. Bian LH, Wang M, Gong J, et al. Comparison of integrated PET/MRI with PET/CT in evaluation of endometrial cancer: a retrospective analysis of 81 cases. PeerJ 2019;7:10.

37. Yu Y, Zhang L, Sultana B, et al. Diagnostic value of integrated 18F-FDG PET/MRI for staging of endometrial carcinoma: comparison with PET/CT. BMC Cancer 2022;22(1).

38. Tsuyoshi H, Tsujikawa T, Yamada S, et al. Diagnostic value of F-18-FDG PET/MRI for staging in patients with endometrial cancer. Cancer Imag 2020;20(1):9.

39. Zhang GM, Chen HY, Liu YY, et al. Is lymph node dissection mandatory among early stage endometrial cancer patients? A retrospective study. BMC Wom Health 2020;20(1):5.

40. Berek JS, Kehoe ST, Kumar L, et al. Cancer of the ovary, fallopian tube, and peritoneum. Int J Gynecol Obstet 2018;143:59–78.

41. Wright AA, Bohlke K, Armstrong DK, et al. Neoadjuvant chemotherapy for newly diagnosed, advanced ovarian cancer: Society of Gynecologic Oncology and American Society of Clinical Oncology Clinical Practice Guideline. Gynecol Oncol 2016;143(1): 3–15.

42. Tsuyoshi H, Tsujikawa T, Yamada S, et al. Diagnostic value of F-18 FDG PET/MRI for staging in patients with ovarian cancer. EJNMMI Res 2020;10(1):14.

43. Jonsdottir B, Ripoll MA, Bergman A, et al. Validation of F-18-FDG PET/MRI and diffusion-weighted MRI for estimating the extent of peritoneal carcinomatosis in ovarian and endometrial cancer -a pilot study. Cancer Imag 2021;21(1):10.

44. Grueneisen J, Beiderwellen K, Heusch P, et al. Simultaneous Positron Emission Tomography/Magnetic Resonance Imaging for Whole-Body Staging in Patients With Recurrent Gynecological Malignancies of the Pelvis A Comparison to Whole-Body Magnetic Resonance Imaging Alone. Invest Radiol 2014;49(12):808–15.

45. Sawicki LM, Kirchner J, Grueneisen J, et al. Comparison of F-18-FDG PET/MRI and MRI alone for whole-body staging and potential impact on therapeutic management of women with suspected recurrent pelvic cancer: a follow-up study. Eur J Nucl Med Mol Imaging 2018;45(4):622–9.

46. Zheng ML, Xie DH, Pan CH, et al. Diagnostic value of F-18-FDG PET/MRI in recurrent pelvis malignancies of female patients: a systematic review and meta-analysis. Nucl Med Commun 2018;39(6): 479–85.

47. Pirasteh A, Lovrec P, Pedrosa I. Imaging and its Impact on Defining the Oligometastatic State. Semin Radiat Oncol 2021;31(3):186–99.

48. Ning MS, Ahobila V, Jhingran A, et al. Outcomes and patterns of relapse after definitive radiation therapy for oligometastatic cervical cancer. Gynecol Oncol 2018;148(1):132–8.

49. Kunos CA, Brindle J, Waggoner S, et al. Phase II clinical trial of robotic stereotactic body radiosurgery for metastatic gynecologic malignancies. Front Oncol 2012;2:6.

Image-Guided Radiotherapy for Gynecologic Malignancies
What the Radiologist Needs to Know

Megan C. Jacobsen, PhD[a], Ekta Maheshwari, MD[b], Ann H. Klopp, MD, PhD[c],
Aradhana M. Venkatesan, MD[d],*

KEYWORDS

- Image-guided radiotherapy • Gynecologic malignancies • Cervical cancer • Endometrial cancer
- Vaginal cancer • Vulvar cancer

KEY POINTS

- Imaging is integral to the management of radiotherapy (RT) candidates with cervical, endometrial, vulvar, and vaginal malignancies, for whom RT with or without platinum-based chemotherapies can be used as a definitive, neoadjuvant, adjuvant, or palliative therapy.
- RT can be delivered using external beam RT or brachytherapy, for which proper positioning of gynecologic applicators is critical. Radiologic reporting of computed tomography (CT) or MR imaging performed following gynecologic brachytherapy implant placement should include a description of the position of uterine tandems, ovoids or rings, cylinders, and interstitial needles relative to the uterus and cervix as well as the bladder, rectum, and sigmoid colon.
- T2-weighted MR imaging provides optimal pretreatment assessment of gynecologic cancers for planning RT, whereas ^{18}F-fluorodeoxyglucose PET/CT is optimal for the detection of metastatic lymphadenopathy and distant disease.
- Diffusion-weighted imaging and early phase postcontrast, fat-saturated T1-weighted MR imaging have high specificity for the detection of residual or recurrent disease following RT.
- Short-term effects of RT include inflammation, edema, and fibrosis of the gynecologic, genitourinary, and gastrointestinal organs. Long-term severe sequelae of gynecologic RT include pelvic fistulas, such as those between the vagina and adjacent organs, as well as pelvic insufficiency fractures that may occur years after RT.

INTRODUCTION

Gynecologic malignancy remains a leading cause of cancer incidence and mortality among women in the United States.[1] Radiotherapy (RT) is an essential modality for the treatment of locally advanced gynecologic malignancy. Imaging is integral to the management of these patients and

---

[a] Division of Diagnostic Imaging, Department of Imaging Physics, The University of Texas MD Anderson Cancer Center, 1400 Pressler Street, Unit 1472, Houston, TX 77030, USA; [b] Division of Abdominal Imaging, Department of Radiology, University of Pittsburgh Medical Center, PUH Suite E204, 200 Lothrop St, Pittsburgh, PA 15213, USA; [c] Department of Radiation Oncology, The University of Texas MD Anderson Cancer Center, 1400 Pressler Street, Houston, TX 77030, USA; [d] Division of Diagnostic Imaging, Department of Diagnostic Imaging, The University of Texas MD Anderson Cancer Center, 1400 Pressler Street, Unit 1473, Houston, TX 77030, USA
* Corresponding author.
E-mail address: avenkatesan@mdanderson.org
Twitter: @megjacobsen (M.C.J.); @dr_ektam (E.M.); @AnnKloppMD (A.H.K.); @AVenkatesanMD (A.M.V.)

Radiol Clin N Am 61 (2023) 725–747
https://doi.org/10.1016/j.rcl.2023.02.012
0033-8389/23/© 2023 Elsevier Inc. All rights reserved.

plays a critical role in candidate selection, RT treatment planning, execution, and follow-up. This review is focused on the role of imaging in the management of RT candidates with cervical, medically inoperable endometrial, vulvar, and vaginal cancers, the primary gynecologic malignancies treated definitively with radiation.

RADIATION THERAPY CONCEPTS

RT is used in conjunction with concurrent chemotherapy in appropriately selected candidates with gynecologic malignancy as part of definitive chemoradiotherapy (CRT). Pelvic radiation treats microscopic disease to minimize the likelihood of recurrence after the initial treatment. RT can be delivered externally using a linear accelerator via external beam radiotherapy (EBRT), or by placing radioactive sources within the patient for set durations, known as brachytherapy (BT). EBRT can be delivered to the whole pelvis or using targeted techniques with intensity modulated radiotherapy (IMRT). IMRT delivers precise radiation doses to tumor with many conformal beams, which results in high dose to tumor while dose to normal tissue and organs at risk (OARs) is minimized. Common OARs for gynecologic cancers include the sigmoid colon, rectum, and bladder. In addition to treating the primary tumor, additional fields to boost dose to involved lymph node basins may be added to treat regional disease.

Imaging is required for RT treatment planning (Fig. 1). It is most frequently performed using computed tomography (CT) but other three-dimensional imaging modalities such as MR imaging and PET/CT are also utilized. T2-weighted MR imaging (T2WI) provides optimal image contrast between tumors and surrounding tissues, allowing for more accurate tumor delineation than CT.[1] Baseline T2WI is frequently used as a reference to guide CT planning. ^{18}F-fluorodeoxyglucose (^{18}F-FDG) PET/CT assesses whole body glucose metabolism, which allows for the detection of regional and distant metastatic sites.

BT for gynecologic malignancies delivers radiation dose to tumor locally using beta-emitting radiation sources, commonly iridium-192, which deposit large amounts of energy over a short range in tissue.[2] Radiation sources are placed into intracavitary applicators (Fig. 2) inserted into the endometrial cavity, vagina, or apposed to the cervix[3] (Boxes 1 and 2). Alternatively, interstitial applicators (needles) can be placed directly into the substance of tumor. CT and MR imaging-based treatment planning has become integral to clinical practice, being able to delineate target tumor, OARs, and the relative position of BT

applicators, leading to treatment regimens associated with lower rates of severe toxicity and improved outcomes.[1,4]

CERVICAL CANCER

Cervical cancer staging is determined by the 2018 International Federation of Gynecology and Obstetrics (FIGO) guidelines (Table 1) and, in contrast to older versions of the FIGO staging system, specifically incorporates MR imaging for tumor staging (Figs. 7 and 8).[5] CRT is the standard of care for locally advanced cervical cancer of stage IB3 or greater. Tumors smaller than 4 cm that remain localized to the cervix are treated surgically but medically inoperable cases of stage IA2-IB2 cervical cancer are also treated with CRT. The RT schema for cervical cancer includes EBRT followed by BT of intact or residual cervical tumors.[6]

Imaging examinations are critical for determining cervical cancer staging at presentation, which has a direct impact on whether patients receive surgery or CRT as their first-line therapy. Nearly all patients receive both baseline MR imaging and ^{18}F-FDG PET/CT. MR imaging is ideal for identifying the extent of local and regional disease, with optimal visualization of tumor extension into the parametrium, vagina, pelvic wall, bladder, and rectum, as well as identification of hydronephrosis (see Figs. 7 and 8).[7–9] Typical imaging sequences for diagnostic MR imaging of cervical cancer and other gynecologic malignancies are summarized in Table 2.[10–12] Acquisition of the T2WI and diffusion-weighted imaging (DWI) acquisitions as oblique axials achieves true axial images through the cervix, enhancing delineation of parametrial tumor extension,[10,12] with some authors advocating acquisition of imaging parallel to the cervical canal to optimize visualization of parametrial invasion.[12,13] Cervical tumors appear moderately hyperintense compared with the hypointense ring of the normal cervix on T2WI (see Fig. 7) and demonstrate restricted diffusion on DWI images (high signal on high b-value images, and low signal on apparent diffusion coefficient maps; Fig. 8). Identification of vaginal involvement is aided by the administration of vaginal gel, which is hyperintense on T2WI.[12,13] Metastatic pelvic and para-aortic lymph nodes can often be visualized with MR imaging and are typically identified using morphology and size thresholds (short axis diameter of >1 cm).

^{18}F-FDG PET/CT is primarily used to identify metabolically active metastatic disease sites (Fig. 9), with a high sensitivity, specificity and accuracy for detecting metastatic pelvic and para-aortic lymph nodes, including those whose size

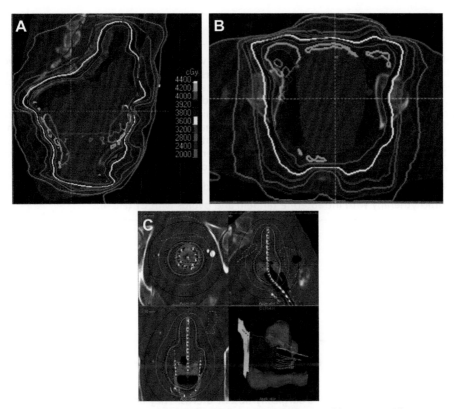

Fig. 1. (A) Sagittal and (B) axial EBRT treatment planning on CT in a 60-year-old woman with FIGO stage IIIB cervical cancer. The primary tumor and high-risk target volume are contoured in solid red and the nodal targets in blue. Isodose lines (unfilled, colored concentric shapes in A, B) connect points receiving an equal radiation dose or equal dose rates; they represent the total dose from EBRT in units of centigray (cGy). (C) Brachytherapy treatment planning in the same patient with a tandem, ovoids, and interstitial needles. Radioactive source dwell locations are represented by red dots, OARs are represented by dotted contours, and the isodose curves are represented as solid lines.

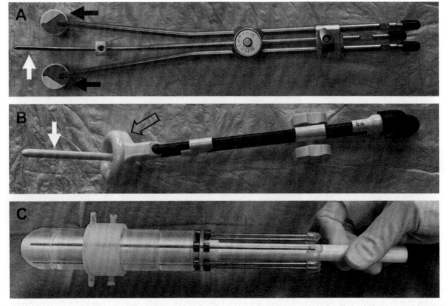

Fig. 2. Examples of gynecologic intracavitary brachytherapy applicators, including (A) an intrauterine tandem (white arrow) and ovoids (black arrows), (B) tandem (white arrow) and ring (open arrow), and (C) a vaginal cylinder.

Box 1
Positioning of the intrauterine tandem

The tip of the intrauterine tandem should be positioned within the endometrial cavity at the level of the uterine fundus, without perforating the myometrium (Figs 3, 4) Sagittal and oblique coronals (aligned with the tandem) are of greatest utility for determining applicator positioning, whether using CT or MR imaging. Real-time ultrasound guidance is recommended during implantation to minimize the risk of uterine perforation. Improper applicator positioning at the time of treatment can result in high-radiation dose to OARs and uterine perforation may increase operating and imaging time, delay treatment, and increase the risk of procedural complications such as hemorrhage or infection.[3,5] Measurement of distance from the tip of the tandem to uterine fundus may be requested by the radiation oncology team to assess applicator movement over time or between treatments.

- MR imaging for brachytherapy with intrauterine tandem and ring (Fig 3)
- CT for brachytherapy with intrauterine tandem and ovoids with CT (Fig 4).

Box 2
Imaging intravaginal cylinders and interstitial needles for brachytherapy

Vaginal cylinders are commonly used for brachytherapy to treat disease that has spread down the vaginal canal or for patients with a surgically absent uterus. They are typically made of high-density plastics or acrylic, and thus many can be imaged on both MR imaging and CT. Intrauterine tandems may be used with many commercial cylinders if the uterus is present

- MR imaging of intravaginal cylinders in patients with an intact uterus (Fig 5)
- MR imaging of intravaginal cylinder in patients with a surgically absent uterus (Fig 6)

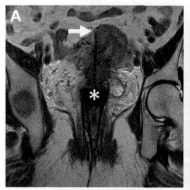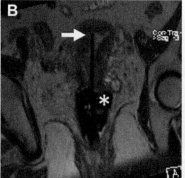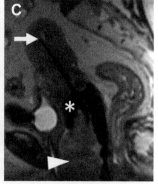

Fig. 3. (*A*) Oblique coronal T2WI in a patient with cervical cancer undergoing brachytherapy demonstrates a hypointense intrauterine tandem (*white arrows*), with the tip located outside the endometrial cavity and embedded in the outer aspect of the fundal myometrium. Intraoperative repositioning was performed, with subsequent MR imaging (*B*) oblique coronal reformat of 3D T2WI and (*C*) sagittal T2WI demonstrate the repositioned tandem properly positioned within the endometrial cavity with the tandem tip positioned near the uterine fundus and with the hypointense ring (*asterisks*) abutting the cervix, with vaginal packing (*arrowhead*) for device immobilization

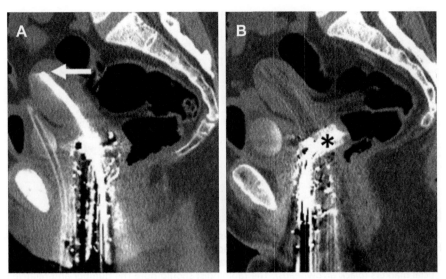

Fig. 4. (*A*) Sagittal CT reformats demonstrating proper positioning of an intrauterine tandem (*white arrow*), which appears hyperdense. Streak artifact may be present due to the use of metallic dummy radiation sources for treatment planning or due to use of metallic applicators. (*B*) Sagittal CT reformat demonstrating proper position of the ovoid (*asterisk*) abutting the cervix. Vaginal packing may also be hyperdense due to insertion of radio-opaque wire impregnated gauze, used both for immobilization, and to visualize the vaginal canal on orthogonal radiographs.

and appearance may not be suspicious on MR imaging.[14] This is particularly important for identifying patients with FIGO stage IIIC1 or IIIC2 disease that may require additional radiation dose to metastatic lymph node basins. Because ^{18}F-FDG PET/CT is typically acquired from the head through the thighs, it is also the optimal modality to detect distant metastases in bone, lungs, liver,

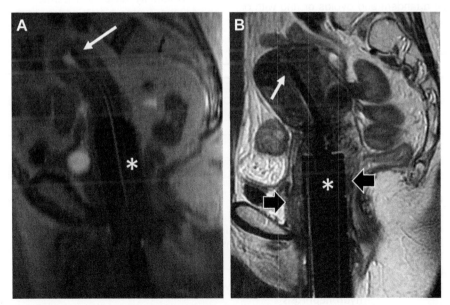

Fig. 5. Sagittal T2WI in patients with: (*A*) Intravaginal cylinder (*asterisk*) in a case of FIGO stage I medically inoperable endometrial cancer. The rounded top of the cylinder is appropriately positioned, abutting the cervix, and the intrauterine tandem with a hyperintense marker defining the radioactive source channel for treatment planning is properly positioned in the endometrial canal with the tip at the fundus. (*B*) Cylinder (*asterisk*) placement in a patient with primary vaginal cancer with a tandem (*white arrow*) and residual tumor (*black arrows*) adjacent to the applicator (**Fig 17**)

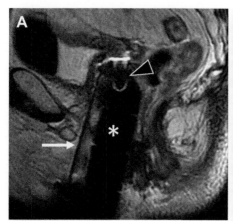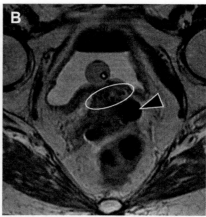

Fig. 6. (*A*) Sagittal T2WI of brachytherapy cylinder (*asterisk*) and interstitial needle (*white arrow*) in a 74-year-old woman with vaginal carcinoma. The needle shown extends into the posterior vaginal cuff lesion. Four additional interstitial needles are visible on (*B*) axial T2WI (*white oval*). The lesion is partially obscured by susceptibility arti-fact from fiducial markers (*black arrowheads*). The radiologist should note the number and relative location of the needles, particularly whether they terminate within or superior to the tumor, and if they are in proximity to organs-at-risk (rectum, sigmoid colon, and bladder).

and distant lymph nodes, which indicate FIGO stage IVB disease.

EBRT simulation for treatment planning is typi-cally performed using CT acquired in the radiation oncology department. Generally, diagnostic MR is acquired following the completion of EBRT to assess treatment response and determine the optimal BT approach. Most cervical cancer BT im-plants utilize a tandem and ovoids or ring with or without interstitial needles (see **Boxes 1** and **2** for positioning and reporting guidelines).

Follow-up imaging for cervical cancer is meant to evaluate the response to CRT and periodically evaluate patients for recurrent disease. The typical imaging schema for posttreatment follow-up in cervical cancer is pelvic MR imaging following EBRT to assess disease before BT, and ^{18}F-FDG PET/CT 3 to 4 months after the completion of CRT to identify residual hypermetabolic sites in the primary tumor, lymph nodes, or distant loca-tions that may represent metastatic disease. In cases where the cervix recovers the normal

Table 1
2018 International Federation of Gynecology and Obstetrics staging guidelines for cervical cancer

Stage	Sub-Stage	Anatomic Involvement	Tumor Size/Extent
I	IA1	Cervix	Stromal invasion <3 mm
	IA2		Stromal invasion 3–5 mm
	IB1		≥5 mm stromal invasion and <2 cm in greatest dimension
	IB2		≥2 and < 4 cm in greatest dimension
	IB3		≥4 cm in greatest dimension
II	IIA1	Upper two-thirds of the vagina,	<4 cm
	IIA2	without parametrial extension	≥4 cm
	IIB	Parametrial extension	Any size
III	IIIA	Lower third of the vagina	Any size
	IIIB	Pelvic wall invasion with or without hydronephrosis	
	IIIC1	Pelvic lymph node metastasis	
	IIIC2	Para-aortic lymph node metastasis	
IV	IVA	Bladder or rectal mucosa	Any size
	IVB	Distant metastases (eg, to lymph nodes, lungs, or bones)	

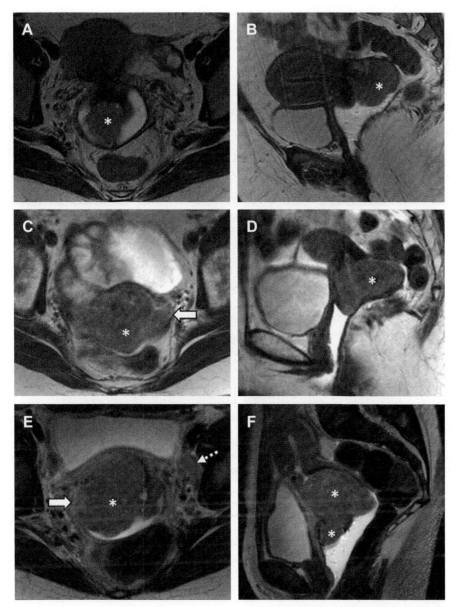

Fig. 7. Cervical cancer stages, on T2-weighted axial (left column) and sagittal (right column) MR imaging. (*A*, *B*) FIGO stage IB3 cervical cancer (*asterisk*) in a 40-year-old woman. Disease is localized to the cervix but measures greater than 4 cm in greatest dimension. (*C*, *D*) A 63-year-old woman with FIGO stage IIB squamous cell carcinoma of the cervix (*asterisk*) with bulky disease extending into the upper third of the vagina and involving the left lateral parametrium (*C*, *arrow*). (*E*, *F*) FIGO stage IIIC1 squamous cell carcinoma in a 36-year-old woman. Parametrial extension (*E*, *solid arrow*), and an enlarged metastatic left external iliac lymph node (*E*, *dotted arrow*) are present, along with disease involving the upper two-thirds of the vagina.

appearance of its zonal anatomy (**Fig. 10**), there is high-negative predictive value for recurrent disease.[15] Additional information regarding the differentiation of residual and recurrent disease on MR imaging is summarized in **Box 3**. The combination of DWI and contrast-enhanced MR imaging enables differentiation of expected postradiation cervical changes (**Fig. 11**) from recurrent disease as recurrent or residual disease will demonstrate enhancement and restricted diffusion (see **Box 3**). Additional MR imaging or ^{18}F-FDG PET/ CT may be obtained if there is clinical evidence

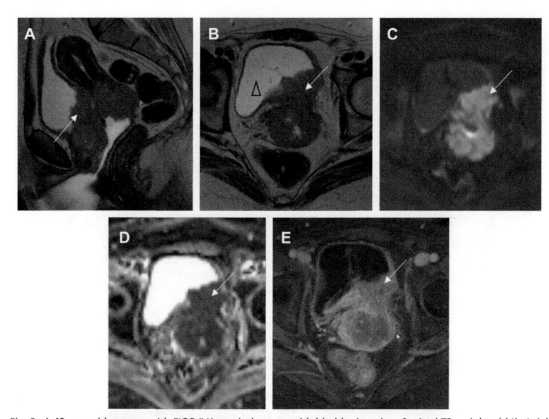

Fig. 8. A 49-year-old woman with FIGO IVA cervical cancer with bladder invasion. Sagittal T2-weighted (*A*), Axial T2-weighted (*B*), axial DWI (*C*) and corresponding ADC map (*D*), and axial T1 fat-saturated post contrast (*E*) images are provided. Gross tumor extension into the bladder lumen is evident (*white arrows*), and the tumor shows characteristic intermediate T2 signal, high DWI signal with low ADC, and enhancement on postcontrast imaging. Double pigtail ureteral stents are partially visualized (*arrowhead* in B).

Table 2
American Brachytherapy Society-Society of Abdominal Radiology suggested MR imaging pulse sequences for imaging of cervical cancer[12]

Dimension/Plane/Contrast	Weighting	Sequence Type
2D Axial/Axial Oblique	T2WI	FSE or FRFSE
2D Sagittal/Sagittal Oblique	T2WI	FSE or FRFSE
2D Coronal/Coronal Oblique	T2WI	ss-FSE
2D Axial	T1WI	FSE
2D Axial/Axial Oblique	DWI	EPI
3D Sagittal Precontrast	T1WI	GRE
3D Sagittal + Contrast	T1WI	GRE
3D Axial Postcontrast	T1WI	GRE

Abbreviations: 2D, two dimensional; 3D, three dimensional; DWI, diffusion-weighted imaging; FRFSE, fast relaxation FSE; FSE, fast spin echo; ss, single-shot; T1WI, T1-weighted; T2WI, T2-weighted.

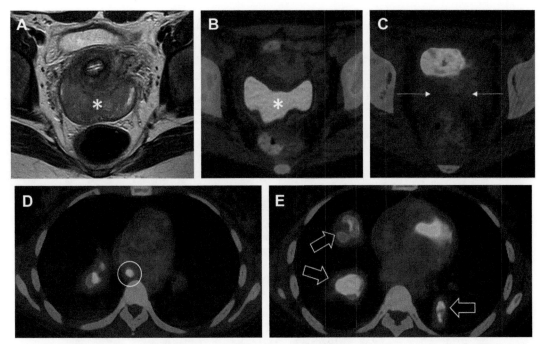

Fig. 9. A 35-year-old woman initially diagnosed with FIGO stage IIB squamous cell carcinoma (*asterisks*), as shown on axial T2-weighted MR imaging (*A*) and baseline ^{18}F-FDG PET/CT (*B*). The patient underwent definitive CRT. On follow-up ^{18}F-FDG PET/CT at 5 months, local disease had resolved, with the treated cervix demonstrating no hypermetabolic activity (*arrows, C*). However, disease had metastasized to the subcarinal lymph nodes (*circle, D*) and lungs (*open arrows, E*).

for disease recurrence or severe RT-induced toxicities (**Box 4**).

ENDOMETRIAL CANCER

Endometrial cancer, also known as cancer of the corpus uteri, develops from the epithelial layer lining the interior of the uterus, and locally extends into the myometrium. Two main subtypes of endometrial cancer have been described by histopathologic criteria. Type I tumors, which are estrogen-dependent include grade 1 and 2 endometrioid adenocarcinomas. Type II tumors are not estrogen-dependent and include the more clinically aggressive grade 3 endometrioid adenocarcinomas, serous papillary adenocarcinomas, and clear cell adenocarcinomas.[16] There are 4 molecular subtypes of endometrial cancers classified by the Cancer Genome Atlas network, ordered here from best to worst prognosis: DNA polymerase ε (POLE) group tumors, comprising exonuclease domain mutations, microsatellite instability hypermutated, low-copy number and and high-copy number tumors, with high copy number tumors presenting with an elevated incidence of TP53 mutations.[16,17] Published studies

have confirmed that these molecular subtypes independently predict clinical outcomes[18] and, as such, help inform risk stratification, particularly when considering whether to utilize adjuvant CRT.

Endometrial cancer is clinically staged using the FIGO classification and staging system, most recently revised in 2009 (**Table 3**). Imaging is not a part of the staging system for endometrial cancer but does influence treatment selection[16] (**Fig. 17**). MR imaging is the preferred imaging modality for preoperative assessment of key prognostic factors, specifically tumor size, depth of myometrial invasion, cervical stromal involvement, extrauterine disease, and nodal involvement.

For localized endometrial cancer, standard therapy is definitive total hysterectomy with bilateral salpingo-oophorectomy with or without lymph node dissection.[19] RT is routinely administered as definitive therapy with EBRT and/or BT and can be used alone or in combination with surgery. Criteria for administration of RT can be found in **Table 4**.

MR imaging is vital to planning definitive, neoadjuvant, adjuvant, and salvage radiation for endometrial cancers.[20] It enables visualization of tumor

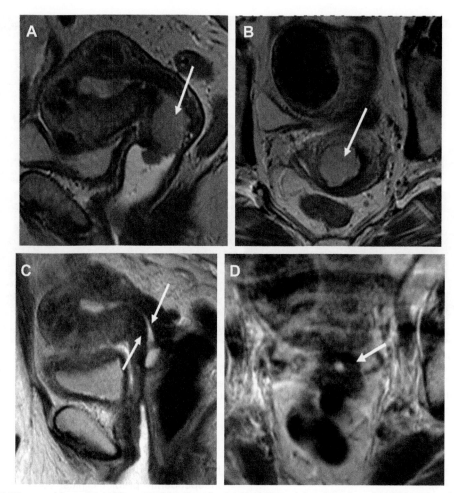

Fig. 10. A 74-year-old woman with sagittal (*A,C*) and axial (*B,D*) T2-weighted MR imaging before (*A, B*) and after (*C, D*) definitive chemoradiotherapy for stage IB3 cervical adenocarcinoma. Pretreatment images demonstrate a T2 hyperintense mass at the level of the cervix (*arrows* in A, B). Posttreatment images demonstrate the resolution of the mass, with restitution of the normal T2 hypointense cervical stroma, apparent as paired linear foci of T2 hypointense signal on the sagittal T2WI (*arrows* in C) and as an intact T2 hypointense ring on the axial T2WI (*arrow* in D).

myometrial depth and local extent, as well as adjacent organ involvement.[21] Endometrial cancer BT frequently utilizes cylindrical applicators (see **Box 2**) for patients who have undergone hysterectomy to treat the vaginal vault but a uterine tandem may be used in cases where the uterus in intact.[22] In the case of endometrial cancers, it is particularly important for the tandem tip to be positioned near the uterine fundus to treat the endometrial cavity[22] (see **Box 1**).

MR imaging following therapy guides subsequent treatment strategy by assessing therapeutic efficacy and evaluating for radiation-resistant or recurrent disease. Published literature demonstrates a high degree of correlation between post-RT response assessment on MR imaging with clinical outcomes in endometrial cancer.[23,24] Expected post-RT findings include decreased uterine and cervical volume (simulating a normal postmenopausal uterus), endometrial thinning, and loss of uterine zonal anatomy definition. The most common sites of endometrial cancer recurrence are the vaginal vault and lymph nodes, with most recurrences occurring within the first 2 years after treatment. MR imaging is vital to assess for recurrent disease, which typically appears as an intermediate or heterogeneous T2 signal intensity mass, with associated restricted diffusion and enhancement (see **Box 3, Fig. 18**). In cases of recurrence, invasion of adjacent organ

Box 3
Identifying residual or recurrent disease on MR imaging following radiotherapy

RT results in posttreatment inflammation and edema, which demonstrate intermediate-to-high signal on T2WI and high-b value MR imaging as well as variable enhancement on postcontrast T1WI. RT-induced fibrosis may also impede visualization of recurrent tumors on T2WI. Therefore, posttreatment changes can be confounders for residual or recurrent disease. DWI and contrast-enhanced T1WI with fat saturation are the MR imaging sequences most sensitive for the detection of recurrent disease following RT.

• Residual endometrial cancer with regions of post-RT tissue changes (**Fig 12**)

• Post-RT tissue changes in the cervix without residual disease (**Fig 13**)

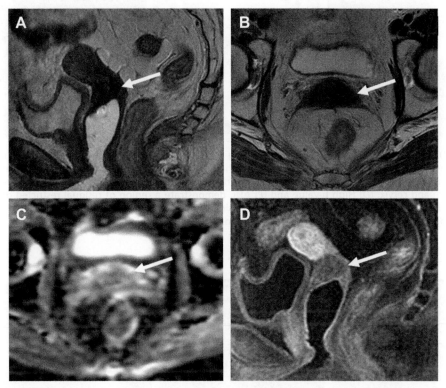

Fig. 11. Post-CRT MR imaging in a 54-year-old woman treated for stage IIB cervical adenocarcinoma. The cervix appears uniformly hypointense (*white arrows*) without return to normal zonal anatomy on sagittal (*A*) and axial T2WI (*B*). The DWI ADC map (*C*) does neither indicate restricted diffusion nor is there significant enhancement on postcontrast sagittal T1WI (*D*), indicating fibrotic cervical tissue.

Box 4
Severe late effects of radiation therapy in gynecologic malignancies

In addition to acute and chronic inflammation and fibrosis, which may occur at the tumor site, in OARs, or surrounding normal tissue exposed to radiation, there are other long-term effects of pelvic RT with severe impacts on patient quality of life, including fistulas, vaginal stenosis, and insufficiency fractures in the pelvis. Vesicovaginal, urethrovaginal, and rectovaginal fistulas are rare complications but are more likely to occur when disease invades or abuts OARs, necessitating high focal radiation dose may be delivered to the region. These complications can occur months to years after initial RT.

• Fistula development in a patient with cervical cancer treated with radiotherapy (**Fig 14**)

• Vesicovaginal and rectovaginal fistulas on MR imaging with vaginal gel (**Fig 15**)

• Pelvic insufficiency fractures following radiotherapy (**Fig 16**)

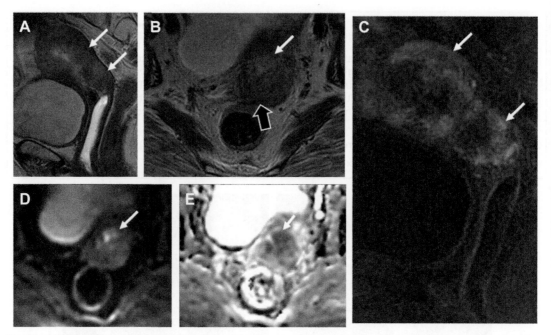

Fig. 12. (A) Sagittal and (B) axial T2WI demonstrating suspected residual endometrial tumor with mixed low (*black arrow*) to intermediate signal (*white arrows*) at the level of the lower uterine segment and cervix. (C) Early phase contrast-enhanced fat-saturated T1WI demonstrates corresponding heterogenous enhancement of the myometrium and cervix. (D) High b-value and (E) ADC demonstrate a region of residual restricted diffusion at the level of the cervix (*white arrow*). Recurrent or residual disease will demonstrate early enhancement with restricted diffusion and is more specific for malignant disease detection than T2WI alone Fig 19.

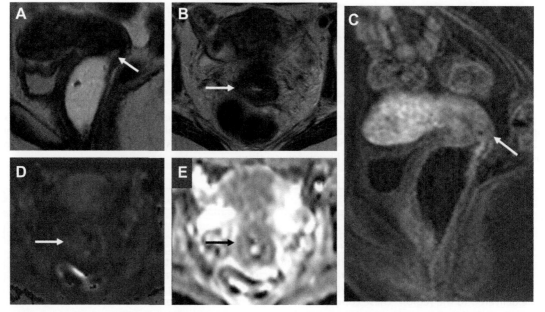

Fig. 13. (A) Sagittal and (B) axial T2WI demonstrating a region of intermediate signal intensity (*white arrow*) in a patient with cervical cancer treated with CRT. (C) Early phase contrast-enhanced fat-saturated T1WI demonstrates subtle cystic changes to the cervix without enhancement (*white arrow*). (D) High b-value and (E) ADC do not demonstrate signs of restricted diffusion, consistent with posttreatment changes. Disease remained stable with no evidence for local recurrence.

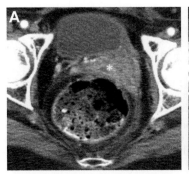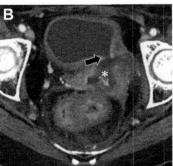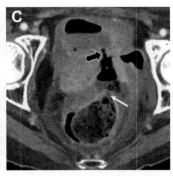

Fig. 14. Contrast-enhanced axial CTs in a patient with recurrent FIGO stage IIIB cervical cancer treated with earlier RT. (*A*) A heterogeneously enhancing mass (*asterisk*) is shown abutting the posterior bladder. (*B*) CT acquired 5 months later shows interval tumor necrosis (*asterisk*) and development of a vesicovaginal fistula (*black arrow*). (*C*) CT obtained 20 months after the CT shown in (*A*) redemonstrates the vesicovaginal fistula (*black arrow*) and interval development of a small rectovaginal fistula tract (*white arrow*).

and pelvic sidewall is evaluated on MR imaging to assess the likelihood of surgical resectability and plan salvage therapy. ^{18}F-FDG PET/CT is helpful to exclude nodal and distant metastases (**Fig. 19**).

VULVAR CANCER

Cancers of the vulva, which include malignancies of the labia majora and minora, clitoris, and vestibular glands, represent 3% to 5% of all gynecologic malignancies.[25] Many lesions present as a lump or sore on the labia with itching, pain, or bleeding. Regional spread occurs through the inguinal and femoral lymph nodes, with the potential for bilateral involvement in large or centrally located tumors. Disease in the pelvic lymph nodes or outside the pelvis indicates metastatic disease.[25]

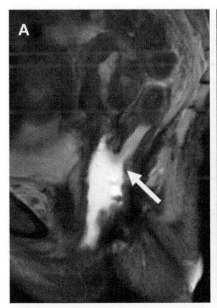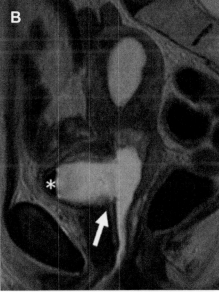

Fig. 15. (*A*) Sagittal T2WI in a patient with cervical cancer treated with CRT showing a large rectovaginal fistula (*arrow*). Vaginal gel demonstrates clear communication between the rectum and vagina. (*B*) Sagittal T2WI in a patient with recurrent cervical cancer treated with definitive CRT with large vesicovaginal fistula (*arrow*), evident as a gross defect between the posterior urinary bladder and anterior vagina. Air (*asterisk*) is seen in the bladder and can be a sign of fistula when the bladder is collapsed at imaging in the absence of recent earlier instrumentation or Foley catheterization. Each of these patients was managed with palliative ostomies and chemotherapy.

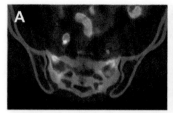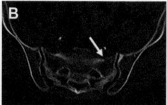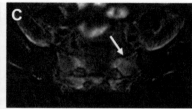

Fig. 16. (*A*) ^{18}F-FDG PET, (*B*) corresponding CT, and (*C*) follow-up fat-saturated T2WI MRI demonstrating pelvic insufficiency fractures following radiotherapy for uterine neuroendocrine carcinoma. ^{18}F-FDG PET demonstrates bilateral heterogeneous FDG uptake of the right and left sacral alae, with the associated CT demonstrating a subtle cortical discontinuity along the anterior left hemisacrum, indicative of an insufficiency fracture (*arrow* in *B*) that was redemonstrated on MR imaging (*arrow* in *C*).

The FIGO staging system for vulvar cancer was revised in 2021[26] (**Table 5**). Analogous to the updated FIGO staging guidelines for cervical cancer, cross-sectional imaging findings have been incorporated into the FIGO staging system for vulvar cancer (**Fig. 20**). Regional lymph node involvement in vulvar cancer is defined as spread to inguinal or femoral nodal basins but there is a debate regarding the staging of patients with limited pelvic nodal metastases because survival outcomes are similar to stage III disease when these nodes are treated with RT.[27,28]

Treatment of vulvar cancer is most frequently surgical but adjuvant and definitive CRT are used in certain circumstances.[25,29,30] BT is theoretically ideally suited to treat medically inoperable cases of vulvar cancer or recurrent tumors via an interstitial approach to deliver high doses to the primary tumor while minimizing dose to OARs, yet survival benefit over EBRT alone is inconclusive.[30] Vaginal cylinders may also be used for intracavitary BT of disease invading the vagina. MR imaging is critical for determining which patients are unlikely to have negative surgical margins and would benefit from definitive or adjuvant RT. Vulvar tumors may be hypointense to intermediate signal on T1WI, are intermediate to hyperintense on T2WI, with restricted diffusion on DWI, and early enhancement on contrast-enhanced fat-saturated T1WI.[14,31] Vulvar carcinoma masses are typically solid, and the radiologist should note any disruption of the hypointense vaginal wall, anal sphincter, or urethra. Fat-saturated T2WI provides optimal visualization of the primary tumor.[32] Disease may extend into the urethra, vagina, and anus in addition to the vulvar anatomy. Although pelvic MR imaging will generally include the inguinal and pelvic nodal basins, ^{18}F-FDG PET/CT is particularly useful for identifying potentially metastatic

Table 3
2009 International Federation of Gynecology and Obstetrics staging guidelines for endometrial cancer

Stage	Substage	Anatomic Involvement	Tumor Size
I	IA1	Corpus uteri	Less than 50% myometrial invasion
	IA2		>50% myometrial invasion
II	II	Cervical stroma, not extending outside uterus	Any size
III	IIIA	Serosa of corpus uteri and/or adnexa	Any size
	IIIB	Vaginal and/or parametrium	
	IIIC1	Pelvic lymph node metastasis	
	IIIC2	Para-aortic lymph node metastasis	
IV	IVA	Bladder and/or rectal mucosa	Any size
	IVB	Distant metastasis in abdomen or other nodal sites	

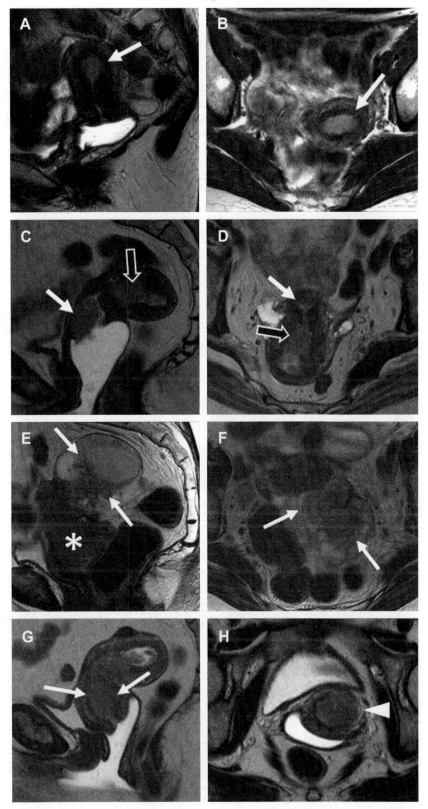

Fig. 17. Sagittal (left column) and axial (right column) T2WI. (*A, B*) MR imaging findings compatible with FIGO stage IA endometrial cancer (*arrows*) with invasion of less than 50% of the myometrium. (*C, D*) MR imaging findings compatible with FIGO stage II endometrial carcinoma (*black arrow*), with invasion of the cervix (*white arrows*). (*E, F*) MR imaging findings compatible with FIGO stage IIIA disease, with a large primary tumor (*asterisk*) and cystic left ovarian metastasis (*arrows*). (*G, H*) MR imaging findings compatible with FIGO stage IIIB endometrial cancer invading the cervix (*arrows* in G) with early left parametrial invasion (*arrowhead* in H).

Table 4
Criteria for treatment modality choice in endometrial cancers

Treatment Modality	Criteria
Surgery alone	• Localized disease
Neoadjuvant radiotherapy + surgery	• Locally advanced disease spread beyond the cervix • Positive pelvic or para-aortic lymph node
Adjuvant radiotherapy + surgery	• Histologic grade 1–2 with deep myometrial invasion • Histologic grade 3 • Clear cell or serous histopathology • FIGO stage III and IV
Definitive chemoradiotherapy	• Early stage disease • Medically inoperable • Patients without upfront adjuvant or neoadjuvant RT

femoral nodes and distant metastases (**Fig. 21**). Ultrasound may also be used to monitor metastatic inguinal or femoral nodes over time given their relatively superficial location.

Follow-up imaging for vulvar cancer is predominantly performed with ¹⁸F-FDG PET/CT and MR imaging, with PET for assessment of nodal and distant metastatic disease and MR to assess for

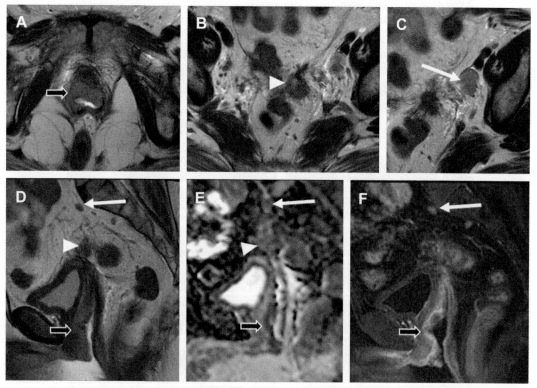

Fig. 18. Recurrent endometrial cancer in a 48-year-old woman following prior hysterectomy. Axial T2WI (*A–C*) demonstrates local recurrence in the vaginal cuff (*black arrow* in A), (*B*) a metastatic implant superior to the vaginal cuff and abutting the sigmoid colon (*arrowhead* in B), and a grossly metastatic left obturator node (*white arrow* in C). (*D*) Sagittal T2WI, (*E*) ADC, and (*F*) early phase contrast-enhanced T1WI with fat saturation demonstrate the superior-inferior extent of the local recurrence (*black arrows*), the metastatic implant (*arrowheads*) also seen in (*B*), and superior rectal adenopathy (*white arrows*).

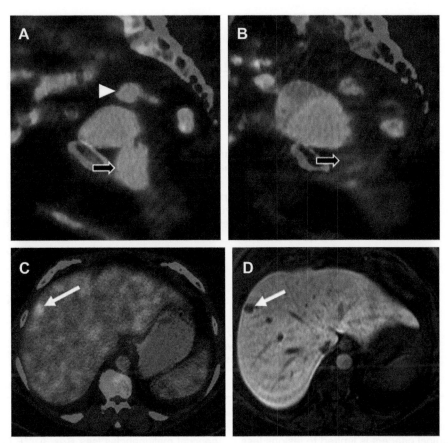

Fig. 19. A 48-year-old patient (same as Fig. 18) with recurrent endometrial cancer of the vaginal cuff. (A) Sagittal ^{18}F-FDG PET/CT demonstrates local recurrence (*black arrow*) and a metastatic implant superior to the vaginal cuff and abutting the sigmoid colon (*arrowhead*). (B) Follow-up sagittal and (C) axial ^{18}F-FDG PET/CT 7 months later after salvage pelvic RT demonstrated resolution of the local recurrence (*black arrow* in B) and pelvic metastatic implant but identified a hypermetabolic focus in the liver (*white arrow* in C), which corresponded to a liver lesion lacking contrast uptake on subsequent T1 fat-saturated postcontrast MR imaging performed with gadoxetaate sodium, imaged at 20 minutes following contrast administration (*white arrow* in D). Subsequent image-guided biopsy of this lesion confirmed hepatic metastatic disease.

local recurrence, which most likely occurs to the perineum or groin. DWI and contrast-enhanced studies are useful for differentiating fibrosis and granulation tissue from recurrent disease because T2WI intermediate signal intensity is less specific after RT.[31]

VAGINAL CANCER

Primary vaginal cancer is rare since approximately 90% of vaginal lesions are metastatic in nature but, when present, these tumors are often associated with high-risk strains of HPV. The most common clinical presentation is vaginal bleeding with odorous discharge, and the

diagnosis is confirmed with biopsy and exclusion of other gynecologic malignancy. As for cervical cancer, approximately 90% of cases are squamous carcinomas, with an additional 10% associated with adenocarcinoma. The disease progresses locally into the paravaginal tissues, with more extensive disease involving the urethra, bladder, or rectum, followed by regional lymphatic spread to the pelvic and groin lymph nodes. Common metastatic sites include lung, liver, and bone.

There are 2 staging systems commonly used to classify vaginal cancers: the American Joint Committee on Cancer (AJCC) TNM classification and the FIGO staging system, although

Table 5
2021 International Federation of Gynecology and Obstetrics staging of vulvar carcinoma

Stage	Sub-stage	Anatomic Involvement	Size or Location Details
I	IA	Vulva	Tumor size ≤2 cm and depth of invasion ≤1 mm
	IB		Tumor size >2 cm or depth of invasion >1 mm
II	None	Extension to any of: • Lower third of urethra • Lower third of vagina • Lower third of anus	Any size
III	IIIA	Extension to upper part of adjacent perineal structures or nonfixed, nonulcerated lymph nodes	Any size, disease extends to upper two-thirds of urethra or vagina, invades the bladder or rectal mucosa, or involves regional (inguinal or femoral) lymph nodes ≤5 mm
	IIIB		Regional lymph node metastases >5 mm
	IIIC		Regional lymph node metastases with extracapsular spread
IV	IVA	Bone lesions of any size, fixed or ulcerated lymph node metastases, distant metastases	Disease fixed to pelvic bone or fixed/ulcerated inguinofemoral lymph node metastases
	IVB		Distant metastases

they are largely similar (**Table 6**). Surgical treatment of vaginal cancers is limited to lesions less than 2 cm deep that do not extend past the vaginal mucosa, or AJCC Stage IA (T1a N0 M0)/FIGO stage I disease.[33] Definitive CRT with EBRT and BT are used to treat the vagina, external iliac and obturator nodes, with fields for the inguinal nodes added if they are metastatic or if the tumor is in the distal vagina. This treatment strategy is largely extrapolated from cervical cancer studies given the rarity of the disease, although some studies have shown a survival benefit for CRT with cisplatin over RT alone.[33,34]

As for cervical cancer, MR imaging is critical for identifying the extent of disease along the vagina, infiltration into the pelvic wall or other organs, and lymphadenopathy. MR imaging is used to identify the depth of invasion and whether tumors are amenable to BT in addition to EBRT. The majority of BT implants for vaginal cancer are cylinders with or without interstitial needles, depending on the extent of disease and proximity to the posterior bladder and anterior rectum. Lesions that are close to the rectum (**Fig. 22**) may be at additional risk for rectovaginal fistulae after CRT if RT is administered in high doses. Recurrent and residual disease are best identified on a combination of T2WI, postcontrast T1WI, and DWI/apparent

diffusion coefficient (ADC) and appear similar to cervical malignancies (see **Box 3**). ^{18}F-FDG PET/CT is used for the identification of distant metastasis or inguinal or pelvic nodal metastases.

PALLIATIVE RADIOTHERAPY FOR GYNECOLOGIC CANCERS

Complications of gynecologic cancers and their therapies can reduce the quality of life for patients and encompass gynecologic, genitourinary, and gastrointestinal symptoms (see **Box 4**). Patients with locally advanced disease and symptomatic but incurable, distant metastases may opt to receive focal palliative radiation to help medically manage their symptoms and improve quality of life. Palliative radiation can be used to reduce bleeding and provide significant pain relief for patients, and it is typically delivered in a short course of high-dose, focal RT.[35] CT and MR imaging are vital to the evaluation of advanced, symptomatic disease that may benefit from palliative RT. Representative imaging findings include bulky disease in the setting of patient pain, tumor associated hemorrhage, and hydronephrosis secondary to genitourinary tract obstruction by retroperitoneal or pelvic adenopathy or implants.

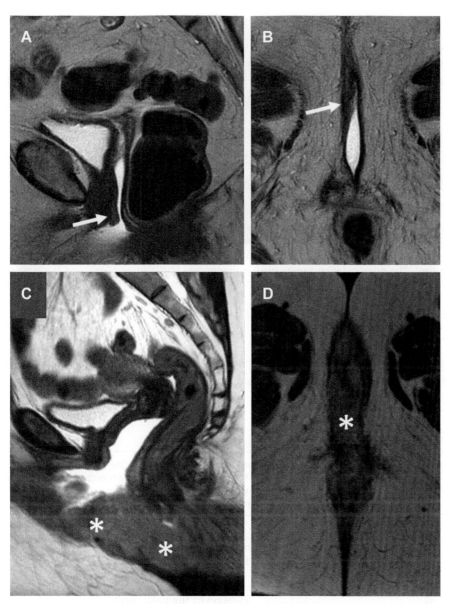

Fig. 20. (*A, B*) Sagittal and axial T2WI of an 83-year-old woman with FIGO stage I vulvar cancer presenting as a nodule of intermediate T2 signal intensity (*arrows*) in the right anterior inner labia. (*C, D*) Sagittal and axial T2WI of a 34-year-old woman with FIGO stage IIIB vulvar cancer presenting with a lobulated mass replacing the vulva (*asterisks*) abutting the clitoris and involving the anus, with spread to the inguinal lymph nodes (not shown).

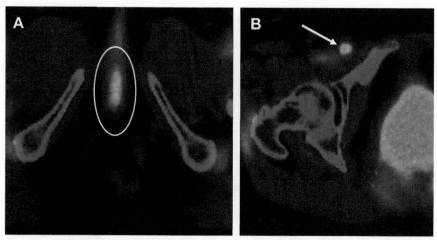

Fig. 21. A 65-year-old woman with FIGO stage IB primary vulvar cancer undergoing ¹⁸F-FDG PET/CT (*A, B*) for the initial assessment. The primary lesion (*white oval*) is moderately FDG-avid and involving the labia majora (*A*), associated with a hypermetabolic right inguinal lymph nodal metastasis on ¹⁸F-FDG PET/CT (*arrow, B*).

Table 6
American Joint Committee on Cancer TNM and International Federation of Gynecology and Obstetrics staging systems for vaginal cancer

AJCC Classification			
Stage	TNM Grouping[a]	FIGO Stage	Description
IA	T1a N0 M0	I	Tumor ≤2 cm localized to the vagina (T1a) without spread to pelvic or inguinal lymph nodes (N0) or distant metastases (M0)
IB	T1b N0 M0		Tumor >2 cm localized to the vagina (T1b)
IIA	T2a N0 M0	II	Tumor ≤2 cm has grown through the vaginal wall without invasion of the pelvic wall
IIB	T2b N0 M0		Tumor >2 cm has grown through the vaginal wall without invasion of the pelvic wall
III	T1-T3 N1 M0	III	Tumor of any size growing into the pelvic wall and/or lower third of the vagina, and/or causing hydronephrosis (T3) or meeting criteria of T1-T2 with spread to pelvic or inguinal lymph nodes (N1)
	T3 N0 M0		Tumor of any size growing into the pelvic wall and/or lower third of the vagina, and/or causing hydronephrosis (T3) without spread to lymph nodes
IVA	T4 Any N M0	IVA	Cancer invading the bladder, rectum, or growing outside the pelvis (T4), with or without spread to any number of pelvic or inguinal lymph nodes (any N) without distant metastasis (M0)
IVB	Any T Any N M1	IVB	Tumor of any size (any T) with spread to distant organs (M1) such as lung or bone, with or without spread to lymph nodes (any N)

[a] T, tumor; N, lymph node; M, metastases.

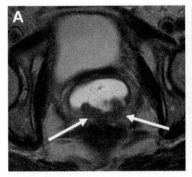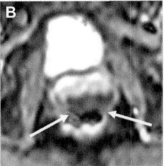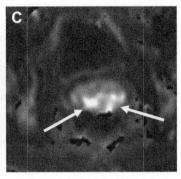

Fig. 22. A 52-year-old woman with FIGO stage II vaginal cancer. Axial (*A*) T2WI, (*B*) ADC, and (*C*) high b-value DWI show a lobulated mass involving the posterior vaginal wall that abuts the rectum without evidence of invasion (*white arrows*).

SUMMARY

Pelvic imaging is integral to the contemporary RT management of gynecologic malignancies. For cervical, endometrial, vulvar, and vaginal cancers, three-dimensional imaging modalities aid in tumor staging and RT candidate selection, confirmation of treatment modality, RT planning, and posttherapy surveillance. State-of-the-art care incorporates MR imaging, ^{18}F-FDG PET/CT, CT and ultrasound to guide EBRT and BT, allowing the customization of RT plans aimed at optimal patient outcomes and minimized treatment-related toxicities.

CLINICS CARE POINTS

- Imaging evaluation of localized gynecologic malignancies in potential radiotherapy candidates should be performed with multiparametric MRI, including T2-weighted, diffusion-weighted, and multi-phase post contrast-enhanced imaging, while evaluation for regional and distant disease is best performed with ^{18}F-FDG PET/CT.

- Imaging of gynecologic brachytherapy applicators for treatment planning is best performed with CT or MR, with T2WI MR providing optimal differentiation of gynecologic tumors from background tissues.

- Assessment of surveillance imaging should include an evaluation for sequelae of radiotherapy, including pelvic visceral inflammation, fibrosis, fistulae, and pelvic insufficiency fractures.

DISCLOSURE

A.H. Klopp is the current president of the American Brachytherapy Society (2021–2022) and Vice Chair of the society's Uterine Corpus Cancer Subcommittee. A.M. Venkatesan receives grant funding from the University of Texas MD Anderson Cancer Center Institutional Research Grant Program, the University of Texas MD Anderson Cancer Center Radiation Oncology Strategic Initiatives Pilot Grant Program, the Oden Institute for Computational Engineering and Sciences, UTMDACC & Texas Advanced Computing Center (TACC) Oncological Data & Computational Sciences Grant Program, and the Department of Defense.

REFERENCES

1. Fokdal L, Sturdza A, Mazeron R, et al. Image guided adaptive brachytherapy with combined intracavitary and interstitial technique improves the therapeutic ratio in locally advanced cervical cancer: Analysis from the retroEMBRACE study. Radiother Oncol 2016;120(3):434–40.

2. Perez-Calatayud J, Ballester F, Das RK, et al. Dose calculation for photon-emitting brachytherapy sources with average energy higher than 50 keV: report of the AAPM and ESTRO. Med Phys 2012;39(5): 2904–29.

3. Bahadur YA, Eltaher MM, Hassouna AH, et al. Uterine perforation and its dosimetric implications in cervical cancer high-dose-rate brachytherapy. J Contemp Brachytherapy 2015;7(1): 41–7.

4. Tan LT, Pötter R, Sturdza A, et al. Change in Patterns of Failure After Image-Guided Brachytherapy for Cervical Cancer: Analysis From the RetroEMBRACE Study. Int J Radiat Oncol Biol Phys 2019;104(4): 895–902.

5. Salib MY, Russell JHB, Stewart VR, et al. 2018 FIGO Staging Classification for Cervical Cancer: Added Benefits of Imaging. Radiographics 2020;40(6): 1807–22.

6. Chino J, Annunziata CM, Beriwal S, et al. Radiation Therapy for Cervical Cancer: Executive Summary of an ASTRO Clinical Practice Guideline. Practical Radiation Oncology 2020;10(4):220–34.

7. Xiao M, Yan B, Li Y, et al. Diagnostic performance of MR imaging in evaluating prognostic factors in patients with cervical cancer: a meta-analysis. Eur Radiol 2020;30(3):1405–18.

8. Woo S, Atun R, Ward ZJ, et al. Diagnostic performance of conventional and advanced imaging modalities for assessing newly diagnosed cervical cancer: systematic review and meta-analysis. Eur Radiol 2020;30(10):5560–77.

9. Woo S, Suh CH, Kim SY, et al. Magnetic resonance imaging for detection of parametrial invasion in cervical cancer: An updated systematic review and meta-analysis of the literature between 2012 and 2016. Eur Radiol 2018;28(2):530–41.

10. Dimopoulos JC, Petrow P, Tanderup K, et al. Recommendations from Gynaecological (GYN) GEC-ESTRO Working Group (IV): Basic principles and parameters for MR imaging within the frame of image based adaptive cervix cancer brachytherapy. Radiother Oncol 2012;103(1):113–22.

11. Haie-Meder C, Pötter R, Van Limbergen E, et al. Recommendations from Gynaecological (GYN) GEC-ESTRO Working Group (I): concepts and terms in 3D image based 3D treatment planning in cervix cancer brachytherapy with emphasis on MRI assessment of GTV and CTV. Radiother Oncol 2005;74(3):235–45.

12. Jacobsen MC, Beriwal S, Dyer BA, et al. Contemporary image-guided cervical cancer brachytherapy: Consensus imaging recommendations from the Society of Abdominal Radiology and the American Brachytherapy Society. Brachytherapy 2022;21(4): 369–88.

13. Manganaro L, Lakhman Y, Bharwani N, et al. Staging, recurrence and follow-up of uterine cervical cancer using MRI: Updated Guidelines of the European Society of Urogenital Radiology after revised FIGO staging 2018. Eur Radiol 2021;31(10): 7802–16.

14. Venkatesan AM, Menias CO, Jones KM, et al. MRI for Radiation Therapy Planning in Human Papillomavirus-associated Gynecologic Cancers. Radiographics 2019;39(5):1476–500.

15. Hricak H, Swift PS, Campos Z, et al. Irradiation of the cervix uteri: value of unenhanced and contrast-enhanced MR imaging. Radiology 1993;189(2): 381–8.

16. Maheshwari E, Nougaret S, Stein EB, et al. Update on MRI in Evaluation and Treatment of Endometrial Cancer. Radiographics 2022;42(7):2112–30.

17. Kandoth C, Schultz N, Cherniack AD, et al. Integrated genomic characterization of endometrial carcinoma. Nature 2013;497(7447):67–73.

18. Cosgrove CM, Tritchler DL, Cohn DE, et al. An NRG Oncology/GOG study of molecular classification for risk prediction in endometrioid endometrial cancer. Gynecol Oncol 2018;148(1):174–80.

19. Koskas M, Amant F, Mirza MR, et al. Cancer of the corpus uteri: 2021 update. Int J Gynaecol Obstet 2021;155(Suppl 1):45–60.

20. Kidd EA. Imaging to optimize gynecological radiation oncology. Int J Gynecol Cancer 2022;32(3): 358–65.

21. Conway JL, Lukovic J, Laframboise S, et al. Brachying Unresectable Endometrial Cancers with Magnetic Resonance Guidance. Cureus 2018;10(3): e2274.

22. Schwarz JK, Beriwal S, Esthappan J, et al. Consensus statement for brachytherapy for the treatment of medically inoperable endometrial cancer. Brachytherapy 2015;14(5):587–99.

23. Otero-García MM, Mesa-Álvarez A, Nikolic O, et al. Role of MRI in staging and follow-up of endometrial and cervical cancer: pitfalls and mimickers. Insights Imaging 2019;10(1):19.

24. Gebhardt BJ, Rangaswamy B, Thomas J, et al. Magnetic resonance imaging response in patients treated with definitive radiation therapy for medically inoperable endometrial cancer-Does it predict treatment response? Brachytherapy 2019;18(4): 437–44.

25. Olawaiye AB, Cuello MA, Rogers LJ. Cancer of the vulva: 2021 update. Int J Gynaecol Obstet 2021; 155(Suppl 1):7–18.

26. Olawaiye AB, Cotler J, Cuello MA, et al. FIGO staging for carcinoma of the vulva: 2021 revision. Int J Gynaecol Obstet 2021;155(1):43–7.

27. Shinde A, Li R, Amini A, et al. Role of Locoregional Treatment in Vulvar Cancer With Pelvic Lymph Node Metastases: Time to Reconsider FIGO Staging? J Natl Compr Canc Netw 2019; 17(8):922–30.

28. Thaker NG, Klopp AH, Jhingran A, et al. Survival outcomes for patients with stage IVB vulvar cancer with grossly positive pelvic lymph nodes: time to reconsider the FIGO staging system? Gynecol Oncol 2015;136(2):269–73.

29. Rao YJ, Hui C, Chundury A, et al. Which patients with inoperable vulvar cancer may benefit from brachytherapy in addition to external beam radiation? A Surveillance, Epidemiology, and End Results analysis. Brachytherapy 2017;16(4): 831–40.

30. Tagliaferri L, Lancellotta V, Casà C, et al. The Radiotherapy Role in the Multidisciplinary Management of Locally Advanced Vulvar Cancer: A Multidisciplinary VulCan Team Review. Cancers 2021; 13(22).

31. Miccò M, Russo L, Persiani S, et al. MRI in the Evaluation of Locally Advanced Vulvar Cancer Treated

with Chemoradiotherapy and Vulvar Cancer Recurrence: The 2021 Revision of FIGO Classification and the Need for Multidisciplinary Management. Cancers 2022;14(16).

32. Kataoka MY, Sala E, Baldwin P, et al. The accuracy of magnetic resonance imaging in staging of vulvar cancer: a retrospective multi-centre study. Gynecol Oncol 2010;117(1):82–7.

33. Adams TS, Rogers LJ, Cuello MA. Cancer of the vagina: 2021 update. Int J Gynaecol Obstet 2021; 155(Suppl 1):19–27.

34. Miyamoto DT, Viswanathan AN. Concurrent chemoradiation for vaginal cancer. PLoS One 2013;8(6):e65048.

35. Skliarenko J, Barnes EA. Palliative pelvic radiotherapy for gynaecologic cancer. Journal of Radiation Oncology 2012;1(3):239–44.

Radiomics and Radiogenomics of Ovarian Cancer

Implications for Treatment Monitoring and Clinical Management

Camilla Panico, MD[a], Giacomo Avesani, MD, MSc[a],*,
Konstantinos Zormpas-Petridis, Bsc, MSc, PhD[a,b], Leonardo Rundo, PhD[c],
Camilla Nero, MD, PhD[d,e], Evis Sala, MD, PhD, FRCR, FRCP[a,e]

KEYWORDS

- Radiomics • Radiogenomics • Ovarian cancer • Tumor heterogeneity • Tumor habitat

KEY POINTS

- Ovarian cancer has high inter- and intra-tumoral heterogeneity that may have implications for response to therapy and prognosis; conventional diagnostic imaging interpretation cannot adequately interrogate these tumor characteristics.
- Radiomics can capture complex patterns related to the microstructure of tissues, providing quantitative data about tumor subvolumes; this allows for the interrogation of whole tumor heterogeneity noninvasively.
- Tracking tumor heterogeneity through the combination of radiomic features, genomic variables and their association with pathology has the potential to enable more effective monitoring of tumor evolution and treatment response compared with conventional approaches.
- Within the same lesion, there are different regions characterized by similar radiomic features, called "habitats," which indicate specific tumor microenvironments and molecular profiles; these can be explored and tracked during treatment noninvasively using virtual biopsy
- Radiomics and multi-omics approaches still need to be standardized and validated before entering the clinical routine, but their promising results may enable more personalized therapy in the future

TUMOR HETEROGENEITY IN OVARIAN CANCER

Ovarian cancer (OC) is the sixth most common cancer and the fifth cause of cancer-related death among women.[1] Many pieces of evidence support that high-grade serous OC (HGSOC) exhibits molecular heterogeneity at both an inter-tumoral level (between patients harboring tumors of the same histologic type) and at an intra-tumoral level (among the tumor cells of a single patient).[2–8] Intratumoral heterogeneity relates to both the different spatial

[a] Dipartimento di Diagnostica per Immagini, Radioterapia Oncologica ed Ematologia, Fondazione Policlinico Universitario "A. Gemelli" IRCCS, Largo A. Gemelli 8, Rome 00168, Italy; [b] Division of Radiotherapy and Imaging, The Institute of Cancer Research, 123 Old Brompton Road, London SW7 3RP, UK; [c] Department of Information and Electrical Engineering and Applied Mathematics (DIEM), University of Salerno, Invariante 12/B, Via Giovanni Paolo II 132, 84084, Fisciano (SA), Italy; [d] Dipartimento di Scienze Della Salute Della Donna, del bambino e di sanità pubblica, Fondazione Policlinico Universitario A. Gemelli IRCCS, Roma, Italy; [e] Università Cattolica Del Sacro Cuore, Largo Francesco Vito, 1, 00168 Roma RM, Italy

* Corresponding author. Dipartimento di Diagnostica per Immagini, Radioterapia Oncologica ed Ematologia, Fondazione Policlinico Universitario "A. Gemelli" IRCCS, Largo A. Gemelli 8, 00168, Rome, Italy
E-mail address: giacomo.avesani@policlinicogemelli.it

Radiol Clin N Am 61 (2023) 749–760
https://doi.org/10.1016/j.rcl.2023.02.006
0033-8389/23/© 2023 Elsevier Inc. All rights reserved.

distribution of subclones across tumor regions and changes in the molecular makeup of a single lesion over time.[2] Despite a general agreement on OC intra-tumoral heterogeneity being driven mainly by structural variants and copy number variations rather than single-gene driver mutations, the existing data evaluating intra-tumoral tumor heterogeneity is limited and differs significantly in methodologies used. Recent results from single-cell sequencing suggest a convergent biological pattern between the primary tumor and matched metastases within the same genetic lineage in the same patient.[9] However, different lineages of cancer cells within one lesion have been shown to display differences in mutations, somatic copy number alterations, gene expression, chromatin accessibility, and DNA methylation, suggesting distinct evolutionary trajectories and intrinsic spatial heterogeneity.[9] Prior work has also shown that lineages with a higher residual DNA methylation level, upregulation of CCN1, HSP90AA1, virus response genes, and angiogenesis are associated with the development of metastatic disease.[9] Among metastatic-specific events, mutations converging at the Wnt/β-catenin signaling pathway have also been also described.[6,7] OC temporal heterogeneity has also been described, with an enrichment of subclones characterized mainly by metabolic and proliferation pathways shown in posttreatment samples, as resistance is acquired to multiple lines of therapy.[10] Larger studies will be required to understand the clinical significance of molecular heterogeneity in OC. However, the available literature suggests that therapeutic decisions based on molecular assessments performed on a single tumor biopsy sample may not be adequate to investigate tumor behavior. A biopsy sample represents only a "snapshot" of tumor at a single time, obtained at a single intratumoral location.

THE CURRENT ROLE OF IMAGING IN OVARIAN CANCER

The presence of intra- and inter-tumor heterogeneity in OC has limited the ability to define specific characteristics of the disease on a per patient basis. This has hampered the development of personalized therapies. Imaging can play a crucial role in the assessment of disease[11] and has been essential in OC management. Ultrasound (US) is the primary imaging modality for detecting and diagnosing OC[12] as it is widely available and cost-effective. Transvaginal ultrasound (TVUS) has a significant role in the initial modality of choice in the assessment of adnexal masses, ruling out malignancy in most cases.[13,14] Risk stratification for malignancies of ovarian masses

on TVUS was first proposed by the International Ovarian Tumor Analysis (IOTA) group in 2008 using a model called the "simple rules." This model, based on five benign features and five malignant features, differentiates benign from borderline/malignant lesions in approximately 77% of masses.[15] Subsequently, a "simple rules risk calculator" was proposed to provide a percentage of risk based on the number of benign and malignant features present in the lesion.[16] The IOTA group also proposed the "ADNEX model" based on clinical and ultrasonographic characteristics.[17] More recently, the American College of Radiology proposed the Ovarian-Adnexal Reporting and Data System for ultrasound (O-RADS US),[18] based on a standardized lexicon,[19] which facilitates risk stratification and management recommendations.

Despite the favorable diagnostic performance of US, 18% to 31% of ovarian masses remain undetermined at TVUS[20] and MR imaging is the second-line imaging technique for further characterization.[21] O-RADS US suggests using MR imaging for those masses classified with a score of 3 or 4 and for a particular subclass of score 2 (unilocular cyst with smooth inner margins between 3 and 10 cm in maximum diameter). MR imaging shows a high sensitivity and specificity for adnexal lesion characterization[22] due to its high contrast and tissue resolution. O-RADS MR imaging was recently published[23]: this classification system provides five risk categories and shows a high performance in differentiating benign and borderline/malignant lesions. Another risk classification system employing non-contrast MR imaging was proposed recently, showing a high performance when used by experienced readers.[24]

Despite its excellent performance in detecting and characterizing primary ovarian lesions, imaging is much less effective in staging peritoneal disease,[25] which is a common clinical scenario, given that approximately 70% of OCs are diagnosed at stages III and IV when the disease has spread outside the pelvis.[26] Computed tomography (CT) is the recommended technique for staging OC.[12] Nevertheless, it has limited accuracy for identifying small implants (less than 1 cm)[27] and peritoneal implants in specific disease locations, such as along the small bowel and mesentery. CT is thus not fully reliable in predicting intraoperative findings.[28] Therefore, laparoscopy remains the gold standard, especially when CT findings are equivocal.[29] MR imaging has been evaluated as an alternative or integrative method for OC staging. Traditional MR imaging has a similar performance compared with CT in detecting peritoneal deposits.[30] Diffusion-weighted imaging (DWI) enhances the diagnostic performance of MR imaging, contributing to a sensitivity and specificity of 94% and 98%, respectively.[31]

The assessment of response to chemotherapy is still limited using conventional imaging techniques and interpretive approaches, and is usually done using CT. The most commonly used response assessment system is Response Evaluation Criteria In Solid Tumors (RECIST), which is based on changes in disease dimensions.[32] However, because of its biology and behavior, OC is typified by peritoneal involvement with varying patterns of disease spread. This includes, frequently, nonmeasurable disease (eg, small, diffuse, linear tumor deposits that may be closely apposed to the surface of viscera), whose quantitative assessment can be challenging, thereby increasing the variability associated with response assessment.

RADIOMICS: PRINCIPLES AND WORKFLOW

Many quantitative semi-automated and automated methods relying upon artificial intelligence (AI) techniques have been developed that can be applied to routine medical images to assess tumor heterogeneity. These quantitative methodologies capture complex patterns related to the microstructure of tissues, referred to as radiomics.[33] The integration of radiomics data into routine practice can augment the information needed to predict important clinical endpoints.[34] The field of radiomics is rapidly evolving (**Fig. 1**) due to the storage of digitalized data that include validated and detailed annotations,[35,36] thus providing information on how the disease can be defined and staged. With this process, subvolumes within a single lesion can be identified which possess distinct morphologic characteristics, called habitats. Habitats may reflect distinct microstructures and, consequently, distinct pathophysiologic processes within a specific tumor subvolume. This is

particularly the case for OCs, for which there is a need to map the characteristics of the primary tumor and the peritoneal implants and for which we know that cellular and genomic heterogeneity is a well-described phenomenon.[37–42] The use of radiomics data to predict disease outcome, optimal therapeutic intervention (ie, surgical or pharmacologic), and to monitor treatment response are all areas of ongoing research.

The typical radiomics process (**Fig. 2**) starts with the identification of qualitative parameters on medical images by a radiologist and culminates with the automated analysis of the microscopic structures.[43,44] This procedure follows a well-established radiomic pipeline, whose steps can be summarized as follows: (a) image acquisition and delineation of a region of interest (ROI) (segmentation); (b) feature extraction; (c) feature selection, dimensionality reduction and definition of a radiomics signature by model construction; and (d) performance assessment and rigorous validation.

The first step is image acquisition; a radiomic pipeline can then be used on the digital images to extract quantitative features from the whole image or, more often, from an ROI. The ROI is outlined through segmentation methods using, if possible, semi-automated or automated tools. The ROI may be further sub-segmented/classified to characterize more distinct areas and tissues better. Automating this process is also essential to save time and money, although the complexity of specific tasks often requires manual adjustment.[39]

From the regions of interest, many different types of radiomic features can be extracted. Each feature reflects a particular characteristic, ranging from simple ones, like volume or shape, to the complex microstructural spatial distribution of pixels. Those features calculated using a predefined algorithm are called "hand-crafted." Radiomics can also be

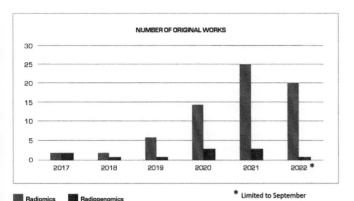

Fig. 1. Bar chart showing the rapid increase in interest in radiomics and radiogenomics. Each bar shows the number of published papers in each year from 2017 to 2022.

RADIOMIC PIPELINE

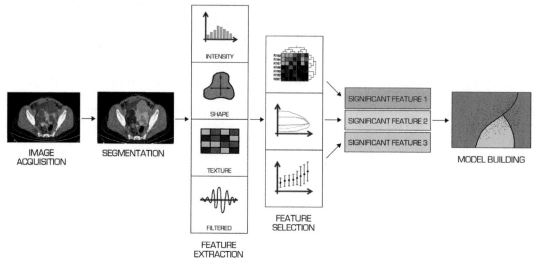

Fig. 2. Schematic of the radiomics pipeline, which starts with image acquisition, followed by the evaluation of the key segments of the images, the selection and extraction of significant features, and the construction of an interpretative model.

deep learning-based, whereby deep neural networks are trained to extract features without a prior external indication.[45]

A large number of features tend to lead to "overfitting," which refers to a model that performs well on training data, but does not perform well on evaluation data, because the model is unable to generalize to unseen examples. To reduce this effect, radiomics signatures can be developed, which consists of a small number of only the most representative and informative features of the essential tumor characteristics. A radiomic signature is a group of weighted features that may help interpret tumor biology and behavior, aiming to answer a significant clinical question, such as diagnosis, risk stratification, treatment response, survival and presence of genetic alterations. These signatures can be developed by selecting independent non-correlated features and using automated analysis techniques such as Least Absolute Shrinkage and Selection Operator (LASSO) regression, recursive feature elimination (RFE) and genetic algorithms. Dimensionality reduction techniques such as principal component analysis (PCA), independent component analysis (ICA), and deep autoencoders can also be applied.

Despite using all these techniques, poor generalization is often observed when radiomics models are applied to data from different institutions or patient sets. Therefore, each model and radiomic signature should be thoroughly validated using a completely independent dataset to assess their generalization capabilities in other clinical scenarios.

INTEGRATION WITH OTHER OMICS DATA AND HABITAT IMAGING

The radiomics pipeline can be complemented with clinical data, biopsy information (conventional sampling or liquid), identification of histopathological biomarkers and the integration of genomic analysis (radiogenomics). Multi-omics data integration can lead to better prediction of treatment response assessment and outcome[46,47] (**Fig. 3**). Adding proteomics information (through mass spectrometry analyses or antibody-based assays of tissue proteomes) allows for a more accurate description of the processes related to cancer development.[48] Proteomics evaluation can quantify the copy number variation, a phenomenon in which sections of the genome are repeated and the number of repeats in the genome varies between individuals. HSGOC has a high degree of copy number variations, which explains the potential advantage of this multi-omics approach, especially for treatment response monitoring.[49] Thus, integrating radiomics, radiogenomics, proteomics and biological correlates could improve clinical management and identify effective therapeutic approaches to HGSOC.

Although radiomic signatures can have high predictive capabilities, they generally ignore the spatial context as the quantitative features extracted usually represent the whole tumor or image. In contrast, habitat imaging, which maps intra-tumoral phenotypically distinct areas, are more appropriate for monitoring tumor microenvironment and structure changes. Current RECIST

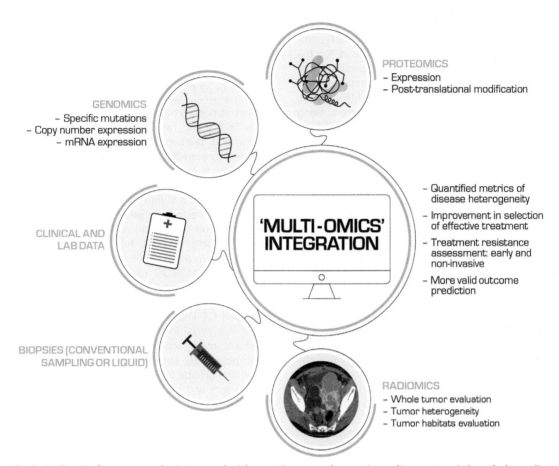

Fig. 3. Radiomics features may be integrated with genetic aspects (genomics and/or proteomics), pathology, clinical and laboratory data to evaluate tumor heterogeneity. The integration of this multi-omics data has the potential to improve the effectiveness of therapy and outcome prediction.

methods, which are essentially based on the evaluation of tumor diameters, are not adequate to monitor the tumor's evolution (ie, after therapy). RECIST reports do not inform on the tumor's characteristics (ie, cystic, necrotic, calcified tissue), underscoring the importance of further segmentation of the lesions[50] and leaving room for machine learning techniques for medical imaging and radiomics to support these procedures. Therapeutic success and prognosis are markedly affected by the heterogeneity detectable in multiple tumor implants in the peritoneal cavity (inter-tumoral heterogeneity).[40–42] Distinct subregions within one single lesion (intra-tumoral heterogeneity) can also be detected.[43,44,50,51] Within this context, treatment response evaluation can be difficult, making assessing the patients' clinical state one of the most challenging tasks.

The biological validation of radiomic-defined habitats via genomic analyses of guided biopsies serves as the basis for the development of "virtual biopsies." Virtual biopsies provide an opportunity to use radiomics signatures to serve as surrogates

for invasive biopsy data.[52] Virtual biopsies not only avoid invasive procedures but also contribute to intratumoral assessment by identifying tumor habitats and delineating their distinct characteristics. This is a crucial step for heterogeneous lesions, as is the case of HGSOC. Monitoring tumor habitats over time may improve the understanding of the effectiveness of therapy within the microenvironment where cancer develops.[52–56]

Having detailed information on tumors and their relationship with molecular traits is also anticipated to improve the effectiveness of screening for OC, as accurate and precise diagnostic information at early cancer stages should inform intervention roadmaps.

RADIOMICS RESEARCH FOR CLINICAL AND TREATMENT MANAGEMENT IN OVARIAN CANCER
Prediction of Cancer Spread at Diagnosis

Chen and colleagues[57] constructed a nomogram derived from portal phase CT images to predict lymph node metastases in HGSOC. The nomogram was found to perform well and was recommended as a new noninvasive method for the clinical decision-making process. Several publications have aimed at predicting the presence of peritoneal carcinomatosis based on the MR imaging characteristics of primary ovarian masses. Song and colleagues[38,58] and Yu and colleagues[59] built two combined models that outperformed conventional clinical assessment in predicting the presence of peritoneal involvement. The former used radiomics features extracted from T2-weighted images (T2WIs), fat-suppressed T2WIs and multi-b-value diffusion-weighted images (DWIs) in 89 patients, whereas the latter also evaluated the post-contrast T1W sequences of 86 patients. The results in terms of accuracy were similar.

CT images at presentation were analyzed to predict the occurrence of metastases in a study of 101 patients. In this study, nine radiomics features and clinical factors were used to classify patients based on whether or not they developed metastases. Age and serum CA-125 levels were identified as the two clinical factors useful in the prediction of metastases. Radiomics features alone and their combination with clinical characteristics were found to be adequate to predict metastatic status.[60]

Li and colleagues[61] built a nomogram based on clinical-radiological characteristics to predict the possibility of residual disease after surgical debulking for HGSOC. They used features from pre- and post-contrast MR sequences of 217 patients. In this study, the radiological model also needed to incorporate clinical information, specifically lactate dehydrogenase (LDH) and CA-125 values, neutrophil-to-lymphocyte ratio and mass characteristics, that is, solid, cystic, or mixed, to perform well in the validation set (Area under the Curve [AUC] = 0.8).

Prediction of Significant Genetic Alterations

Regarding the ability of radiomics features to predict BRCA mutational status, conflicting results are reported. Meier and colleagues[62] tested the correlation between inter-site heterogeneity and BRCA mutational status and found no significant association. In a study on Chinese patients, three different radiomics models were found to be able to predict BRCA mutational status, with no statistically significant differences between them.[63] However, in a recent multicentric study, the authors tested both radiomics and deep learning models' ability to predict BRCA mutational status, with the only model achieving acceptable prediction of BRCA mutation status being one that

combined radiomics signatures with clinical information, like age and family history of ovarian or breast cancer.[64]

Prediction of Recurrence

Numerous papers have focused on the integration of radiomics and radiogenomics data to predict progression-free survival (PFS) and overall survival (OS) and to identify patients at increased risk of recurrence, to inform personalized therapies. In a study of 101 patients with HGSOC, Rizzo and colleagues[65] found a significant 14% increase in the accuracy of predicting disease progression when the model combined both radiomics and clinical data, including residual tumor at surgery, as compared with a radiomics model alone.

To predict HGSOC clinical outcomes, other radiomics-based models were developed by Hu and colleagues[66] using preoperative contrast-enhanced CT images. Predictive models for OS and PFS survival in patients with HGSOC based on stable radiomics features were constructed, which accurately stratified patients into high-risk or low-risk groups for cancer-related death within 2 to 6 years and recurrences within 1 to 5 years. These radiomics models can potentially facilitate patient-specific prognostication schemes as well as more appropriate clinical decision-making for patients with HGSOC.

In another study performed on patients with advanced HGSOC, a combined model was developed based on a radiomics score and a model based on independent clinical factors, specifically International Federation of Gynecology and Obstetrics (FIGO) stage at diagnosis and presence of residual disease after surgery. The AUC was higher using the radiomics score alone than the model using only clinical factors. The real advantage was found using the combined model, for which AUC was significantly better. Patients categorized as high risk by the integrated model showed a shorter PFS as compared with low risk patients.[67]

Despite these promising findings, radiomics findings are not easy to introduce in clinical practice. In a recent multicentric study using a real-life dataset, including CTs from many vendors and centers, radiomics and deep learning models could not reliably predict PFS in the validation sets.[64]

In a sample of 286 patients, a radiomics score was calculated based on radiomic multisequence features detected on MR imaging that identify high-risk patients, that is, those with a four-fold higher risk of recurrence.[68] Similarly, an MR imaging-derived radiomic model employing data from 117 patients to identify high-risk features for HGSOC recurrence showed a significantly shorter PFS in those patients with high-risk features for recurrence compared with low recurrence risk patients.[69]

A radiomic-clinical nomogram was used to identify patients with a high risk of recurrence, including radiomic features and clinical information at the diagnosis, specifically age, CA-125 values, FIGO stage and Ki-67 levels, to predict PFS (dichotomized).[70] In an MR imaging study of 141 patients, radiomics features from different sequences were used to build a mixed nomogram with radiomics and clinical variables (ie, CA-125 and HE4 levels, FIGO stage, the presence of peritoneal metastases, type of treatment, and presence of residual tumor) to predict recurrence. The model had good performance in identifying patients at risk for recurrence, which was confirmed by Kaplan–Meier survival curves.[71] In an effort to integrate these analyses with clinical parameters, the authors correlated radiomics features with fibrinogen level and neutrophil-to-lymphocyte ratio (thought to be risk factors in OC), finding no significant relationships.

18F-fluorodeoxyglucose (^{18}F-FDG) PET-CT has also been investigated to predict recurrence in patients with HGSOC. Two cohorts were evaluated (training and validation) using different combinations of models and clinical or metabolic variables obtained from PET and CT. The addition of PET radiomic features to the model improved prognostic accuracy as compared with combined clinical and CT radiomics features.[72]

Fewer studies have focused on OS. A study by Lu and colleagues[73] used a machine learning radiomics analysis in 364 patients with primary ovarian tumors. Four descriptors derived from 42 features were evaluated. Preoperative CT images of the primary tumor were used to generate an algorithm able to identify the 5% of patients with a median OS of fewer than 2 years, thus potentially informing patient prognostication. The analysis was also evaluated using an external validation cohort, which confirmed the prognostic significance of the radiomic model for PFS[74] although not for OS as described in this group's prior publication.[73]

A radiomics-clinical nomogram to evaluate OS post-surgery in patients with HGSOC was developed in two cohorts (training and validation). The proposed radiomics-clinical nomogram based on a radiomics signature and four clinical predictors (age, tumor size, pathologic staging, and tumor grade) was found to increase the predictive accuracy of OS in these patients after surgery, thereby contributing to clinical decision-making.[75]

Studies that have evaluated genetic intra-lesion heterogeneity HGSOC have also shown significant associations between genetic heterogeneity and the likelihood of tumor recurrence. Prior work has shown that poorer survival is associated with higher heterogeneity.[76] In a study on 75 patients, an integrated intra-site and inter-site radiomics-clinical-genomic marker of HGSOC was developed. This combination predicted outcomes better than radiomics measures alone.[77]

In two other studies, inter-site texture heterogeneity parameters derived from CT were associated with lower OS and PFS.[62,78] Specifically, higher inter-site cluster variance was associated with both lower PFS and OS. Higher inter-site cluster prominence, an indicator of asymmetry in the distribution of intensity levels in an image, was associated only with lower PFS while higher inter-site cluster entropy (an indicator of the amount of variation in the similarities between the different sites) correlated with lower OS. These findings indicate the potential of radiomics to predict patient outcome and improve treatment effectiveness via noninvasive assessment. A recent systematic review evaluating six radiomics studies found a significant association between the heterogeneity of radiomics features and OS for HGSOC between 6 and 36 months, with similar results achieved for PFS.[79] So far, we have had limited knowledge of the genomic heterogeneity in HGSOC as we rely only on single biopsies, which provide little meaningful information concerning the mechanisms of tumor invasion and clonal expansion occurring at the cellular level, thereby limiting a comprehensive assessment of tumor biology across tumor sites.[76,80–84]

Response to Treatment

Response to neoadjuvant chemotherapy (NACT) in HGSOC patients has been studied using the chemotherapy response score for omental tumor deposits, thereby informing the utility of upfront cytoreductive surgery. Prior work has found that combining pre-NACT radiomics with tumor volumetry predicted response in a timely fashion and was robust in the face of external testing.[85]

An analysis of heterogeneity in patients undergoing immunotherapy suggested that lower intra- and inter-tumor heterogeneity may predict a better response to immunotherapy.[86]

In this study, radiogenomic biomarkers enabled the pretreatment prediction of hypoxia patterns in cancer cells and tissues, with a hypoxic microenvironment thought to play an essential role in tumorigenesis.[87] The authors extracted optimal radiogenomics biomarkers for predicting the risk status of patients using machine learning algorithms. The prediction of hypoxia patterns may further inform personalized therapies.

Proteomics analyses integrated with CT-derived radiomics features have identified proteins associated with intra-tumoral heterogeneity.[56] This study suggests the potential utility of standard-of-care CT as a prognostic indicator, given the association between CT radiomics features and proteome status, which may be beneficial in monitoring response to treatment.

Radiomics features integrated with clinical and genomic variables were used to facilitate intervention in high-risk patients, by predicting resistance to platinum-based chemotherapy.[77] Platinum resistance was also predicted in a study for which Sulfatase 1 (SULF1) polymorphism was incorporated into a CT-based radiomics model.[88]

Additional work correlating MR imaging, tumor histologic, and genomic characteristics has corroborated the importance of assessing tumor habitats. Weigelt and colleagues[84] used *in vivo* multiparametric imaging derived from MR imaging and 18F-FDG PET-CT to identify distinct tumoral habitats, which showed distinct histologic and genomic features after surgical removal and *ex vivo* analysis. Tardieu and colleagues[89] used high field 9.4 T MR to obtain microstructural information and evaluated correlations between these MR microscopy (MRM)-derived radiomics features and tumor histologic characteristics.

Challenges and Future Perspectives

A major issue in radiomics research is the lack of generalization. The overall evidence for OC reflects an abundance of AI-based models, each able to improve prediction or response to therapy interpretation on single datasets, but with a scarce possibility to generalize well-developed models that can make robust predictions generalizable to unseen, independent data. The lack of detailed documentation and data-sharing restrictions inherent in contemporary radiomics research make comparing a large number of methodologies challenging. The Cancer Genome Atlas (TCGA)[90] and The Cancer Imaging Archive (TCIA)[91] can serve as valuable resources for the independent validation of radiomics-based models.

One of the leading causes for the lack of generalization is the absence of a standard protocol for image acquisition. There are several parameters in image acquisition and reconstruction, which vary widely in clinical practice and are specific for each imaging technique, thereby affecting the robustness of features extracted. This caveat is particularly prominent for MR imaging data, where even the use of scanners produced by different vendors downgrades the generalization of AI models.[92,93] The repeatability of radiomic features still needs to be adequately studied and understood.

Another issue that hinders clinical adoption is the lack of interpretability of complex mathematical features with deep-learning features, which are generally regarded as a "black box." The spatial histologic and genomic validation of radiomic-defined tumor habitats resulting from genomic analyses could shed light on the inner workings of underlying tumor biology pathways and provide more confidence in the predictive models. The advantages of such approaches may positively impact not only prediction but also inform the design of prospective clinical trials and their endpoints.[76,81–83]

The clinical application of models derived from research settings is still far from being a common approach. Their integration into routine clinical workflow will be facilitated when the methods proposed are proven to be easily useable, generalizable, economically sustainable, and time-effective.

SUMMARY

The precision of diagnostic and therapeutic approaches for OC has the potential to improve considerably in the future, paving the way for better-personalized treatments. As such, the tracking of tumor heterogeneity using a combination of radiomic features, genomic variables and knowledge of their association with pathology has the potential to inform more effective monitoring of tumor evolution and treatment response thereby informing the refinement of personalized therapeutic strategies. The identification of distinct imaging phenotypes (habitats), which reflect specific tumor microenvironments and molecular profiles can also inform future experimental trial design by defining novel endpoints. The integration of spatially validated radiomics, histopathology and genomic data[94] can yield noninvasive "virtual biopsy" data that may alleviate the need for successive invasive serial procedures post-therapy.[55]

CLINICS CARE POINTS

- Tumor heterogeneity can be evaluated noninvasively by imaging and quantitative radiomics features can be extracted to derive tumor habitats that in the future might serve as virtual biopsies.

- Integration of radiomics with other omics data such as genomics and proteomics and with histopathological and clinical data, may be an effective way to obtain new predictive and prognostic biomarkers in ovarian cancer, potentially leading to personalized treatment.
- Radiomics and multi-omics approach still needs standardization and validation to be generalized and used in routine clinical practice.

DISCLOSURE

E. Sala: co-founder and shareholder, Lucida Medical. Research support, GEHC, Canon, Netherlands. Speakers' bureau, GEHC, Canon. C. Nero: Travel support by MDS, United States and Illumina, United States. The other Authors have nothing to disclose.

ACKNOWLEDGMENTS

The authors would like to thank Alberto Panico and Carolina Scarpetta for creating and formatting the images of the paper.

REFERENCES

1. Siegel RL, Miller KD, Fuchs HE, et al. Cancer statistics, 2022. CA A Cancer J Clinicians 2022;72(1): 7–33.
2. Dagogo-Jack I, Shaw A. Tumour heterogeneity and resistance to cancer therapies. Nat Rev Clin Oncol 2018;15:81–94.
3. Bashashati A, Ha G, Tone A, et al. Distinct evolutionary trajectories of primary high-grade serous ovarian cancers revealed through spatial mutational profiling. J Pathol 2013;231:21–34.
4. Network CGAR. Integrated genomic analyses of ovarian carcinoma. Nature 2011;474:609.
5. Verhaak RG, Tamayo P, Yang J-Y, et al. Prognostically relevant gene signatures of high-grade serous ovarian carcinoma. J Clin Invest 2013;123:517–25.
6. Hao Q, Li J, Zhang Q, et al. Single-cell transcriptomes reveal heterogeneity of high-grade serous ovarian carcinoma. Clin Transl Med 2021;11(8):e500.
7. Masoodi T, Siraj S, Siraj AK, et al. Genetic heterogeneity and evolutionary history of high-grade ovarian carcinoma and matched distant metastases. Br J Cancer 2020;122(8):1219–30.
8. Yin X, Jing Y, Cai M-C, et al. Clonality, heterogeneity, and evolution of synchronous bilateral ovarian cancer. Cancer Res 2017;77:6551–61.
9. Wang Y, Xie H, Chang X, et al. Single-cell dissection of the multiomic landscape of high-grade serous ovarian cancer. Cancer Res 2022;82(21):3903–16.
10. Nath A, Cosgrove PA, Mirsafian H, et al. Evolution of core archetypal phenotypes in progressive high grade serous ovarian cancer. Nat Commun 2021; 12(1):3039.
11. European Society of Radiology. Medical imaging in personalised medicine: a white paper of the research committee of the European Society of Radiology. Insights Imaging 2015;6:141–55.
12. Forstner R, Sala E, Kinkel K, et al. ESUR guidelines: ovarian cancer staging and follow-up. Eur Radiol 2010;20(12):2773–80.
13. Meys EMJ, Kaijser J, Kruitwagen RFPM, et al. Subjective assessment versus ultrasound models to diagnose ovarian cancer: A systematic review and meta-analysis. European Journal of Cancer 2016; 58:17–29.
14. Froyman W, Landolfo C, De Cock B, et al. Risk of complications in patients with conservatively managed ovarian tumours (IOTA5): a 2-year interim analysis of a multicentre, prospective, cohort study. Lancet Oncol 2019;20(3):448–58.
15. Timmerman D, Testa AC, Bourne T, et al. Simple ultrasound-based rules for the diagnosis of ovarian cancer. Ultrasound Obstet Gynecol 2008;31(6): 681–90.
16. Timmerman D, Van Calster B, Testa A, et al. Predicting the risk of malignancy in adnexal masses based on the Simple Rules from the International Ovarian Tumor Analysis group. Am J Obstet Gynecol 2016; 214(4):424–37.
17. Van Calster B, Van Hoorde K, Valentin L, et al. Evaluating the risk of ovarian cancer before surgery using the ADNEX model to differentiate between benign, borderline, early and advanced stage invasive, and secondary metastatic tumours: prospective multicentre diagnostic study. BMJ 2014; 349(oct07 3):g5920.
18. Andreotti RF, Timmerman D, Strachowski LM, et al. O-RADS US Risk Stratification and Management System: A Consensus Guideline from the ACR Ovarian-Adnexal Reporting and Data System Committee. Radiology 2020;294(1):168–85.
19. Andreotti RF, Timmerman D, Benacerraf BR, et al. Ovarian-Adnexal Reporting Lexicon for Ultrasound: A White Paper of the ACR Ovarian-Adnexal Reporting and Data System Committee. J Am Coll Radiol 2018;15(10):1415–29.
20. Mohaghegh P, Rockall AG. Imaging Strategy for Early Ovarian Cancer: Characterization of Adnexal Masses with Conventional and Advanced Imaging Techniques. Radiographics 2012;32(6):1751–73.
21. Thomassin-Naggara I, Aubert E, Rockall A, et al. Adnexal Masses: Development and Preliminary Validation of an MR Imaging Scoring System. Radiology 2013;267(2):432–43.
22. Hu X, Li D, Liang Z, et al. Indirect comparison of the diagnostic performance of 18F-FDG PET/CT and

MRI in differentiating benign and malignant ovarian or adnexal tumors: a systematic review and meta-analysis. BMC Cancer 2021;21(1):1080.

23. Thomassin-Naggara I, Poncelet E, Jalaguier-Coudray A, et al. Ovarian-Adnexal Reporting Data System Magnetic Resonance Imaging (O-RADS MRI) Score for Risk Stratification of Sonographically Indeterminate Adnexal Masses. JAMA Netw Open 2020;3(1):e1919896.

24. Sahin H, Panico C, Ursprung S, et al. Non-contrast MRI can accurately characterize adnexal masses: a retrospective study. Eur Radiol 2021;31(9): 6962–73.

25. van 't Sant I, Engbersen MP, Bhairosing PA, et al. Diagnostic performance of imaging for the detection of peritoneal metastases: a meta-analysis. Eur Radiol 2020;30(6):3101–12.

26. Konishi I, Abiko K, Hayashi T, et al. Peritoneal dissemination of high-grade serous ovarian cancer: pivotal roles of chromosomal instability and epigenetic dynamics. J Gynecol Oncol 2022; 33(5):e83.

27. Coakley FV, Choi PH, Gougoutas CA, et al. Peritoneal Metastases: Detection with Spiral CT in Patients with Ovarian Cancer. Radiology 2002;223(2):495–9.

28. Avesani G, Arshad M, Lu H, et al. Radiological assessment of Peritoneal Cancer Index on preoperative CT in ovarian cancer is related to surgical outcome and survival. Radiol Med 2020;125(8): 770–6.

29. Fagotti A, Ferrandina G, Fanfani F, et al. Prospective validation of a laparoscopic predictive model for optimal cytoreduction in advanced ovarian carcinoma. Am J Obstet Gynecol 2008;199(6):642.e1–6.

30. Qayyum A, Coakley FV, Westphalen AC, et al. Role of CT and MR imaging in predicting optimal cytoreduction of newly diagnosed primary epithelial ovarian cancer. Gynecol Oncol 2005;96(2):301–6.

31. Michielsen K, Dresen R, Vanslembrouck R, et al. Diagnostic value of whole body diffusion-weighted MRI compared to computed tomography for preoperative assessment of patients suspected for ovarian cancer. European Journal of Cancer 2017; 83:88–98.

32. Eisenhauer EA, Therasse P, Bogaerts J, et al. New response evaluation criteria in solid tumours: Revised RECIST guideline (version 1.1). European Journal of Cancer 2009;45(2):228–47.

33. Gillies RJ, Kinahan PE, Hricak H. Radiomics: Images Are More than Pictures, They Are Data. Radiology 2016;278(2):563–77.

34. Lambin P, Leijenaar RTH, Deist TM, et al. Radiomics: the bridge between medical imaging and personalized medicine. Nat Rev Clin Oncol 2017;14:749–62.

35. Ravì D, Wong C, Deligianni F, et al. Deep Learning for Health Informatics. IEEE J. Biomed. Health Inform. 2017;21(1):4–21.

36. Shaikhina T, Khovanova NA. Handling limited datasets with neural networks in medical applications: a small-data approach. Artif Intell Med 2017;75: 51–63.

37. Nougaret S, Tardieu M, Vargas HA, et al. Ovarian cancer: An update on imaging in the era of radiomics. Diagn Interv Imaging 2019;100(10):647–55.

38. Nougaret S, McCague C, Tibermacine H, et al. Radiomics and radiogenomics in ovarian cancer: a literature review. Abdominal Radiology 2021;46: 2308–22.

39. Skubitz AP, Pambuccian SE, Argenta PA, et al. Differential gene expression identifies subgroups of ovarian carcinoma. Transl Res 2006;148:223–48.

40. Stanescu AD, Ples L, Edu A, et al. Different patterns of heterogeneity in ovarian carcinoma. Rom J Morphol Embryol 2015;56:1357–63.

41. Zangwill BC, Balsara G, Dunton C, et al. Ovarian carcinoma heterogeneity as demonstrated by DNA ploidy. Cancer 1993;71:2261–7.

42. Globocan - Global Cancer Observatory. International Agency for Research on Cancer. Available at. https://gco.iarc.fr/-. Accessed 24 November 2022.

43. Nougaret S, Tibermacine H, Tardieu M, et al. Radiomics: an Introductory Guide to What It May Foretell. Curr Oncol Rep 2019;21(8):70.

44. Lubner MG, Smith AD, Sandrasegaran K, et al. CT Texture Analysis: Definitions, Applications, Biologic Correlates, and Challenges. Radiographics 2017; 37(5):1483–503.

45. Afshar P, Mohammadi A, Plataniotis KN, et al. From Handcrafted to Deep-Learning-Based Cancer Radiomics: Challenges and opportunities. IEEE Signal Process Mag 2019;36(4):132–60.

46. Sala E, Mema E, Himoto Y, et al. Unravelling tumour heterogeneity using next-generation imaging: radiomics, radiogenomics, and habitat imaging. Clin Radiol 2017;72:3–10.

47. Mazurowski MA. Radiogenomics: what it is and why it is important. J Am Coll Radiol 2015;12(8):862–6.

48. Zhang H, Liu T, Zhang Z, et al. Integrated proteogenomic characterization of human high grade serous ovarian cancer. Cell 2016;166(3):755–65.

49. McCague C, Beer L. Radioproteomics in patients with ovarian cancer. Br J Radiol 2021;94:20201331.

50. Rundo L, Beer L, Ursprung S, et al. Tissue-specific and interpretable sub-segmentation of whole tumour burden on CT images by unsupervised fuzzy clustering. Comput Biol Med 2020;120:103751.

51. Litjens G, Kooi T, Bejnordi BE, et al. A survey on deep learning in medical image analysis. Med Image Anal 2017;42:60–88.

52. Beer L, Martin-Gonzalez P, Delgado-Ortet M, et al. Ultrasound-guided targeted biopsies of CT-based radiomic tumour habitats: technical development and initial experience in metastatic ovarian cancer. Eur Radiol 2021;31(CP 21 6):3765–72.

53. Crispin-Ortuzar M, Sala E. Precision radiogenomics: fusion biopsies to target tumour habitats in vivo. Br J Cancer 2021;125(6):778–9.

54. Zhang B, Whiteaker JR, Hoofnagle AN, et al. Clinical potential of mass spectrometry-based proteogenomics. Nat Rev Clin Oncol 2019;16(4):256–68.

55. Martin-Gonzalez P, Crispin-Ortuzar M, Rundo L, et al. Integrative radiogenomics for virtual biopsy and treatment monitoring in ovarian cancer. Insights Imaging 2020;11(1):94.

56. Beer L, Sahin H, Bateman NW, et al. Integration of proteomics with CT-based qualitative and radiomic features in high-grade serous ovarian cancer patients: an exploratory analysis. Eur Radiol 2020; 30(8):4306–16.

57. Chen HZ, Wang XR, Zhao FM, et al. The Development and Validation of a CT-Based Radiomics Nomogram to Preoperatively Predict Lymph Node Metastasis in High-Grade Serous Ovarian Cancer. Front Oncol 2021;11:711648.

58. Song XL, Ren JL, Yao TY, et al. Radiomics Based on Multisequence Magnetic Resonance Imaging for the Preoperative Prediction of Peritoneal Metastasis in Ovarian Cancer. Eur Radiol 2021;31:8438–46.

59. Yu XY, Ren J, Jia Y, et al. Multiparameter MRI Radiomics Model Predicts Preoperative Peritoneal Carcinomatosis in Ovarian Cancer. Front Oncol 2021;11: 765652.

60. Ai Y, Zhang J, Jin J, et al. Preoperative Prediction of Metastasis for Ovarian Cancer Based on Computed Tomography Radiomics Features and Clinical Factors. Front Oncol 2021;11:610742.

61. Li H, Zhang R, Li R, et al. Noninvasive Prediction of Residual Disease for Advanced High-Grade Serous Ovarian Carcinoma by MRI-Based Radiomic-Clinical Nomogram. Eur Radiol 2021;31:7855–64.

62. Meier A, Veeraraghavan H, Nougaret S, et al. Association between CT-texture-derived tumor heterogeneity, outcomes, and BRCA mutation status in patients with high-grade serous ovarian cancer. Abdom Radiol (NY) 2019;44(6):2040–7.

63. Mingzhu L, Yaqiong G, Mengru L, et al. Prediction of BRCA gene mutation status in epithelial ovarian cancer by radiomics models based on 2D and 3D CT images. BMC Med Imaging 2021;21(1):180.

64. Avesani G, Tran HE, Cammarata G, et al. CT-Based Radiomics and Deep Learning for BRCA Mutation and Progression-Free Survival Prediction in Ovarian Cancer Using a Multicentric Dataset. Cancers 2022; 14(11):2739.

65. Rizzo S, Botta F, Raimondi S, et al. Radiomics of high-grade serous ovarian cancer: association between quantitative CT features, residual tumour and disease progression within 12 months. Eur Radiol 2018;28(11):4849–59.

66. Hu J, Wang Z, Zuo R, et al. Development of survival predictors for high-grade serous ovarian cancer based on stable radiomic features from computed tomography images. iScience 2022;25(7):104628.

67. Chen HZ, Wang XR, Zhao FM, et al. A CT-based radiomics nomogram for predicting early recurrence in patients with high-grade serous ovarian cancer. Eur J Radiol 2021;145:110018.

68. Zhang H, Mao Y, Chen X, et al. Magnetic Resonance Imaging Radiomics in Categorizing Ovarian Masses and Predicting Clinical Outcome: A Preliminary Study. Eur Radiol 2019;29:3358–71.

69. Li HM, Gong J, Li RM, et al. Development of MRI-Based Radiomics Model to Predict the Risk of Recurrence in Patients With Advanced High-Grade Serous Ovarian Carcinoma. Am J Roentgenol 2021;217:664–75.

70. Wang T, Wang H, Wang Y, et al. MR-Based Radiomics-Clinical Nomogram in Epithelial Ovarian Tumor Prognosis Prediction: Tumor Body Texture Analysis across Various Acquisition Protocols. J Ovarian Res 2022;15(1):6.

71. Li C, Wang H, Chen Y, et al. A Nomogram Combining MRI Multisequence Radiomics and Clinical Factors for Predicting Recurrence of High-Grade Serous Ovarian Carcinoma. J Oncol 2022; 2022:1716268.

72. Wang X, Lu Z. Radiomics Analysis of PET and CT Components of (18)F-FDG PET/CT Imaging for Prediction of Progression-Free Survival in Advanced High-Grade Serous Ovarian Cancer. Front Oncol 2021;11:638124.

73. Lu H, Arshad M, Thornton A, et al. A mathematical-descriptor of tumor-mesoscopic-structure from computed-tomography images annotates prognostic- and molecular-phenotypes of epithelial ovarian cancer. Nat Commun 2019;10(1):764.

74. Fotopoulou C, Rockall A, Lu H. Validation analysis of the novel imaging-based prognostic radiomic signature in patients undergoing primary surgery for advanced high-grade serous ovarian cancer (HGSOC). Br J Cancer 2022;126:1047–54.

75. Hong Y, Liu Z, Lin D, et al. Development of a radiomic-clinical nomogram for prediction of survival in patients with serous ovarian cancer. Clin Radiol 2022;77(5):352–9.

76. Bashashati A, Ha G, Tone A, et al. Distinct evolutionary trajectories of primary high-grade serous ovarian cancers revealed through spatial mutational profiling. J Pathol 2013;231:21–34.

77. Veeraraghavan H, Vargas HA, Jimenez-Sanchez A, et al. Integrated Multi-Tumor Radio-Genomic Marker of Outcomes in Patients with High Serous Ovarian Carcinoma. Cancers 2020;12(11):3403.

78. Vargas HA, Veeraraghavan H, Micco M, et al. A novel representation of inter-site tumour heterogeneity from pre-treatment computed tomography textures classifies ovarian cancers by clinical outcome. Eur Radiol 2017;27:3991–4001.

79. Rizzo S, Manganaro L, Dolciami M, et al. Computed Tomography Based Radiomics as a Predictor of Survival in Ovarian Cancer Patients: A Systematic Review. Cancers 2021;13(3):573.

80. Schwarz RF, Ng CK, Cooke SL, et al. Spatial and temporal heterogeneity in high-grade serous ovarian cancer: A phylogenetic analysis. PLoS Med 2015; 12:e1001789.

81. Zhang AW, McPherson A, Milne K, et al. Interfaces of malignant and immunologic clonal dynamics in ovarian cancer. Cell 2018;173:1755–69.

82. McPherson A, Roth A, Laks E, et al. Divergent modes of clonal spread and intraperitoneal mixing in high-grade serous ovarian cancer. Nat Genet 2016;48:758–67.

83. Jimenez-Sanchez A, Memon D, Pourpe S, et al. Heterogeneous tumor-immune microenvironments among differentially growing metastases in an ovarian cancer patient. Cell 2017;170:927–38.

84. Weigelt B, Vargas HA, Selenica P, et al. Radiogenomics Analysis of Intratumor Heterogeneity in a Patient With High-Grade Serous Ovarian Cancer. JCO Precis Oncol 2019;18:410.

85. Rundo L, Beer L, Escudero Sanchez L, et al. Clinically interpretable Radiomics-Based Prediction of Histopathologic Response to Neoadjuvant Chemotherapy in High-Grade Serous Ovarian Carcinoma. Front Oncol 2022;12:868265.

86. Himoto Y, Veeraraghavan H, Zheng J, et al. Computed Tomography-Derived Radiomic Metrics Can Identify Responders to Immunotherapy in Ovarian Cancer. JCO Precis Oncol 2019;3:38.

87. Feng S, Xia T, Ge Y, et al. Computed Tomography Imaging-Based Radiogenomics Analysis Reveals Hypoxia Patterns and Immunological Characteristics in Ovarian Cancer. Front Immunol 2022;13:868067.

88. Yi X, Liu Y, Zhoug B, et al. Incorporating SULF1 polymorphisms in a pretreatment CT-based radiomic model for predicting platinum resistance in ovarian cancer treatment Biomed. Pharmacother 2021;133: 111013.

89. Tardieu M, Lakhman Y, Khellaf L, et al. Assessing Histology Structures by Ex Vivo MR Microscopy and Exploring the Link Between MRM-Derived Radiomic Features and Histopathology in Ovarian Cancer. Front Oncol 2022;11:771848.

90. The future of cancer genomics. Nat Med 2015;21(2): 99.

91. Clark K, Vendt B, Smith K, et al. The Cancer Imaging Archive (TCIA): maintaining and operating a public information repository. J Digit Imaging 2013;26(6): 1045e57.

92. Yan W, Wang Y, Gu S, et al. The Domain Shift Problem of Medical Image Segmentation and Vendor-Adaptation by Unet-GAN. In Medical image computing and computer assisted intervention –. MICCAI 2019;623–31. https://doi.org/10.1007/978-3-030-32245-8_69.

93. Bluemke DA, Moy L, Bredella MA, et al. Assessing Radiology Research on Artificial Intelligence: A Brief Guide for Authors, Reviewers, and Readers-From the Radiology Editorial Board. Radiology 2020; 294(3):487–9.

94. Crispin-Ortuzar M, Gehrung M, Ursprung S, et al. Three-Dimensional Printed Molds for Image-Guided Surgical Biopsies: An Open Source Computational Platform JCO. Clin Cancer Inform 2020;4: 736–48.

Moving?

Make sure your subscription moves with you!

To notify us of your new address, find your **Clinics Account Number** (located on your mailing label above your name), and contact customer service at:

Email: journalscustomerservice-usa@elsevier.com

800-654-2452 (subscribers in the U.S. & Canada)
314-447-8871 (subscribers outside of the U.S. & Canada)

Fax number: 314-447-8029

Elsevier Health Sciences Division
Subscription Customer Service
3251 Riverport Lane
Maryland Heights, MO 63043

*To ensure uninterrupted delivery of your subscription, please notify us at least 4 weeks in advance of move.

Printed and bound by CPI Group (UK) Ltd, Croydon, CR0 4YY

08/05/2025

01864717-0005